Instructors's Resource Manual And Test Bank

to accompany

Potter • Perry

Basic Nursing

A Critical Thinking Approach

Fourth Edition

Instructor's Resource Manual And Test Bank

to accompany
Potter • Perry

Basic Nursing

A Critical Thinking Approach

Fourth Edition

Instructor's Resource Manual by
Patricia A. Castaldi, RN, BSN, MSN
Associate Dean
Elizabeth General Medical Center
School of Nursing
Elizabeth, New Jersey
A Cooperative Program with Union County College

Test Bank by
Rick Daniels, RN, BSN, MSN, PhD
Associate Professor of Nursing
Oregon Health Sciences University at Southern
Ashland, Oregon

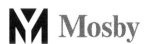
Mosby

St. Louis Baltimore Boston Carlsbad Chicago Minneapolis New York Philadelphia Portland
London Milan Sydney Tokyo Toronto

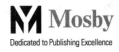

Mosby
Dedicated to Publishing Excellence

A Times Mirror
Company

Publisher: Sally Schrefer
Senior Editor: Susan Epstein
Developmental Editor: Billi Carcheri
Project Manager: Gayle May Morris
Manufacturing Manager: Linda Ierardi
Cover Designer: Brian Salisbury

Composition by Black Dot Group
Printing/Binding by Plus Communications, Inc.

Mosby, Inc.
11830 Westline Industrial Drive
St. Louis, Missouri 63146

ISBN: 0-323-00103-3

98 99 00 01 02 / 9 8 7 6 5 4 3 2 1

PREFACE

This Instructor's Resource Manual and Test Bank to accompany the fourth edition of *Basic Nursing* is designed to coordinate with the text and provide support to instructors teaching the fundamentals of nursing. Although differences exist in the implementation of fundamentals nursing courses, this manual should provide assistance in the selection and planning of learning activities for students.

Each chapter of the manual contains a topical outline of the content in the text chapter, critical thinking activities and suggested answers (also from the text), educational strategies, and recommended multimedia resources, including videotapes, computer-assisted instruction, and interactive video programs. The educational strategies that are identified in this manual may also serve as stimuli for additional experiences for the presentation and application of the subject matter. Where a class discussion may be suggested, the same information may be elicited from the students through quizzes, essays, or post-clinical meetings.

New additions to each chapter of the manual include the student resources (study charts and various tools) and independent learning activities that are found in the Student Study Guide. Students may be encouraged to use the study charts for organization and documentation of the major points identified in each chapter. The assessment tools and forms may be used in classroom or clinical situations. In addition, a cross curriculum guide provides suggestions for the application of fundamentals content to other nursing courses or experiences.

The Test Bank questions, prepared in line with the NCLEX format, may be used or adapted for use in student testing. The answers are keyed to the page in the text where the material is covered.

It is hoped that this Instructor's Manual and Test Bank, in coordination with the Student Study Guide, will be a valuable resource in the preparation and offering of a beginning nursing course.

CONTENTS

Instructors's Resource Manual And Test Bank

to accompany

Potter • Perry

Basic Nursing

A Critical Thinking Approach

Fourth Edition

UNIT 1

The Client and the Health Care Environment

CHAPTER 1

Health and Wellness

CRITICAL THINKING ACTIVITIES AND ANSWERS

1. How would you describe your current state of health: excellent, good, fair, or poor? What definition of health did you use to make this judgment? List the current health promotion, wellness, and illness prevention activities in which you regularly engage. Are there any areas that need to be improved or changed? What will influence your ability to adopt any needed changes?

Answer: I would describe my current state of health as good based on the World Health Organization's definition of health ("a state of complete physical, mental, and social well-being, not merely the absence of disease or infirmity," 1947) and my individual view of health. One active health promotion activity in which I engage is regular exercise–walking 3 miles three times a week. I regularly integrate principles of wellness living into my lifestyle by incorporating what I have learned about stress management. An illness prevention strategy that I practice is obtaining a flu shot each fall. I would like to exercise more and eat more nutritious foods. Internal barriers to a better diet are my fondness for sweet foods, and external barriers include my limited cooking skills and the minimal time I allow for meal preparation.

2. Assess the lifestyle patterns of someone you know. Identify risk factors that increase his or her vulnerability to illness or susceptibility to disease. Are there risk factors present that could be modified?

Answer: I have chosen an older uncle for the risk factor profile. Risk factors:
Genetic and Physiological: Overweight by 100 pounds, strong family history of cardiovascular disease (several family members have high blood pressure, mother died of a stroke, father died of heart attack).
Age: 64
Environment: Still working 5 full days a week, managing an independent corporation. No industrial or home environment risk factors known.
Lifestyle: Poor nutrition (overeating foods high in cholesterol and fat—red meat, fried foods), although he does not smoke or drink alcohol. Hobbies include golf and fishing (outdoor activities that include risk of overexposure to the sun and possible shoulder and arm injury). Occupation is stressful (may interfere with ability to implement any needed lifestyle modifications). Comparisons of the individual's weight and nutritional intake were made using the standard height-weight chart and food pyramid.

3. Using the same individual as above, how could you approach the subject of risk-factor modification? What influences exist that will assist the individual in making a change? What barriers exist that may prevent maintenance of a change in health behavior? What is the major nursing implication in the maintenance stage of health behavior change? What resources are available to you and to this individual that may assist in the change process?

Answer: Open discussion and identification of risk factors is the first step in health promotion, wellness education, and illness prevention activities. The client must be allowed to decide if he or she wants to maintain or improve health status. My uncle has a strong desire to lead a healthier life; this will assist him in implementing the required changes. The major barrier for him is his busy work schedule. The major nursing implication for the maintenance stage of health behavior changes is that the changes need to be integrated into the client's lifestyle. Community resources can be explored, such as the local library (book, journal, and video series on health improvement programs), local schools or community colleges (classes or workshops on health-related topics), local health care agencies, and on-site corporate activities in the workplace.

EDUCATIONAL STRATEGIES

1. Review the definitions of health and illness. Ask students to identify their perceptions of health/wellness and illness, citing specific personal examples.

2. Discuss Healthy People 2000 and its potential impact on overall health care delivery and nursing practice.

3. Use the Healthy People 2000 priority areas to discuss how they might be addressed in the community, what specific health care activities might be planned, and what the role of the nurse may be in their implementation and evaluation.

4. Discuss the models of health and illness. Using a case study example, have students apply the different models and identify the advantages and limitations of each one.

5. Ask students to identify possible internal and external variables that influence health beliefs and practices.

6. Discuss risk factors that can have an impact upon health. Have students perform an assessment on themselves, their peers, their family members, and/or a client in order to determine the presence of risk factors.

7. Use the stages of Health Behavior Change to have students identify how risk behaviors can be altered or eliminated in themselves, their peers, their family members, and/or the client.

8. Review the levels of prevention. Have students identify examples of health care activities for each level. Provide students with the following, or similar, examples and ask them to identify client and nursing behaviors (as applicable) for primary, secondary, and tertiary levels of prevention:
   a. Hypertension
   b. Diabetes
   c. Skin cancer
   d. Sexually transmitted disease

9. Assign students to investigate an actual health need in their own community (students may be provided with specific problems for follow-up). Have students report on their findings and identify a possible community-based health care response to the need.

10. Review holistic nursing interventions. Have students, individually or in small groups, plan creative strategies for clients with the following, or similar, difficulties:
    a. Headaches
    b. Gastric upset
    c. Arthritic pain
    d. Fatigue/sleep pattern disruption

11. Discuss the possible impact of illnesses on clients and their significant others. Ask students to share personal illness-related experiences as appropriate. Have students draw their current family relationships, using circles to represent the hierarchy and interactions among the members. Ask students if and how the drawing will change if one of the family members were to become ill.

12. Ask students to identify how illness behavior might be demonstrated in clients of different ages and sociocultural backgrounds. Correlate changes in body image and self-concept that can occur with specific illness experiences.

INDEPENDENT LEARNING

1. Students can investigate available health resources in a community, such as a Women's and Infant's Center or a public health agency, and develop a reference book of phone numbers and contact persons.

2. Students can complete a risk-factor assessment for family or friends, and discuss their findings with them.

STUDENT RESOURCES

Health Models

	Health-Illness Continuum	Agent-Host Environment	Health Belief	Health Promotion	Basic Human Needs	High-Level Wellness	Wellness-Illness	HEALTH-Healing/Disordering
Key concepts								
Meaning of health								
Meaning of illness								
Client's perception/role								
Nurse's role								

Levels of Prevention

	Primary Prevention	Secondary Prevention	Tertiary Prevention
Client activities			
Nursing activities			

Risk Factor Assessment Tool

Risk Factors	Specific Behaviors/Activities
Smoking	
Nutritional intake	
Alcohol/drug use	
Exercise	
Occupational hazards/stress	
Sleep patterns	
Sexuality	
Family history	
Other (e.g., cultural practices/beliefs)	

CROSS-CURRICULUM GUIDE

General information on health and illness models and practices and the levels of prevention are applicable to client situations throughout the curriculum in all specialty areas and clinical locations.

CHAPTER 2

The Health Care Delivery System

CRITICAL THINKING ACTIVITIES AND ANSWERS

1. Consider Mr. Wilson, a 62-year-old man who will have major surgery to replace the joint in his hip. He is married and employed at a chemical company. The doctor is concerned that he is about 20 pounds overweight. Before discharge from the hospital, what type of health care referrals might be appropriate in planning Mr. Wilson's care?

Answer: Mr. Wilson will most likely need physical therapy to help him regain range of motion, strength, and mobility following the hip replacement. Referral to a dietitian can help in giving Mr. Wilson an appropriate nutritional dietary plan. Because of potential limitation in his mobility, a home health referral might be useful in helping the client and his family anticipate the necessary adjustments in the home. The client may be discharged to a rehabilitation or extended care unit prior to returning home.

2. Mrs. Ramirez is a 42-year-old woman who is employed as an advertising agent for a large corporation. She travels 65% of the time. Her business requires her to have a physical exam every 2 years. During a recent checkup, Mrs. Ramirez was found to have elevated cholesterol and triglyceride levels. Her blood pressure was 134/84, up from 2 years ago. The nurse who conducted a health history learned that Mrs. Ramirez eats "on the go" and only exercises when at home. She also smokes 2 packs of cigarettes a day. What level of health care should Mrs. Ramirez pursue?

Answer: Preventive care.

3. Ms. Yim is a 65-year-old woman who experienced a stroke 4 days ago. She has lost movement on her left side but is able to speak clearly. Mr. Rogers is a 60-year-old man who has been coming to the neighborhood clinic regularly for the last 5 years for ongoing monitoring of his diabetes. Which of these clients would benefit most from case management, and why?

Answer: Ms. Yim has the greater immediate need for case management because a stroke predisposes her to numerous complications requiring continual health care. She will most likely be moved to a rehabilitation facility before being sent home. A case manager can help to coordinate the transition to each of these services to limit any unnecessary delays and ensure that Ms. Yim receives the right level of care.

Mr. Rogers may not need case management presently. However, diabetes is a chronic disease. If the disease becomes uncontrolled, complications may arise that require hospitalization and home care. The nurse responsible for Mr. Rogers' care, if not a formal case manager, should be sure that information about Mr. Rogers' situation is communicated to the hospital. Similarly, there should be continued coordination once Mr. Rogers returns home.

4. There are two clients that Don Jones, the evening nurse, is preparing to assess. One is Mr. Seguera, who experienced a myocardial infarction 4 days ago and will ambulate down the hall for the first time this evening. The other is Mrs. Lennox, who was newly admitted with gastrointestinal bleeding. Don finds that Mr. Sequera is resting comfortably and talking to his daughter. He is anxious to start walking. Mrs. Lennox is very restless and is experiencing discomfort from her nasogastric tube. The physician has ordered stool specimens to be collected. Which of these two clients should Don delegate to Linda, the nurse technician?

Answer: The answer is neither client. Unlicensed assistive personnel should be delegated tasks, not clients. Don would appropriately want to ambulate Mr. Seguera for the first time to ensure that he experiences no heart irregularities. If Mr. Seguera does well, future ambulation can probably be supervised by Linda. In Mrs. Lennox's case, Linda can be very helpful in assisting Don in positioning and making her more comfortable. Linda can also obtain stool specimens.

EDUCATIONAL STRATEGIES

1. Discuss the different types of health care financing, their eligibility criteria, and the health care services that are covered.

2. Ask students to share their opinions on how health care delivery has been and might continue to be affected by managed care and the capitated payment structure.

3. Assign students to observe and report on items presented in the media on the current health care delivery system.

4. Invite a case manager and/or discharge planner to discuss his or her role in a health care agency.

5. Provide students with examples of different insurance brochures and claim forms. Have them practice filling out the forms and then discuss how easy or difficult the process was for them to accomplish.

6. Review the wide variety of health care agencies and the types of health care services that might be offered by each agency. Ask students to identify the level of prevention and the role of the nurse in each agency or location.

7. Arrange for students to visit different community health care agencies and report on the following:
   a. Client access to the agency
   b. Environment within and surrounding the agency
   c. Client population and eligibility
   d. Nurse's role
   e. Fee structure
   f. Services offered

8. Have students develop an actual "game" that represents client access to a health care agency, including what is required to move into and out of the system (e.g., financing, level of wellness).

9. Provide students with a list of activities and ask them to identify what they believe may or may not be delegated to unlicensed assistive personnel.

10. Stimulate a discussion on the students' career interests in nursing. Have students obtain an article from a nursing journal that relates to their area of interest (e.g., community health, pediatrics).

11. Ask students to identify the types of services and referrals that are available to the following clients:
    a. Juvenile diabetic
    b. Pregnant teenager
    c. Young adult with human immunodeficiency virus (HIV)
    d. Client on dialysis
    e. Older adult with a cerebrovascular accident (CVA) (stroke)

12. Have students, working in small groups, discuss the type of health care services that might be sought by the following individuals:
    a. A mother with a 2-year-old who has a fever of 102° F and is vomiting at 2 AM on Sunday
    b. The daughter of an 85-year-old man who has Alzheimer's disease and has been found wandering around the neighborhood
    c. A 16-year-old football player who has an apparent fracture
    d. A 50-year-old who is experiencing severe chest pain after doing some yard work
    e. The parents of a newborn who will require immunizations
    f. A young man who needs a physical examination for his new job
    g. A 20-year-old who suspects that she has a sexually transmitted disease

13. Discuss the concept of work redesign. Ask students about the possible advantages and disadvantages of this process.

14. Have students discuss the necessary education and experience for the nurse to practice in the following health care environments: adult day care center, neonatal intensive care unit, nursing home, grammar school, and company health office.

INDEPENDENT LEARNING

1. Students can investigate an area of interest in the health care delivery system and determine the education and experience that is necessary for the nurse to practice in that area.

2. Students can determine the type of health care coverage that they or their families possess and what inpatient and outpatient services are covered by the plan.

STUDENT RESOURCES

Health Care Financing

	Private Insurance	Government Programs	Managed Care	Long Term and Catastrophic
Description of programs				
Eligibility and coverage				

Health Care Delivery Agencies

	Primary Health Care	Secondary/Tertiary Health Care	Restorative Care	Continuing Care
Examples of types of agencies providing care				
Health services provided				
Nursing roles/activities				

CROSS-CURRICULUM GUIDE

Information in this chapter may be applied to all areas of practice. The nurse may act as an advocate by assisting the client to navigate through the health care delivery system and its rules and regulations of eligibility, coverage and financing, and referral. Students may also be exposed clinically to a variety of different health care agencies, client populations, and nursing roles throughout their program of study.

MULTIMEDIA RESOURCES

Mosby's Community Health Nursing Video Series:
Set 1: *Community Assessment*
Set 2: *This Is Community Health Nursing*

Nursing Management of Client Care

CRITICAL THINKING ACTIVITIES AND ANSWERS

1. Tina has worked on the general surgical unit for about 15 months. A client is transferred to the unit from the trauma intensive care unit. The client has had abdominal surgery for removal of a ruptured spleen and laceration of the liver. In addition, the client has the left leg suspended in traction for immobilization of a fracture. The surgeon arrives and finds Tina handling the traction incorrectly. Although Tina says she is unfamiliar with traction, the surgeon complains to the head nurse. If you were the head nurse, what approach to situational leadership would you use in this case?

Answer: Coaching. Tina obviously has had experience with general surgery clients but is less familiar with orthopedic clients. Coaching provides direction and support. The head nurse should stress to Tina the importance of seeking assistance when she is unfamiliar with any nursing procedure. At the same time the head nurse should stay with Tina and review the principles of traction care and maintenance.

2. Mr. Tanaka is scheduled for surgery at 1 PM to repair torn ligaments in the knee. It is the first time that Mr. Tanaka has had surgery. It is now 11:30 AM and the operating room personnel have notified nursing that they will pick up Mr. Tanaka in 30 minutes. Mr. Lines, the nurse, enters the room to complete the preoperative checklist for Mr. Tanaka and to make final preparations for surgery. He finds the client moving about restlessly in bed and reluctant to talk. What would be Mr. Lines' priority in this situation to continue preparation for surgery, perform an assessment of the client, or call the operating room to delay pickup?

Answer: The nurse's focus in this situation must be the client. Even though the time for surgery is quickly approaching, Mr. Lines knows that Mr. Tanaka must be prepared, both physically and mentally. An assessment must be made of the cause of Mr. Tanaka's restlessness and reluctance to communicate. Mr. Lines should consider pain in the injured knee, anxiety about the impending surgery, or some other physical factor that may be causing restlessness.

3. Lisa is a student nurse assigned to two clients. She begins her afternoon by checking first on Mrs. Rhodes, who is being discharged in approximately 2 hours, after a right lumpectomy this morning for breast cancer. She examines the surgical site and begins to take Mrs. Rhodes' blood pressure. The call light at the bedside comes on to let Linda know that her second client, Mr. Sawyer, has finished lunch and wants to ambulate down the hall. Mr. Sawyer had surgery just 2 days ago for acute pancreatitis. Lisa lets Mrs. Rhodes know that she will return in just a moment and leaves to check Mr. Sawyer. Once she arrives in Mr. Sawyer's room, Lisa learns that he wants a pain medication. While preparing the medication, Lisa notices that Mrs. Rhodes' blood pressure should have been checked 10 minutes ago. How might Lisa have managed her time more wisely?

Answer: Lisa would have benefited from better planning and prioritizing care. Mrs. Rhodes is in the postoperative period and should be monitored closely. Before assessing Mrs. Rhodes, Lisa could have checked on Mr. Sawyer and told him that they would plan his ambulation after mealtime. Lisa could have given him a pain injection before seeing Mrs. Rhodes so that the medication would have time to be effective before Mr. Sawyer ambulated. In addition, Lisa could have asked a staff member to assist Mr. Sawyer in ambulating after the pain medication had some effect. (Ambulation may not be appropriate immediately after certain pain medications.) This would have prevented Lisa from being interrupted while caring for Mrs. Rhodes.

EDUCATIONAL STRATEGIES

1. Compare and contrast the concepts of leadership and management in nursing.

2. Review the different styles of leadership, identifying the advantages and limitations of each style. Ask students to provide examples of how each style of leadership can be implemented in clinical situations.

3. Divide the students into small groups and provide them with a problem-solving scenario (e.g., airplane crash in the desert with minimal resources). Have students identify the leaders who emerge in the groups and the style of leadership that is exhibited. Follow up with students completing a self-assessment of their perceived leadership styles.

4. Present the nursing care delivery models, including total patient care, functional nursing, team nursing, primary nursing, and case management. Provide students with sample client care units and agencies and have them propose the delivery model that will be most effective.

5. Assign students to observe nurses in leadership positions in order to determine their styles of leadership and management. Discuss the students' observations, including positive and negative behaviors demonstrated by the nurse leader. Ask students how their perceived style of leadership might have changed a situation.

6. Review principles of time management and their importance in clinical decision making. Provide students with a sample multiple client assignment and ask them to prioritize their activities for the day.

7. Invite a nurse manager to speak to the class about his or her role, educational preparation, and experience.

INDEPENDENT LEARNING

1. Students can review situations that they have encountered to determine which leadership styles have been adopted.

2. Students can observe individuals in diverse leadership positions to identify which styles are being used and if the styles differ with the circumstances.

3. Students can keep a record of their activities for a week in order to see where their time management is most and least effective. They can try to prioritize their activities in order to improve upon their use of time.

STUDENT RESOURCES

Leadership Styles

Leadership Style	Description	Advantages/Limitations
Autocratic		
Democratic		
Laissez-faire		
Situational		

Nursing Care Delivery Models

Model	Description of the Model	Role of the Nurse	Delegation of Activities
Total patient care			
Functional nursing			
Team nursing			
Primary nursing			
Case management			

CROSS-CURRICULUM GUIDE

Principles of leadership, management, delegation, and nursing care delivery are woven throughout the nursing curriculum. As students progress through their educational program and are exposed to diverse client care situations, they may build upon their knowledge and application of these principles. Students who are just about to graduate and enter the profession may benefit from a classroom review of this information along with clinical experiences that allow them to test their leadership and management abilities.

MULTIMEDIA RESOURCES

Mosby's Nursing Leadership and Management Video Series
  Leadership
  Delegating Effectively and Appropriately
Mosby's Nursing Leadership and Management Interactive Videodisc Series
  Problem Solving and Decision Making
  Assigning and Delegating Client Care Activities

UNIT 2

Critical Thinking in Nursing Practice

Critical Thinking and Nursing Judgment

TOPICAL OUTLINE

CRITICAL THINKING ACTIVITIES AND ANSWERS

1. Put yourself in John's position as he completes a day on a busy medical nursing unit. John was involved with a medication error. At 10 AM he had just completed a bedbath for one of his clients. He then went to the medication room to prepare the medications for his four clients. Just before John finished this, a nurse told him that Mr. Williams in room 10 was requesting a pain medication. John saved some time and prepared the 10 mg of morphine ordered for Mr. Williams. He gathered the medications he had prepared and went to room 10 first, giving Mr. Lazar his ordered medications and then giving Mr. Williams the requested injection of morphine. After administering all the medications, John looked at Mr. William's chart and discovered that he had received morphine only 2 hours ago. The medication is be given no more than every 4 hours. Within 15 minutes of receiving the morphine, Mr. William's vital signs were stable. As a follow-up, John completed an incident report describing the medication error.

   Reflect upon this experience while considering the errors that were made and describe what John might learn from the experience.

Answer: The experience can be helpful in several ways. John failed to follow a standard of always checking to see when a medication (especially a p.r.n.) was last given. In an effort to save time, he took the other RN's report for granted. Even though Mr. Williams wanted something for pain, John should have assessed the client's condition first in case something else was occurring. There are standard evaluation criteria to use when assessing pain, which can be symptomatic of many conditions. John was not methodical in his thinking. The next time he attempts to organize care for four clients he should be responsible for assessing each client's needs, use complete information, and then plan his actions logically. He showed responsibility for his actions by completing the incident report.

2. A staff nurse, Maria, tells the evening shift during report that no matter what she tries to do, she cannot get a client, Mrs. Lee, to do her postoperative exercises. Mrs. Lee had abdominal surgery just 24 hours ago. Maria reports, "The woman is just unwilling to do anything for herself. I have told her that she can develop pneumonia if she fails to cough routinely." What approach to problem solving might you take to understand Mrs. Lee's situation better?

Answer: Problem solving begins with assessment. When entering Mrs. Lee's room, watch her behavior closely. Is she hesitant to move, or does she move spontaneously? Does she hold her incisions guardedly? Sit down for just a moment and let her know you have heard that she is having difficulty doing her breathing exercises. Encourage her to express the reasons for her difficulty. She may be afraid, for some unexplained reason, or she may not have been instructed properly in the first place. Do not simply assume that she in uncooperative. Learn what factors are preventing her from performing the exercises correctly. Work with Mrs. Lee to find a way that will succeed.

3. Select a recently assigned client. Reflecting on your actions during that experience, prepare an outline that describes your plan of care for future clients with similar health care needs. As you complete the plan, consider these questions: What might you do differently? What might you do in the same way? How might you improve the client's participation in your plan?

Answer: As you reflect upon the experience, consider the nursing interventions that were successful and those that were not successful. What were the reasons for your outcomes? Consider whether you performed all nursing activities competently. How would you evaluate your relationship with the client? Consider whether you established trust and were able to work collaboratively with the client.

EDUCATIONAL STRATEGIES

1. Discuss the concept and process of critical thinking and its application to nursing practice. Ask students to provide examples of activities that might occur with each level of the critical thinking process.

2. Share personal nursing experiences with the class, focusing on the use of critical thinking in providing client care.

3. Lead the class in the application of the decision making process for resolution of a common, non-medical situation, such as buying a new car, choosing an apartment to rent, or selecting a bank.

4. Divide the class into small groups and have students work through the problem-solving process with an actual or simulated client scenario.

5. Ask students what problems might be anticipated and what further information will be required from clients who are experiencing the following:
   a. Elevated blood pressure
   b. Fever
   c. Difficulty walking
   d. Disorientation to time, place, and persons
   e. Joint pain

6. In a post-clinical or classroom discussion, have students use the technique of reflection to self-assess their behaviors.

7. Have students apply the critical thinking skills to an actual or simulated client care situation.

8. Using the case study presented in the text (Mrs. Bryan), ask students to speculate on how the situation might be altered if there is no nearby neighbor for support, the relationship with her daughter is strained, or her health status diminished drastically.

9. Define and describe the steps of the nursing process, incorporating the concept of critical thinking.

10. Ask students to begin to develop creative strategies for the following, or similar client situations:
    a. A homeless individual who requires dressing changes
    b. An older adult, living alone, who has poor vision and needs daily insulin injections
    c. First-time parents of quadruplets
    d. An active adolescent with a broken arm

11. Set up a client simulation in a classroom or nursing lab and have individuals or groups of students enter the room, observe for a brief period (e.g., 30 seconds to 1 minute), and then discuss their observations. Focus the "debriefing" on what their perceptions were, along with what may have been wrong with the scenario.

INDEPENDENT LEARNING

1. Students can determine how the outcome of previous decision-making experiences may have been improved with the use of critical thinking.

2. Students can apply the critical thinking process to a current problem, writing out the necessary steps to take and evaluating the outcome of their decision making.

STUDENT RESOURCES
Levels of Critical Thinking

Levels of Critical Thinking	Nursing Behaviors/Thought Processes

Comparison of the Scientific Method and Nursing Process

	Similarities	Differences
Scientific method		
Nursing process		

CROSS-CURRICULUM GUIDE

Critical thinking and the nursing process are applied in all nursing situations, with clients of diverse ages and backgrounds. This information is relevant in discussions throughout the curriculum, with the complexity and sophistication of its application increasing as students progress in the program. Early exposure of students to the process of critical thinking may promote its effective use in subsequent client interactions.

MULTIMEDIA RESOURCES

Mosby's Nursing Leadership and Management Video Series
> *Problem Solving and Decision Making: Critical Thinking in Action*

Mosby's Nursing Leadership and Management Interactive Videodisc Series
> *Problem Solving and Decision Making*

5

Nursing Assessment

TOPICAL OUTLINE

CRITICAL THINKING ACTIVITIES AND ANSWERS

1. Develop examples of closed and open-ended questions that you would use to determine Mrs. Byran's health care needs. Practice using them on a classmate and compare the information you gather.

Answer: Ask Mrs. Byran what she feels she needs. Identify her resources, limitations, and concerns. Ask how she is able to do activities of daily living. If possible, observe Mrs. Byran performing these activities. Ask her what type of help does she think she needs. Ask her some questions to determine her perception of the care she is receiving and whether it meets her needs.

2. You greet Mrs. Jacob on your first home visit following her major abdominal surgery. You introduce yourself, your role, and the physician's post-operative orders. What aspect of the interview has taken place? What will you do next?

Answer: The orientation phase has taken place. Next you should obtain assessment data regarding physical aspects, incision site, activity level, comfort level, comfort measures, and Mrs. Jacob's expectations for this aspect of care.

3. Take the following narrative and identify subjective and objective data. Mr. Kantor is lying on his side, grimacing and rubbing his abdomen, moaning, and complaining of pain. His vital signs are as follows: blood pressure 140/100, pulse 120, respiration 22. He is pale, diaphoretic, and his skin is warm to touch. Oral temperature is 102° F.

Answer: *Subjective data:* Mr. Kantor is moaning and complaining of pain. *Objective data:* He is lying on his side, grimacing, and rubbing his abdomen. His vital signs are as follows: blood pressure 140/100, pulse 120, respirations 22. He is pale, diaphoretic, and his skin is warm to touch. His oral temperature is 102° F.

EDUCATIONAL STRATEGIES

1. Identify the components of assessment within the nursing process.

2. Discuss techniques for data collection, including client interviews and physical assessments.

3. Describe the difference between objective and subjective data. Provide students with a list of client signs, symptoms, and statements and have students identify the objective and subjective data.

4. Review basic communication techniques and the phases of the interview. Have students role play an interview with a peer (videotape the experience, if possible, for later review and critique by the students).

5. Ask students to identify the possible sources of data and how data can best be validated.

6. Provide students with copies of different assessment tools. Review the types of client data that can be obtained with the use of closed and open-ended questions.

7. Using photos and/or student "actors," have the class do quick assessments of situations (e.g., a client grimacing, limping, or coughing).

8. Ask the students how the initial nursing assessment of a client may be altered in the following circumstances:
   a. An individual who is admitted to the medical center in severe pain
   b. An adolescent who comes to the clinic with an overly enthusiastic parent
   c. A client who comes to the psychiatric outpatient center and is hallucinating and acting aggressively

9. Describe and demonstrate the techniques of physical assessment. Ask students what type of data might be obtained with the use of inspection, palpation, percussion, and auscultation. Have students practice the basic techniques on their peers or a practice mannequin.

10. Provide students with an actual or simulated case study and have them identify and cluster the objective and subjective data. (Refer to the case studies in the text and student study guide.)

11. Assign students to complete a basic client history (provide an assessment tool). After the experience, ask students to share the information they obtained and their feelings about the experience, including how they could have improved upon their communication.

INDEPENDENT LEARNING

1. Students can practice assessment techniques with their friends and family members. General observations may be made of individuals in the community while shopping, waiting in line for a movie, and so on.

2. Students can research articles in nursing journals on specific areas of client assessment.

STUDENT RESOURCES
Approaches to Data Collection

Comprehensive Data Base	Problem-focused Data Base

Organization of Data

	Subjective Data	Objective Data
Methods to obtain data		
Sources to obtain data		

Nursing Health History

Biographical Information

Name _____ Sex _____ Date _____

Address _____

Family member or significant-other name _____

Address & phone number _____

Marital status _____ Religious preference/practices _____

Occupation _____

Length of occupation _____

Health care provider _____

Insurance _____

Reason for seeking health care _____

Present Illness

Onset _____ Sudden or gradual_____

Duration _____

Symptoms _____

Precipitating factors _____

Relief measures _____

Expectations of health care providers _____

Past History

Illness: Childhood _____

            Illnesses & hospitalizations _____

            Operations _____

            Major illnesses _____

Allergies: Type _____

            Reaction _____

            Treatment _____

Immunizations: _____

Habits: Ethanol _____ Smoking _____ Drugs _____

            Duration _____

Medications: Prescribed _____

               Self-medicated _____

Sleep patterns _____

Exercise patterns _____

Nutritional patterns _____

Work patterns _____

Family History

Health of parents, siblings, spouse, children _____

Risk-factor analysis: cancer, heart disease, diabetes mellitus, kidney disease, hypertension,
      mental disorders:
_____

Environmental History

Cleanliness _____

Hazards _____

Pollutants _____

Psychosocial & Cultural History

Primary language _____

Cultural activites social group _____

Community resources _____

Mood _____

Development stage _____

Review of Systems

Head:	Headaches _____	Dizziness _____
Vision:	Last eye exam _____	
	Glasses _____	Contacts ____ (hard, soft, how long wearing)
	Blurring _____	Double vision _____
	Pain _____	Inflamation _____
Hearing:	Impairment_____	Type of hearing aid _____
		Date of new batteries _____
	Discharge, pain _____	
Nose:	Allergic rhinitis _____	Type of allergen _____
		Relief meassures _____
	Frequency of colds/year _____	
	History of polyps, fracture, surgery _____	
	Sinuses _____	
	Nose bleeds_____	
Throat & mouth	Last dental exam _____	
	Dentures _____	
	Pain, Bleeding _____	
	Speech disorders _____	
	Swallowing prolems _____	
Respiratory:	Cough _____	Sputum, hemoptysis _____
	Dyspnea _____	Dyspnea on exertion _____
	Pain _____	
	Activity tolerance _____	
	Last chest x-ray _____	

Circulatory:	Pain _____	Palpitations _____
	Edema _____ Numbness _____	Tingling _____
	Changes in color, hair of extremities _____	
	Syncope _____	Dizziness _____
Nutritional:	Appetite _____	
	Nausea _____	Vomiting _____
	Weight loss or gain _____	
Elimination:		
Bowel:	Pattern _____	Use of laxatives _____
	Constipation or diarrhea _____	
	Bleeding _____	Ostgomy _____
Urine:	Pattern _____	Medications _____
	Incontinence _____	Infections _____
Reproductive:	Pregnancies _____	Children _____
	Last Pap test _____ Results _____	LMP _____
	Bleeding or discharge _____	
	Self breast or testicular exam _____	
Neurological:	Orientation _____	Convulsions _____
	Paralysis or paresthesia _____	Weakness _____
	Incoordination _____	Headaches _____
Musculoskeletal:	Pain _____	Stiffness _____
	Deformity _____	
	Exercise patterns _____	
Integument:	Color _____	Turgor _____
	Texture _____	Temperature _____
	Rashes or lesions _____	
Vital Signs:	Temperature _____	Pulse _____
	Respirations _____	BP _____

CROSS-CURRICULUM GUIDE

Critical thinking and the nursing process are applied in all nursing situations, with clients of diverse ages and backgrounds. Information on client assessment is relevant in discussions throughout the curriculum, with the approaches increasing in complexity and sophistication as students progress in the program. Accurate assessment is critical in order that subsequent interactions with clients and significant others be as effective as possible in the acute, extended care, or home care setting.

Nursing Diagnosis

CRITICAL THINKING ACTIVITIES AND ANSWERS

1. Describe the relationship of the nursing diagnosis to the other steps of the nursing process.

Answer: Nursing diagnoses must be supported by assessment data; changes in assessment result in modifications of nursing diagnoses; nursing diagnoses provide direction for the care plan.

2. During an assessment the nurse notes that the client reports an increase in the number of colds, that sputum is thick and yellow, and that there is an increase in shortness of breath. Which step of the diagnostic process is taking place?

Answer: Analyzing, validating, and clustering data.

3. These three nursing diagnoses are worded incorrectly. What is wrong?
   a. High risk of ineffective airway clearance due to pneumonia
   b. Body disturbance due to anorexia nervosa
   c. Fatigue and sleep disturbance related to interrupted sleep pattern

Answer:
   a. Etiology is described with a medical diagnosis.
   b. Etiology is described with a medical diagnosis.
   c. Two diagnostic labels are used and the etiology repeats a diagnostic label.

EDUCATIONAL STRATEGIES

1. Describe what a nursing diagnosis is and how it fits into the nursing process.

2. Correlate the process of critical thinking with the identification of nursing diagnoses.

3. Review the NANDA-approved nursing diagnostic labels and statements.

4. Provide examples of how data clustering and analysis lead to the formulation of nursing diagnoses. Give students different sets of client data and defining characteristics; have them cluster the data and then begin to identify possible nursing diagnostic labels.

5. Discuss the components of the nursing diagnosis, including the diagnostic label or statement and etiology. Ask students how the nursing approach might vary for the same diagnostic label but with a different etiology for the following, or similar, statements:
   a. Knowledge deficit related to. . .
   b. Immobility related to. . .
   c. Constipation or diarrhea related to. . .
   d. Fluid volume deficit related to. . .

6. Compare and contrast the different types of nursing diagnoses: actual, risk, possible, syndrome, and wellness. Provide, or ask students to provide, examples of each type of diagnosis.

7. Review possible errors that can be made in the identification and formulation of nursing diagnoses. Provide examples of erroneous diagnostic statements and ask students to suggest corrections for the errors.

8. Compare and contrast medical and nursing diagnoses.

9. Discuss how nursing diagnoses and care plans are individualized and prioritized for the client.

10. Ask students to identify the advantages and limitations of the use of nursing diagnoses.

11. Have students, working individually or in small groups, take sample client situations, identify, cluster, and analyze the client data, and formulate nursing diagnoses.

INDEPENDENT LEARNING

1. Students can practice assessment on classmates, family members, or friends and write nursing diagnoses for identified needs (e.g., altered sleep patterns).

2. Students can take diagnostic labels and statements and see how the nursing approach may vary when the etiology is different.

STUDENT RESOURCES

Nursing Diagnosis Worksheet

Assessment Data	Diagnostic Label	Related Factors

Nursing Diagnosis Errors and Corrections

Common Errors	Corrections

CROSS-CURRICULUM GUIDE

Critical thinking and the nursing process are applied in all nursing situations, with clients of diverse ages and backgrounds. Information on client assessment and nursing diagnosis is relevant in discussions throughout the curriculum, with the approaches increasing in complexity and sophistication as students progress in the program. Accurate assessment and diagnosis is critical in order that subsequent interactions with clients and significant others be as effective as possible in the acute, extended care, or home care setting.

CHAPTER 7

Planning for Nursing Care

CRITICAL THINKING ACTIVITIES AND ANSWERS

1. How are the goals and expected outcomes of nursing care linked to nursing diagnoses?

Answer: Measurable criteria determine when the client's need or problem that generated the nursing diagnosis is resolved. Nursing diagnoses form the basis for the goals of care.

2. What criteria are used to determine expected outcomes for a given set of client-centered goals?

Answer: Expected outcomes are the measurable responses of the client to nursing care. Expected outcomes are directed toward goal attainment and are important in client evaluation.

3. What information is necessary to plan nursing interventions for your clients? If you had nursing assistants, how would you plan the nursing strategies that could be delegated to these persons?

Answer: Necessary information includes available resources, client's resources, client's level of care, preparation of nursing assistance, client's assessment, changes in client's status, and discharge planning activities. Upon determining the strategies to be implemented for the client, the nurse should decide which ones are appropriate for delegation to a nursing assistant.

EDUCATIONAL STRATEGIES

1. Discuss how goals, outcomes, and nursing interventions stem from client assessment and nursing diagnosis.

2. Discuss the concept of mutually designed goals and outcomes and priorities.

3. Compare and contrast long- and short-term goals, and goals and expected outcomes. Ask students to identify where and how long- and short-term goals might be most effectively utilized.

4. Provide the guidelines for stating goals and expected outcomes. Ask students to identify goals and outcomes for different nursing diagnoses. Give students examples of properly and improperly written goals and outcomes and ask them to critique and correct the statements.

5. Discuss the process of selecting nursing interventions and the necessary competencies of the nurse in their implementation.

6. Identify the three types of interventions (nurse-initiated, physician-initiated, and collaborative) and ask students to provide examples for each type.

7. Review the purpose and different types of care plans and critical pathways. Provide examples of available formats for students to use to practice documentation of the nursing process. Ask students to provide the possible rationale for differences in care plan formats from agency to agency.

8. Compare and contrast traditional and computerized care plans and critical pathways.

9. Present the criteria for writing nursing interventions. Discuss possible errors in formulating the nursing intervention statement. Provide examples of properly and improperly written nursing interventions, and ask students to critique and correct the statements.

10. Review the steps of the consultation process. Provide students with different client scenarios and ask them to identify possible consultants who may be contacted.

11. Have students, working individually or in small groups, identify goals, expected outcomes, and nursing interventions for an actual or simulated client situation.

INDEPENDENT LEARNING

1. Students can identify nursing diagnoses for themselves, family members, or friends. They can practice writing long- and short-term goals, expected outcomes, and possible nursing interventions. Provide students with a sample agency care plan for practice in documentation.

2. Students can investigate the different types of consultants that are available in the health care delivery system.

3. Students can research articles in nursing journals on the use of care plans and/or critical pathways.

STUDENT RESOURCES

Seven Guidelines for Goals/Outcomes

Guidelines	Description
1. Client-centered factors	
2. Singular factors	
3. Observable factors	
4. Measurable factors	
5. Time-limited factors	
6. Mutual factors	
7. Realistic factors	

Types of Nursing Interventions

Nursing Interventions	Specific Examples
Nurse-initiated	
Physician-initiated	
Collaborative	

Sample Agency Care Plan

Nursing Diagnosis or Client Problem	Expected Outcomes	Nursing Interventions

Multidisciplinary Critical Pathway

Medical diagnosis (code): _____ Expected length of stay: _____

Nursing diagnostic or client need: _____

Expected outcomes: _____

INTERVENTIONS	1ST DAY - (DATE)	2ND DAY - (DATE)	3RD DAY - (DATE)
Nursing			
Treatments			
Medications			
Diagnostic tests			
Diet therapy			
Consults or referrals			
Teaching or discharge needs			

CROSS-CURRICULUM GUIDE

Critical thinking and the nursing process are applied in all nursing situations, with clients of diverse ages and backgrounds. Information on prioritizing care, identifying goals and expected outcomes, and selecting nursing interventions is relevant in discussions throughout the curriculum, with the focus increasing in complexity and sophistication as students progress in the program. Accurate determination of goals, outcomes, and nursing interventions is critical in order that interactions with clients and significant others be as effective as possible in the acute, extended care, or home care setting.

Implementing Nursing Care

TOPICAL OUTLINE

CRITICAL THINK-ING ACTIVITIES AND ANSWERS

1. Mr. Clark is a 45-year-old man admitted with congestive heart failure. His lung sounds are clear; his blood pressure is 130/88, his pulse is 112, and his respirations are 24. His nursing history reveals that he does not consistently take all his medications nor does he follow a low-sodium diet, which was designed to reduce fluid retention. List the types of interventions that you might select to assist in resolving Mr. Clark's present illness and prevent further complications.

Answer: *Direct care activities:* grooming, hygiene
Assistive care activities: ambulating
Teaching: medications and diet
Counseling: adapting to chronic illness

2. You are assigned to administer all medications. What measures will you take to reduce the incidence of adverse reactions in clients who receive piggyback intravenous medications?

Answer: Knowledge of medications; determination of appropriate equipment; ensuring patency of IV and compatibility of IV solutions; assessment for medication allergy; knowledge of five rights of medication administration

3. Mrs. Jones is a 240-pound comatose client. You assign the nursing assistant to provide skin and hygiene care. What type of help do you anticipate that the nurse assistant will need in order to provide safe care and reduce the risk of pressure ulcers to Mrs. Jones?

Answer: Knowledge of skin care–general hygiene and perineal care; knowledge of the hazards of immobility; determination of personnel needed to turn and position the client; use of time management skills to plan for assistance with care

EDUCATIONAL STRATEGIES

1. Describe the implementation phase and its integration in the nursing process.

2. Discuss the nurse's role with standing orders and protocols.

3. Discuss and apply the information-processing model to a nursing situation, such as with a diabetic client.

4. Review the implementation process: reassessment, reviewing and revising the care plan, organizing resources and care delivery, and implementing and communicating nursing interventions. Provide students with, or ask them to provide, examples for each part of the process.

5. Review the formulation of the nursing care plan or pathway. Share actual client experiences and have students suggest how the care plan might have to be altered depending on the client's current status.

6. Discuss the implementation methods used in nursing. Have students identify, verbally or in writing, specific nursing interventions for the following implementation methods:
   a. Assistance with performing activities of daily living
   b. Counseling
   c. Teaching
   d. Providing direct care
   e. Achieving the goals of care
   f. Delegating, supervising, and evaluating the work of others

7. Provide the students with a client-specific situation that may arise in an acute care, a home care, or an extended care agency and ask them to identify the equipment and resources (including staff) that must be organized in order to effectively deliver client care.

8. Assign students to observe or participate in the communication of nursing interventions at a change-of-shift report, conference, or staff meeting.

9. Provide students with examples of different types of documentation and discuss how the nursing interventions are communicated to other members of the health care team.

10. Discuss the nursing skills necessary for implementation of care–cognitive, interpersonal, and psychomotor. Have students provide specific examples of each. Give students specific nursing interventions and ask them to identify which skill is being used by the nurse.

11. Review the provision of direct nursing care and have students provide examples of each of the following:
    a. Compensation for adverse reactions
    b. Preventive measures
    c. Preparation for procedures
    d. Lifesaving measures

12. Stimulate a discussion on how nursing implementation measures might differ depending on the physical location or type of agency.

13. For the following situations, ask students to identify what further information or preparation is required before implementing nursing interventions:
    a. An older client who is 2 days postoperative with a repair of a fractured left hip
    b. An infant who will be receiving intravenous fluids
    c. An adult client who has an order for an antihypertensive medication
    d. A newly diagnosed diabetic client, with a hearing impairment, who will require daily insulin injections

14. Review delegation of client care activities. Have students identify which activities might be delegated, to whom they may be delegated, and how their performance will be evaluated.

15. Assign students to observe or participate in selected client care activities in an agency. In a post-care discussion, have students identify the implementation methods that were used by the nurses and any adaptations in care that were made according to the clients' conditions.

16. Discuss, generally, how the client's (and nurse's) age and developmental status may alter the nurse's implementation of nursing interventions.

INDEPENDENT LEARNING

1. Students can inquire how nurses in different health settings have altered their care in order to meet a client's changing needs.

2. Students can research articles in nursing journals on particular implementation methods.

STUDENT RESOURCES
Implementation Methods

Implementation Methods	Description
1.	
2.	
3.	
4.	
5.	
6.	

CROSS-CURRICULUM GUIDE

Critical thinking and the nursing process are applied in all nursing situations, with clients of diverse ages and backgrounds. Information on the implementation of care and the adaptation of the care plan or pathway is integral to discussions throughout the curriculum, with the focus increasing in complexity and sophistication as students progress in the program. Accurate selection of nursing interventions is critical in order that clients and significant others are able to achieve expected outcomes and goals in the acute, extended care, or home care setting.

Chapter 9

Evaluation

TOPICAL OUTLINE

CRITICAL THINKING ACTIVITIES AND ANSWERS

1. Mr. Vacaro has been visiting the clinic for more than a month on a weekly basis for follow-up care for a chronic venous stasis ulcer of the left leg. The nurse's note at the time of his first visit contained the following information: "Ulcer with irregular margins, 4 cm wide by 5 cm long, approximately 1/2 cm deep, with foul-smelling purulent yellowish drainage. Only subcutaneous tissue visible. Skin around ulcer brownish rust in color. Zinc oxide and calamine gauze applied to ulcer; Ace bandage applied to gauze. Client instructed to return in 2 weeks."

   As the nurse who is caring for the client on the follow-up visit, what expected outcomes would you anticipate for the goal of "Wound will demonstrate healing within 4 weeks?" What evaluative measures would you use to determine if the wound is healing?

Answer: The goal of "wound will demonstrate healing in 4 weeks" will most likely have outcomes that include the following: "Wound margins will decrease 1 cm in width and length within 2 weeks" and "Depth of wound will decrease 1/4 cm within 2 weeks" with "Wound drainage absent within 4 weeks." The nurse will evaluate the client's status and progress by measuring the size and depth of the wound as well as observing the amount of drainage found on the dressing at the time of dressing change.

2. Mr. Chu is a 50-year-old man with chronic obstructive pulmonary disease (COPD) with hypoxemia, fatigue, and dyspnea. He is to be discharged with home oxygen at 2 L. His primary nurse has identified the need to teach Mr. Chu information about home oxygen. Mr. Chu will probably be in the hospital for 2 more days. Explain why evaluation is important in this case example. How will the nurse's evaluation of Mr. Chu's learning influence the plan of care at discharge?

Answer: It is important to know Mr. Chu's progress in learning. The nurse must evaluate specific evidence of content learning. For example, does Mr. Chu know what kind of oxygen he is using? Can he describe how to administer his oxygen at home? Does he know how to use the portable oxygen canister? How often is he to use his oxygen? Does he know whom to call if there are problems with the equipment? Evaluation will determine if reinstruction is needed or if the staff can move to other topics. Evaluation will also determine if Mr. Chu will need continued instruction or home care after discharge.

3. As a nurse on a general medicine unit you care for a number of clients who receive central line intravenous (IV) therapy. Over the last month, three client's central IV lines have developed an infection at the line insertion site. Develop a quality indicator and monitoring criteria to measure this clinical practice problem.

Answer: The quality indicator would be the incidence of central line infections in clients receiving IV therapy. Staff would monitor over a period of time the number of clients receiving central line IV therapy who developed an infection at the insertion site. Criteria to measure to understand the nature of this problem might include time of central catheter insertions, type of infection, type of IV fluids and medications, frequency and type of dressing change, and location of infection. Should the incidence of infections continue or increase, staff will be able to identify potential actions based on the criteria that contribute to the infections.

EDUCATIONAL STRATEGIES

1. Discuss evaluation and its focus in the nursing process and overall health care delivery.

2. Review how goals and expected outcomes determine evaluative measures. Provide examples to students of goals and outcomes and ask them to identify how and when the nurse may evaluate their achievement by the client.

3. Review methods of evaluation that might be used for health care delivery, such as the use of JCAHO guidelines and PSROs.

4. Identify the steps of the evaluation process:
   a. Examination of the goal statement
   b. Assessment of client behaviors and responses
   c. Determination of the degree of agreement between the outcome criteria and the client behaviors and responses
   d. Investigation of possible factors when there is no agreement with the outcome criteria

   Provide students with client examples and have them go through the evaluation process to determine if goals were achieved.

5. Discuss how assessment skills (e.g., physical and psychosocial assessment) are also used in evaluating the client's status.

6. Provide examples of how evaluation of the client might be documented in different agencies, including flow sheets, and care plans/pathways (as available). Have students practice documenting examples of actual or simulated client evaluations on sample agency records.

7. Provide examples of how care plans/pathways can be modified according to the evaluation and reassessment of the client's status.

8. Define the concept of and describe the process of Quality Improvement (QI) in health care, including its multidisciplinary approach. Discuss the dimensions of performance and the JCAHO 10 Steps for Quality Improvement.

9. Discuss the formation of QI teams. Ask students to identify how a team might be organized to meet the following agency needs:
    a. Keeping a large facility neat and clean
    b. Increasing the speed of meal delivery to clients
    c. Preventing client falls

10. Have students provide the rationale for QI, including its relationship to cost, and client and staff satisfaction.

11. Describe and identify the focus of the quality indicators–structure, process, and outcome. Ask students to provide examples of each type of quality indicator.

12. Review actual QI projects that have been implemented in health care agencies.

13. Assign students to select an area to assess for QI. Have them specify the quality indicators, sample thresholds for compliance, and process for evaluation and communication of results.

14. If possible, have students participate in the QI process within the educational or health care institution. Assign them to attend a QI conference or meeting, and have students report back on the process observed and information received.

15. Invite a Quality Improvement director or manager to speak to the class about his or her role in the overall enhancement of health care delivery.

16. Apply the Focus-PDCA approach to a client management situation.

17. Have students identify possible evaluative measures for the following client goals:
    a. Client will maintain a reduced sodium diet.
    b. Client will self-catheterize for residual urine.
    c. Client will demonstrate a reduced level of anxiety.
    d. Client will perform postoperative exercises.

INDEPENDENT LEARNING

1. Students can research articles in nursing journals on the QI process and its application to a client care situation.

2. Students can complete self-evaluations of attainment of personal or academic goals, identifying areas that might be reassessed and enhanced for the future.

3. Students can practice documentation of the nursing process, using actual or simulated client situations and trying different types of care plan formats.

STUDENT RESOURCES
Steps in Evaluating Goal Achievement

Steps	Client Example
1.	
2.	
3.	
4.	
5.	

JCAHO Ten Steps for Quality Improvement

Steps for QI	Description and/or Example
1. Establish responsibility for QI program.	
2. Define the scope of service for a clinical area.	
3. Define the key aspects of service for a clinical area.	
4. Develop quality indicators.	
5. Establish thresholds for evaluation of indicators.	
6. Collect and analyze data.	
7. Evaluate the results of monitoring activities.	
8. Resolve problems by developing action plans.	
9. Reevaluate to determine success of plan.	
10. Communicate QI results to organization.	

Agency Care Plan Sample

Client name:

DATE AND INITIALS	NURSING DIAGNOSIS	SHORT-TERM GOALS AND OUTCOMES	RESOLVED OR REVISED (DATE AND INITIALS)	NURSING ACTIONS OR ORDERS

Discharge planning:

Student Care Plan

SUPPORTING DATA	NURSING DIAGNOSIS	GOALS AND OUTCOMES	NURSING INTERVENTION	SCIENTIFIC RATIONALE	EVALUATION MEASURES

CROSS-CURRICULUM GUIDE

Critical thinking and the nursing process are applied in all nursing situations, with clients of diverse ages and backgrounds. The evaluation of client care, reassessment of the client, and the modification of the care plan or pathway is integral to discussions throughout the curriculum, with the focus increasing in complexity and sophistication as students progress in the program. Accurate evaluation of the client's achievement of goals is critical in order that clients and significant others are able to achieve an optimum level of wellness in the acute, extended care, or home care setting.

The QI process is an essential component of the health care delivery system. Students need to become aware of how it is integrated into all aspects of client care and implementation of nursing interventions. Students may be involved in QI studies that focus on reducing client falls in an extended care agency, improving the identification of child abuse in a school setting, or determining the cost of home visits and medical supplies.

UNIT 3

Professional Standards in Nursing Practice

CHAPTER
10

Professional Nursing Roles

CRITICAL THINKING ACTIVITY AND ANSWER

1. You are assigned eight surgical clients to care for on the day shift. Two clients are to have surgery today; one at 8 AM and the other to follow. Three clients will be discharged by noon, and one is a postoperative client that had surgery during the night. Two clients are admitting and are having procedures that will require overnight observation. You will have an LPN and unlicensed assistive personnel (UAP) to assist you with providing care. How will you utilize the personnel you will be working with to care for these clients? What tasks are appropriate to delegate to the UAP? How can you best utilize the LPN?

Answer: The UAP would be best utilized in obtaining vital signs, providing morning care, helping the clients who will be going home to pack, and assisting clients who will be admitted following a procedure. The LPN will be helpful in managing the short-stay clients, assisting with patient and family education for the clients to be discharged today, and helping with administration of pain medications as needed. The RN will focus care on assessing the postoperative client and developing a plan of care. The RN needs to evaluate the clients to be discharged, determine if the goals and outcomes were met, and coordinate any home care activities with the social worker or case manager. The RN will be able to assess and develop a plan of care for the two short-stay clients and those who may be returning from the operating room on this shift. Collaboration with the surgeons, case manager, and social worker, and appropriate allied health professionals will be critical to developing an appropriate plan of care. Communication with the LPN and UAP will be critical to ensure that the client's care is well coordinated, compassionate, and up to the client's expectation. Making sure that the LPN and UAP know the goals and outcomes of care will increase the success of meeting them.

EDUCATIONAL STRATEGIES

1. Discuss the historical background of the nursing profession, including its development in relation to societal and economic changes and needs.

2. Assign students to select a major figure in the history of nursing and have them report, verbally and/or in writing, on the influence of that individual on past or current nursing practice.

3. Discuss current nursing practice and present different definitions of "nursing." Ask students to share their own definition or philosophy of nursing.

4. Discuss the standards of practice and how they contribute to nursing as a profession. Provide specific examples of how the standards are used in nursing practice.

5. Identify the difference between the standards of care and the standards of practice. Discuss how the standards of care correlate with the nursing process.

6. Identify the different nursing organizations that exist, their different objectives, and their role in professional practice.

7. Discuss the different types of educational programs that prepare nurses for entry into practice. Ask students to identify the advantages and disadvantages of the different programs for LPNs/LVNs and RNs.

8. Discuss graduate nursing education and the preparation for advanced nursing practice roles.

9. Invite an advanced practice nurse to speak to the class about his or her role and educational background.

10. Ask students to share their individual nursing career goals, including the experience and education they believe they will need to achieve these goals. Have students interview a nurse working in their area of interest in order to determine the specific educational preparation and scope of practice required for the position.

11. Compare and contrast different nurse practice acts. Identify the legal parameters outlined within the acts for licensure, nursing practice, standards of care, and disciplinary responsibility.

12. Ask students to investigate and share their information on nursing roles in their local community.

13. Review different practice settings and roles for nurses.

14. Assign students to research a past year of a selected professional nursing journal. Have them share, verbally and/or in writing, the focus of the journal articles and advertisements for that year. Ask them to compare the focus of the selected year to the current practice of nursing.

15. Ask students to identify the members of the health care team. Review delegation in nursing practice and name the appropriate members of the team to whom the nurse may delegate responsibility.

16. Discuss potential challenges for the profession of nursing in the future. Stimulate a discussion on what nursing might be like 20 years from now.

17. Use educational media to demonstrate the portrayal of nurses in the media, such as clips from different television shows or news broadcasts. Have students bring in examples from newspapers and radio or television broadcasts on nurses or nursing.

INDEPENDENT LEARNING

1. Students can write their own definition or philosophy of nursing, put it aside, and refer back to it before graduation from the program to see if their ideas have changed throughout their educational experience.

2. Students can review the conceptual and theoretical models of nursing and select one that they would like to apply to their own practice.

3. Students can research an article in a nursing journal on trends in current nursing practice and/or educational requirements for practice.

4. Students can think about their career interests and investigate the education and experience that is necessary to follow that path.

STUDENT RESOURCES

ANA Standards of Practice

ANA Standard	Specific Practice Example
I. Quality of care	
II. Performance appraisal	
III. Education	
IV. Collegiality	
V. Ethics	
VI. Collaboration	
VII. Research	
VIII. Resource utilization	

CNA Standards of Practice

Standards of Practice	Specific Practice Example
Nursing practice requires that a conceptual model(s) for nursing be the basis of practice.	
Nursing practice requires the effective use of the nursing process.	
Nursing practice requires that the helping relationship be the nature of the client-nurse interaction.	
Nursing practice requires nurses to fulfill professional responsibilities.	

Entry Level Nursing Education

	LPN	Diploma	Associate	Baccalaureate
Average time needed to complete the program.				
Degree or credential received.				
Primary focus of the graduate.				
Usual setting for the program.				

Nursing Roles

Nursing Roles	Specific Nursing Interventions
Direct care provider	
Protector and client advocate	
Case manager	
Patient/family educator	

Career Nursing Roles

Career Roles	Educational Preparation & Additional Credentialing	Practice Setting
Nurse educator		
Advanced practice nurse		
Nurse administrator		
Nurse researcher		

CROSS-CURRICULUM GUIDE

Concepts of professionalism may be woven throughout the curriculum. Students beginning in a program will benefit from discussions on the historical development of the nursing profession, entry into practice, licensure requirements, ongoing educational requirements, the elements of professionalism, and current nursing roles and career opportunities.

CHAPTER 11

Ethics and Values

CRITICAL THINKING ACTIVITIES AND ANSWERS

1. Complete the Cultural Values Exercise with your classmates or with members of another class of professionals. Compare the answers and discuss the differences.

Answer: No "right" answers exist to this exercise. One goal is to provide a structured experience for the students that illustrates how varied personal values may be. A second goal is to encourage the students to practice tolerance, even in the presence of difference. It is important to guide discussion toward the differences that exist with the group, even if many similarities exist.

2. You are caring for a 17-year-old client who has been admitted for treatment of sickle cell crisis. She needs fluid management and comfort management. Even though she is receiving narcotics around the clock, she continues to complain of pain. She also complains about her roommate, the food, and the intravenous (IV) device. She comes from a community far from the hospital, and her mother cannot visit every day. She has an older brother who has been convicted of possession of illegal drugs. Discuss your approach to this client. Rank her needs. What is your priority action, based on what you know so far? Examine and describe your opinions about pain, pain management, and addiction.

Answer: Clients who live with sickle cell disease experience acute exacerbations of pain. Management of the pain requires large doses of narcotics, in addition to other management modalities. Especially in large metropolitan communities, the fact that sickle cell clients are mostly African American renders them vulnerable to stereotyping as poor or addicted. The point of this exercise is to help the student understand how easy it is to classify clients in error and how the consequences of the error might include inadequate care. A common misconception about pain management includes the idea that too much medication will produce a drug addict. The students should be encouraged to express this and other ideas about pain, narcotics, cultural biases, and stereotyping. The common event of mislabeling sickle cell clients as malingering or manipulative provides an excellent opportunity for the exploration of values, values clarification, ethical standards of care, and critical thinking.

3. You are a clinic nurse in a small community clinic. A 45-year-old man has been coming to the clinic for several years for treatment and support of his acquired immune deficiency syndrome (AIDS). In recent months he lost his long-term companion to AIDS. In addition, both his parents died many years ago. His clinical condition has deteriorated. His vision is failing, his nutritional status is difficult to maintain, and he has been hospitalized three times in the past 3 months for pneumonia. He asks for your help in planning his suicide. Discuss your response to his request. Begin by examining your personal feelings about assisted suicide. Include a discussion about your understanding of AIDS: where it comes from, who gets the disease, why, and what your feelings and opinions are about people with AIDS. Construct your response keeping in mind the ethical principles of fidelity, autonomy, and beneficence. Since all these principles collide in this example, it will be necessary to rank them according to your feelings and then according to how you imagine the client would rank them. For the sake of this discussion, it is illegal in your state for nurses to prescribe medications. What are your possible courses of action?

Answer: The goal in this discussion is to challenge the student with a situation where caring and compassion may conflict with personal philosophy. The student should work to articulate personal opinions about assisted suicide and about persons with AIDS, a client population that has experienced marginalization and discrimination, which is unacceptable in a health care setting. In the end, the answer should include some reference to hospice care or other kinds of comfort and support, regardless of personal opinions about assisted suicide. In answering these questions, the student will have the opportunity to utilize an ethic of care to construct both a personal and a professional plan of management.

EDUCATIONAL STRATEGIES

1. Define ethics and values, identifying the difference between these concepts and legal issues. Differentiate morals and ethics, providing examples of each.

2. Discuss the criteria for professions. Ask students how nursing meets these criteria.

3. Review the Code of Ethics and its purpose within a profession.

4. Discuss the basic principles inherent in a Code of Ethics (responsibility, accountability, competence, and judgment) and ask students to provide examples of how they might be demonstrated in nursing.

5. Have students identify how the nurse may act as a client advocate.

6. Identify the basic standards of ethics in health care: autonomy, justice, fidelity, and beneficence. Have students provide examples of how each standard might be met by the nurse.

7. Define values and discuss the process of values formation. Ask students to share some of their own personal values. Discuss situations where personal and professional values can come into conflict.

8. Present the process of values clarification. Have students complete a values clarification exercise and discuss their findings.

9. Demonstrate how communication techniques assist in sharing values and feelings.

10. Discuss the following theories of ethics that might be applied in nursing practice: deontology, utilitarianism, feminist ethics, and the ethics of care. Provide possible situations where these theories can be applied.

11. Review the steps for processing an ethical dilemma. Ask students to provide an example of current events that can be viewed and processed as an ethical dilemma.

12. Assign students to attend and report on, if possible, a meeting of an agency's ethics or bioethics committee.

13. Provide students with, or ask them to provide, examples of possible ethical situations in nursing practice for the following:
    a. Ambulatory care settings
    b. Acute care/managed care settings
    c. Restorative care settings
    d. Multidisciplinary collaboration
    e. Cost containment
    f. Cultural sensitivity
    g. Delegation

14. Ask students to discuss their feelings on "hot" topics in health care, such as abortion, assisted suicide, euthanasia, fetal tissue research, "do not resuscitate" orders, and transplants.

15. Have students respond to the following, or other similar, situations where values clarification can be implemented. Ask students how their own values might be in conflict with those of the client.
    a. A client who elects not to receive lifesaving treatment because of religious beliefs.
    b. A client who opts to have an abortion or who chooses to give the child up for adoption.
    c. An adult who places his or her parent in a nursing home.
    d. A middle-age adult client with severe multiple sclerosis who is pursuing assisted suicide.

INDEPENDENT LEARNING

1. Students can think about issues that they have strong feelings about in relation to health care and nursing. They can begin to identify when and where they might be faced with an ethical dilemma as a result of their own belief systems and how they might respond in that situation.

2. Students can complete the following exercises in the text to assist them in gaining greater self-awareness:
   a. Values clarification
   b. Cultural values

STUDENT RESOURCES

Fundamental Principles of Codes of Ethics

Principles	Specific Examples of Their Application
Responsibility	
Accountability	
Competence	
Judgment	

Ethical Theories and Concepts

Ethical Theory/Concept	Description of Theory/Concept	Relation to Health Care and Nursing

STRATEGIES FOR VALUES CLARIFICATION

SENTENCE COMPLETETION

Complete the following sentences. Use them to examine your feelings and values.

I feel I succeed in caring for a client when . . .

A Client has a right to . . .

I wish my clinical supervisor would . . .

I fail in caring for a client if I cannot . . .

The most difficult client is one who . . .

RANK ORDERING

The following questions require you to make value judgments. Rank the choices to the questions according to your value preferences. Write the number 1 to the left for the most important value. Continue in the same manner until all four values are ranked. Discuss your preferences with a colleague and examine the alternatives.

If I had the time, money, and skill to solve problems for nurses, I would

____ Increase nurses' salaries

____ Enhance staff education

____ Increase the number of nurses to staff the division

____ Give staff more positive feedback

In developing a professional relationship with a physician, I believe a student or nurse should

____ Respond promptly to all requests

____ Demonstrate knowledge of the clients assigned to the physician

____ Look attractive and be neatly dressed

____ Share ideas about the clients' needs

When assigned to a client's care, the nurse should

____ Make him or her as physically comfortable as possible

____ Let him or her know you are interested in his or her ideas and feelings

____ Be competent and skilled in the performance of all procedures

____ Allow the client to make decisions about his or her care

If I had a serious health problem, I would prefer to

____ Not be told

____ Be told immediately by the physician

____ Learn by accident

____ Keep it secret from my family

HEALTH VALUE SCALE

Below you will find 10 values listed in alphabetical order. Arrange the values in order of their importance as guiding principles in your life. Study the list carefully and choose the value that is most important to you. Write the number 1 in the space to the left of that value. Write the number 2 for the value that ranks second in importance. continue in the same manner for the remaining values until you have included all ranks. Each value will have a different rank.

____ A comfortable life (a prosperous life)

____ An exciting life (a stimulating, active life)

____ A sense of accomplishment (lasting contribution)

____ Freedom (independence, free choice)

____ Happiness (contentedness)

____ Health (physical and mental well-being)

____ Inner harmony (freedom from inner conflict)

____ Pleasure (an enjoyable, leisurely life)

____ Self-respect (self-esteem)

____ Social recognition (respect, admiration)

Modified from Uustal DB: *Am J Nurs* 78:2058, 1978

CULTURAL VALUES EXERCISE

If people from a variety of cultures were given this questionnaire some would stongly agree with the beliefs listed on the left, and others would strongly agree with the opposite viewpont listed on the right. Circle 1 if you strongly agree or 2 if you moderately agree with the statement on the left. Circle 3 if you moderately agree or 4 if you stongly agree with the statement on the right.

1. Preparing for the future is an important activity and reflects maturity.	1	2	3	4	Life has a predestined course that the individual should follow.
2. Vague answers are dishonest and confusing.	1	2	3	4	Vague answers are sometimes preferred bcause they prevent embarrassment and confrontation.
3. Punctuality and efficiency are characteristics of a person who is both intelligent and concerned.	1	2	3	4	Punctuality is not as important as maintaining a relaxed atomosphere, enjoying the moment, and being with family and friends.
4. When in severe pain, one should remain strong and not complain too much.	1	2	3	4	When in severe pain, one should talk about the discomfort and express frustration.
5. It is self-centered and unwise to accept a gift from someone you do not know well.	1	2	3	4	It is an insult to refuse a gift when it is offered.
6. Addressing someone by first name shows friendliness.	1	2	3	4	Addressing someone by first name is disrespectful.
7. Direct questions are usually the best way to gain information.	1	2	3	4	Direct questioning is rude and could cause embarrassment.
8. Direct eye contact shows interest.	1	2	3	4	Direct eye contact is intrusive.
9. Ultimately, the independence of the individual must come before the needs of the family.	1	2	3	4	The needs of the individual are always less important than the needs of the family.

CROSS-CURRICULUM GUIDE

The principles of ethics and values are valid in discussions throughout the curriculum. There are current issues in obstetrics, pediatrics, gerontology, and other fields of medicine that will influence the practice of nursing. Students will be exposed to a wide variety of situations where they will need to respond to clients from diverse backgrounds. It is important to assist students in recognizing their own value systems so that they may be more aware and nonjudgmental of their clients' values. The role of the nurse as a client advocate may be identified in all content areas (e.g., assisting the client to obtain cost-effective supplies for colostomy care). Having students present possible ethical dilemmas in different practice settings may assist in their understanding of the nurse's role and responsibility in these "gray" areas.

CHAPTER 12

Legal Concepts in Nursing Practice

CRITICAL THINKING ACTIVITIES AND ANSWERS

1. Mrs. Smith is an 80-year-old client with a fractured hip. Dr. Jones writes a pain medication order for Mrs. Smith that reads: "Morphine sulfate 50 mg IM every 6 hours." You transcribe that order and note that 50 mg of morphine is an extremely large dose. In fact, you know that the normal dose of morphine is less than 10 mg.
   a. What risk do you face if you follow the doctor's order?
   b. What should you do?
   c. If you cannot get Dr. Jones on the phone, may you give a smaller dose of morphine?

Answer:
   a. If 50 mg of morphine is given to Mrs. Smith and she suffers harm, the nurse would be liable.
   b. The nurse should call the doctor and clarify the order.
   c. No. The nurse should administer nothing until the order is clarified. The problem with giving a smaller dose of the morphine based on an erroneous order is that the doctor could have meant "Demerol 50 mg" instead of morphine because Mrs. Smith is allergic to morphine.

2. Mrs. Brown is expecting her first baby. She and her husband have arrived at the labor and delivery suite. You have a copy of Mrs. Brown's prenatal record, which indicates that she has had two elective abortions. When you are filling out the history on the labor and delivery record, Mrs. Brown states in the presence of her husband that this is her first and only pregnancy.
   a. How should the nurse handle the situation?
   b. What is the nurse's legal obligation regarding confidentiality of the client's previous elective abortions?
   c. What is the nurse's legal responsibility for sharing the client's pregnancy information with her husband?

   Answer:
   a. If the nurse needs to question Mrs. Brown about her medical history, the nurse should ask that Mr. Brown leave the room.
   b. The information is confidential unless Mrs. Brown gives consent.
   c. The nurse would be liable for any harm.

3. Mr. Adams is hospitalized for congestive heart failure. He is occasionally confused and tries to get out of bed without assistance. The physician orders side rails up at all times and restraint of the patient if necessary. While you are bathing Mr. Adams you remove the restraint and put the side rails down. When you run out of the room for a second to get another washcloth, Mr. Adams falls out of bed and fractures his hip. Identify the elements of negligence and use this scenario to apply those elements.

   Answer: The nurse owes a duty of care to Mr. Adams to make sure that he is restrained and the side rails are up when the nurse leaves the room. The nurse breached that duty by leaving Mr. Adams unattended. Mr. Adams suffered a fractured hip that was caused by the nurse's breach of duty.

4. Miss Smith, a 16-year-old, brings her newb baby to the hospital emergency room with high fever. The physician wants to perform lumbar puncture on the baby and advises I Smith of the risks involved. Since Miss Sm a minor, who can sign the consent form for baby?

Answer: Miss Smith can sign the consent form because she is an emancipated minor. Minors v are married or are parents are emancipated.

EDUCATIONAL STRATEGIES

1. Discuss the sources of law, including the d ences between civil and criminal law.

2. Define torts and provide examples of their application to nursing situations.

3. Review the unintentional tort of negligence practice. Describe the criteria necessary for ligence/malpractice to be established. Provi examples of negligent care.

4. Review the standards of care, where they nate, and how they are legally applied to n ing practice.

5. Discuss the purpose of and the protection offered through the Good Samaritan Laws

6. Review the role of the Board of Nursing i licensure and disciplinary action. If possibl have students attend and report on a Boar meeting or disciplinary hearing.

7. Discuss the Patient's Bill of Rights. Have s dents identify examples of how nursing pr. is influenced by this document.

8. Ask students to identify the legal liability student nurse compared to a licensed nurs and an instructor.

9. Describe the role of the nurse in relation to physician's orders and client consent. Ask students to provide examples of how nurses should respond to the following situations:
   a. Obtaining consent for a minor who requires care
   b. Implementing physician's orders that are illegible or possibly incorrect
   c. Dealing with a client who refuses treatment

10. Identify the legal issues relating to death and dying, organ/tissue donation and transplants, advance directives (Patient Self-Determination Act), and nursing employment. Stimulate class discussions on these topics.

11. Invite a nurse attorney or a risk-management nurse to speak to the class about his or her role and situations in nursing practice where legal issues come into play.

12. Review strategies for minimizing liability in nursing practice. Ask students how they should respond to the following situations:
   a. Working on a unit that is short-staffed
   b. Floating to a unit where they are unfamiliar with the client population and treatment needs
   c. Completing an incident report for a client who is found on the floor of his room
   d. Identifying a potential child abuse case

13. Review the legal issues that relate to the specialty areas in nursing.

14. Discuss legal guidelines that might be specific to different health care agencies.

15. Organize a role-playing experience where the students act out a possible courtroom scene, with a nurse being questioned about his or her care of a client. Provide students with the general case information and have them develop the questions to ask the witnesses.

16. Discuss the legal implications involved in nursing documentation, including general guidelines for written and computerized client records.

INDEPENDENT LEARNING

1. Students may review the Patient's Bill of Rights to see how nursing practice might be influenced.

2. Students should obtain detailed information on their own nursing malpractice insurance, including any limitations of coverage.

3. Students can research an article in a nursing journal on a legal issue that affects current nursing practice.

STUDENT RESOURCES

Intentional and Unintentional Torts

Torts	Description
Intentional: Assault	
Battery	
Invasion of privacy	
Defamation of character	
Unintentional: Negligence	
Malpractice	

Legal Responsibilities of the Nurse

	Description	Nursing Responsibilities
Doctor's orders		
Consent		
Death and dying issues		
Employment issues		

Minimizing Liability

Situations	Description	Nursing Actions to Minimize Liability
Short staffing		
Floating		
Incident reports		
Risk management		
Reporting		

CROSS-CURRICULUM GUIDE

Students must learn how to practice nursing within legal guidelines. Legal concepts may be integrated throughout the curriculum, but introduction of this material should begin early in the educational program in order to provide parameters for the student. Content may become more sophisticated and specific as the student progresses through the program. For example, discussions on assessment of the pediatric client should include the legal responsibility of the nurse in reporting suspected child abuse. Clinical experiences in critical care or hospice should prompt questions about legal issues relating to death and dying.

CHAPTER 13

Communication

CRITICAL THINKING ACTIVITIES AND ANSWERS

1. Walter Jordan is a 34-year-old who was brought to the emergency room with crushing chest pain, shortness of breath, and exercise intolerance. His wife is at his side, in tears, moaning, "He's dying." What factors influencing communication are present in this scenario, and how would they affect the nurse's communication?

Answer: The situation is an emergency, so the nurse must set priorities for getting and giving information. The setting is high-stress and technical, so the nurse must explain things to the Jordans, such as the ECG monitor. Because the client-nurse relationship has no history, the nurse should take extra care to be polite, introduce oneself, and quickly establish caring and competency. The wife feels extremely anxious and fearful, so the nurse should acknowledge these feelings, repeat things, and use short, simple, direct explanations.

2. The nurse takes Mrs. Jordan's arm to escort her to the waiting room. Mrs. Jordan reacts angrily, wrenching her arm out of the nurse's grasp. What should the nurse do now?

Answer: Acknowledge Mrs. Jordan by using her name. Empathize with her: acknowledge what a stressful time it is, say that you can see she doesn't want to leave, and apologize for upsetting her further. Give her information: tell her firmly but gently that the team can concentrate on her husband better when the family is not present. Reassure her: "I'll come let you know what's going on whenever I possibly can." Keep telling her that the staff will do all they can to help him. Offer her your hand.

3. The couple's child, a 4-year-old boy, is in the emergency room. His eyes are wide open, his skin is pale, and his eyes are tearing. How would you explain to him what is happening with his father?

Answer: Get down on the child's level. Be simple and direct: "Your Daddy needs to see the doctor now. Help him feel safe: "You can stay here with your sister." Give him an explanation: "Your Mommy is scared, and I'm going to help her." Provide a play outlet for his feelings: get him a toy, a book, or crayons and paper.

4. The Jordan's 16-year-old daughter is pacing and picking at her nails. Construct a way to establish a helping-trust relationship with her.

Answer: Be empathetic: "I know it's a frightening situation for your family right now." Be informative: "Your Dad might be having a heart attack, and we will do the best we can to help him." Answer her questions honestly but with a sense of hope. Involve her: tell her she can help by taking care of Danny, and give her something to do. Encourage use of resources: ask her if there is anyone who might be called to come and stay with the family while they wait. Accept her behavior: teens vacillate between adult and childlike reasoning and behavior, and when frightened they may react with sullenness, sarcasm, or other unexpected responses.

5. The nurse notices Emily, a team member, going into the bathroom in tears. How can the nurse offer help without invading her privacy?

Answer: Make an observation: "I noticed you were in tears awhile ago." Offer to listen: "Want to talk about it?" Use touch if appropriate: lay a hand on her hand or forearm. Offer professional advice and help: "Sometimes it helps to talk about things that are bothering you." Suggest collaboration: "Maybe if we take a minute and talk, we can get a different perspective on the situation." Encourage evaluation: "Whatever happened to upset you, maybe you can figure out why you had such a strong reaction."

EDUCATIONAL STRATEGIES

1. Define and describe communication and the communication process.

2. Discuss Watson's caring/carative factors and their relationship with communication.

3. Discuss how critical thinking is applied to the communication process.

4. Ask students how communication might be a positive or a negative influence in a client situation.

5. Discuss and provide examples of perceptual bias. Have students identify how they can recognize and overcome this bias.

6. Organize role-playing experiences where students act out and respond to the Challenging Communication Situations (box in text).

7. Discuss and provide examples of the levels of communication (intrapersonal, interpersonal, and public).

8. Describe verbal and nonverbal communication. Ask students to identify how both can be used and interpreted in the communication process. Use the following, or similar, situations and ask how the nurse might interpret verbal and nonverbal communication:
   a. A client experiencing pain
   b. An adolescent who is anxious
   c. An adult client who is angry
   d. An infant or child who is hungry
   e. A child who is frightened
   f. A young adult who is grieving over the loss of a spouse

9. Identify the zones of personal space and demonstrate how the zones are approached during nurse-client interactions.

10. Describe the factors that can influence communication: psychophysiological, relational, situational, environmental, and cultural.

11. Discuss how cultural background and values can influence nurse-client communication. Ask students to share personal examples of how they might have been misinterpreted because of their backgrounds.

12. Identify how the developmental status of the individual influences communication. Have students provide communication techniques that might be used for clients of different ages.

13. Review the phases of the helping relationship and identify how effective communication is integral to the process.

14. Describe in depth the principles and guidelines for effective communication. Give examples of negative communication techniques and ask students to respond in the appropriate manner.

15. Review how communication is used throughout the nursing process. Ask students to give examples of situations where opportunities are provided for client communication (e.g., during the client's bath).

16. Ask students to identify how physical communication barriers can interfere with the communication process. Use the following, or similar, examples to have students provide nursing interventions that might facilitate communication:
   a. A client who has had a laryngectomy
   b. An individual who speaks another language
   c. An individual who is deaf or has a hearing impairment
   d. A client who is hallucinating
   e. An older individual with diminished sensory capacity
   f. An unconscious client

17. Provide students with simulated client data (different ages and backgrounds) and have them interview each other in order to compile a nursing history. If possible, videotape or audiotape the experience for later critique by the students themselves. (Students can save the tapes to view before graduation in order to see how they have progressed.)

18. Assign students to observe or participate in client care experiences. Have them keep a written log of their interactions with clients for discussion in post-care conference. Based on their interactions, ask students how they might improve or alter their communication techniques for future experiences.

19. Have students complete a plan or care for a client with a nursing diagnosis of ineffectual or impaired communication.

INDEPENDENT LEARNING

1. Students can use the Challenging Communication Situations (refer to text) to think about and practice how they should respond in similar circumstances.

2. Students can observe communication patterns between nurses and other health care providers and their clients. They can then compare their observations with communications observed in social and business situations.

3. Students can practice effective communication techniques with their peers, friends, and family members to see if overall communication is changed/improved.

STUDENT RESOURCES

Verbal and Nonverbal Communication

Verbal Communication	Influence on Nurse-Client Interaction
Vocabulary	
Denotative and connotative meanings	
Pacing	
Intonation	
Clarity and brevity	
Timing and relevance	

Nonverbal Communication	Influence on Nurse-Client Interaction
Personal appearance	
Posture and gait	
Facial expression	
Eye contact	
Gestures	
Sounds	
Territoriality and space	

Effective Communication Techniques

Techniques	Application Within a Caring Relationship
Professionalism	
Courtesy	
Confidentiality	
Trust	
Availability	
Empathy	
Sympathy	
Listening and responding	
Acceptance and respect	
Silence	
Socializing	
Assertiveness and autonomy	
Humor	
Touch	
Cultural sensitivity	
Gender sensitivity	

CROSS-CURRICULUM GUIDE

Review of information about therapeutic communication, along with practice and critique of simulated or actual client interactions, will assist students in preparing for clinical experiences in all types of health settings. Because communication is such an integral part of nursing, reinforcement of information and techniques is valuable for students at all levels of nursing education. Techniques should be adapted as appropriate for clients of different ages, developmental status, and sociocultural background. Specific guidelines and practice sessions for communication with clients in a psychiatric setting are recommended.

MULTIMEDIA RESOURCES

Mosby's Communication in Nursing Video Series:
    Basic Principles for Communicating Effectively in Nursing
    Communicating with Clients and Colleagues: Effectiveness in the Caring Environment
    Communicating with Clients and Colleagues from Different Cultures
    Communicating with Difficult Clients and Colleagues
    Communicating with Clients with Mental Disorders or Emotional Problems
    Communicating across the Lifespan: Children, Families, and the Elderly

Mosby's Nursing Leadership and Management Video Series:
    Effective Communication

Whaley and Wong's Pediatric Nursing Video Series:
    Communicating with Children and Families

TOPICAL OUTLINE

CRITICAL THINKING ACTIVITIES AND ANSWERS

1. Obtain a client care record in a nursing setting and find examples that follow guidelines for good documentation of factual basis, accuracy, completeness, currentness, organization, and confidentiality. Write out the actual examples and provide your critique of their content.

   Answer: While at your clinical agency, identify yourself as a nursing student, wearing appropriate clinical uniform, and secure a client chart. Then examine the various chart forms, including the nursing notes section of the chart. Make a list of the guidelines for good documentation and write examples for each.

2. Personally observe a change-of-shift report at a health care facility and critique it in a clinical conference.

Answer: The instructor should arrange for your attendance at a change-of-shift report. Take notes on the report and critique it according to the guidelines given in the textbook. For example, if the report is given in person, does the nurse clearly introduce the client in an organized fashion? If the nurse reports on multiple clients, is there an obvious pattern that is followed (e.g., background information, primary problem, nursing diagnoses). Then critique whether the reporting nurse is concise, objective, professional, and verbalizes only those items that are pertinent to the client.

3. Document client care performed in the clinical setting using two of the following formats: charting by exception, narrative documentation, focus charting, and SOAP charting.

Answer: Provide client care as prescribed in your clinical setting. Then review the care of the day, choose two of the methods of charting, and write examples of each. For example, narrative documentation would involve writing specific sentences or phrases describing the care provided during a clinical shift. It would include the times of the care and the specific interventions of the nurse. Focus charting, on the other hand, would be narrowed to the data, actions, and responses of the nursing care. It would be organized in a very specific manner and interesting to compare to the information given in narrative charting.

4. Participate in a client interview and separate observations into objective versus subjective data.

Answer: Provide client care and set aside time to interview the patient. Follow the guidelines you have been given in your nursing school in the interview. Then make two columns with the headings *objective* and *subjective*. Write out as accurately as possible example statements that the client makes under the subjective list. Then assess the client for objective data and write those items under the objective list. Compare and contrast how the subjective data entries could be assessed for objective data and vice versa.

EDUCATIONAL STRATEGIES

1. Discuss the purpose of documentation and the regulations that influence its content and format, such as diagnosis-related groups (DRGs) and the Joint Commission on Accreditation of Healthcare Organizations (JACHO).

2. Review the guidelines for recording. Provide students with examples of documentation errors/problems and ask them for the corrections that should be made in the record.

3. Discuss how information is communicated to other members of the health care team through recording, reporting, and consultation.

4. Discuss the information that is usually found in a client's record. Demonstrate the differences in documentation formats (e.g., flowsheets, nurses' notes, clinical pathways) as available and show how they might be used in various health care settings.

5. Review the different methods of documenting, including POMR (SOAP/SOAPIE, PIE), focus (DAR), and narrative styles. Provide students with actual and/or simulated client interactions and have them practice documentation using different methods and recording formats.

6. Ask students to compare the positive and negative characteristics of the different documentation styles and formats.

7. Describe how client acuity levels can influence documentation and staffing. Provide students with examples of documentation that is based on client acuity or diagnosis.

8. Discuss and demonstrate, if available, computerized documentation. Have students identify the advantages and disadvantages of a computerized record keeping system.

9. Review the general guidelines for information that should be included in the following reports: change-of-shift, telephone, incident, and transfer.

10. Have students observe or give a report, with supervision, on the client's status.

11. Assign students to participate in the care of clients in a health care setting. Have students keep a record of times and nursing/client activities throughout the experience, then have them document their interactions. Students may initially practice documentation on a sample paper for instructor review before actual written or computerized recording.

12. Have students provide their responses to the following situations that might be encountered in relation to client documentation:
    a. Another nurse asks you to record some client information for him or her
    b. A mistake is made when writing on the client's record
    c. A student is making copies of the client's record to take home for reference

13. Invite a quality assurance nurse and/or nurse attorney to speak to the class about the legal implications of nursing documentation.

14. Review the importance of the use of correct medical terminology, spelling, and grammar in client documentation.

15. Use the following, or a similar, situation to have students practice documentation in POMR, focus, and/or narrative styles:

A client is admitted to the coronary care unit at 11 PM. He is having chest pain that is going along his left arm, and he is sweating. The nurse has taken his vital signs and found the following: temperature 98.8° F; pulse 102; respirations 32; and blood pressure 210/100. The client looks nervous and upset, saying that he's never experienced anything like this before. His family is waiting outside to talk to the physician. The client is currently having an electrocardiogram (ECG) done by the technician.

INDEPENDENT LEARNING

1. The students can practice different types of documentation for actual or simulated client situations.

2. The students should review medical terminology in order to improve the accuracy of their documentation.

STUDENT RESOURCES

*Use of available blank records from affiliating agencies for student review and practice of documentation.

Purpose of Records

Purpose of Records	Explanation

Guidelines for Documenting and Reporting

Guidelines	Description
Factual basis	
Accuracy	
Completeness	
Currentness	
Organization	
Confidentiality	

CROSS-CURRICULUM GUIDE

Documentation of client assessments and evaluations and nursing interventions is critical in all areas of practice. Whether documentation is completed in handwritten form or by computer input, nurses are responsible in all health care settings to record pertinent observations and activities. Different types of documentation, depending on the clinical focus, the agency's policy or external regulation, may be discussed throughout the curriculum. For example, an inpatient pediatric unit may have more flowsheets in the record for documentation of the child's intake and output, play activities, and developmental assessment.

CHAPTER 15

Client Education

CRITICAL THINKING ACTIVITIES AND ANSWERS

1. Mr. Clifford is a 75-year-old widower who was diagnosed with uncontrolled Type II diabetes mellitus and now requires insulin institution. He is hard of hearing, has poor eyesight and lives alone although he does have a daughter who lives nearby. Mr. Clifford has the dexterity necessary to manipulate a syringe. Design a teaching plan, including appropriate resources and modifications, for Mr. Clifford to monitor his blood glucose and administer his insulin.

Answer: A teaching plan for Mr. Clifford may be as follows:

Nursing diagnosis: Knowledge deficit (cognitive, psychomotor) regarding diabetes self-care related to inexperience.

Goals	Expected Outcomes	Interventions
1. Mr. Clifford will participate in diabetes self-care at discharge.	1a. Mr. Clifford will draw up and self-inject insulin before breakfast and before dinner. 1b. Mr. Clifford will monitor blood glucose levels before each meal and at bedtime using his own blood glucose meter. 1c. Mr. Clifford will carry a treatment for low blood sugar reactions with him at all times.	1a. The nurse will demonstrate, for Mr. Clifford, insulin preparation and administration with the next insulin dose. Mr. Clifford will be allowed to return demonstrate drawing and administering insulin with all subsequent injections. A syringe magnifier will be obtained from a pharmacy to aid Mr. Clifford in visualizing the syringe, and a pictorial brochure outlining the steps of the injections will be provided. 1b. Mr. Clifford will return demonstrate the finger stick procedure and operation of the meter with each blood glucose reading. 1c. Mr. Clifford will be instructed on signs, symptoms, and treatment of low blood sugar. 1d. Mr. Clifford's daughter will be instructed on the above diabetes care activities in order to assist her father after discharge. 1e. Mr. Clifford will follow up at the Diabetes Education Center 2 weeks after discharge for reinforcement and evaluation.

2. Mr. Taylor, who is 53 years old, has a cast on his right leg after repair of a fractured ankle. He is to begin crutch walking tomorrow and must learn about cast care. You ask Mr. Taylor to read the cast-care pamphlet and discuss its content with you. You discover that he is unable to read and comprehend the information in the brochure. Describe the interventions you would employ in developing a teaching plan for this client.

Answer: Interventions necessary in teaching a client of low literacy, such as Mr. Taylor, include the following:
   a. Using simple terminology to enhance the client's understanding
   b. Frequently asking for feedback and return demonstration
   c. Providing time for frequent review of procedures
   d. Utilizing teaching materials written with short words and sentences, large type, and simple format
   e. Including family or significant others in the teaching plan

3. Mrs. Sanchez, who is 38 years old, is scheduled for a breast biopsy. Her mother and her sister have a history of breast cancer. They are both currently in remission and in their sixth and seventh year after initial diagnoses. Mrs. Sanchez has never had surgery. She is nervous and "scared of the diagnosis." List your teaching priorities for this client.

Answer: Teaching priorities for Mrs. Sanchez include alleviating her anxiety by providing her with accurate and clear information about the biopsy procedure and the preparation involved. It is imperative, however, that Mrs. Sanchez be allowed to verbalize her feelings about the biopsy procedure and possible diagnosis as well as her feelings about the diagnoses of her mother and sister. Mrs. Sanchez should be encouraged to ask any questions and discuss her fears and concerns.

4. Joey Carter is a 4-year-old recently diagnosed with asthma. He and his parents are being taught to use an inhaler and nebulized bronchodilator. Describe the teaching methods that are effective with a preschool-age child.

Answer: A preschool child often expresses feelings during play, more through actions than words. The nurse should use role playing, imitation, and play to make it fun for Joey to learn about asthma and its treatment. Joey should also be encouraged to ask questions, and the nurse should provide simple explanations and demonstrations of bronchodilator use. A coloring book describing lung function and asthma treatment would be an effective teaching tool for Joey.

EDUCATIONAL STRATEGIES

1. Identify the standards in place regarding client education. Ask students how these standards influence the nurse's role in client education.

2. Discuss the purpose of client education in promoting, maintaining, and restoring health. Have students provide specific examples for each area.

3. Describe the concepts of teaching and learning and the role of the nurse.

4. Compare the teaching and communication processes. Provide students with a client example and have them carry it through all steps of the teaching process.

5. Identify the domains of learning and how they influence the way in which different concepts are taught to clients. Provide students with the following examples and have them identify the associated domain(s) of learning for each:
   a. Client is to have diagnostic testing tomorrow and has never had this experience.
   b. Self-injection of medication is required.
   c. Client is not following the treatment plan.
   d. A class on personal hygiene is being offered to 7 year olds.

6. Discuss the principles of learning in client education. Relate the principles to the examples in strategy 5.

7. Compare the teaching and nursing processes. Ask students how the focus of the nursing process is placed on the learning needs of the client.

8. Describe the variety of teaching approaches that might be used by the nurse in client education. Ask students what methods they believe may be most effective in the client situations presented in strategy 5.

9. Discuss the role of positive and negative reinforcement in the educational process.

10. Review the preparation of a teaching plan for a client, including the incorporation of the client's learning needs and capabilities, psychophysiological and cultural considerations, and the nursing approaches used in the process.

11. Invite a client educator to speak to the class about his or her role in preparing clients to meet their health needs.

12. Have students prepare and present a brief teaching plan for their peers on the performance of a simple household activity, such as making a cup of coffee. Ask the class to provide feedback on each student's presentation.

13. Assign students to prepare a teaching plan for one or more of the following:
    a. A lesson on fire safety for a third-grade class
    b. Newborn care for a group of new parents
    c. A class on general driving safety for adolescents
    d. An information session on insurance coverage for a group of older adults in a senior citizen center
    e. A client, newly diagnosed with diabetes, who will require insulin injections

14. Assign students to observe or participate in the care of clients in a variety of clinical settings. Have them identify the learning needs and abilities of their clients and prepare appropriate teaching plans to share in post-care discussions. Provide feedback to the group on areas for alteration in the plan. With approval, have students implement their teaching plans with their clients, document the process, and evaluate their clients' goal achievements.

INDEPENDENT LEARNING

1. Students can identify the types of teaching methods that they believe have most effectively helped them to learn different information or skills.

2. Students can research an article in a nursing journal on specific strategies that may be implemented for client education.

3. Students can select a basic nursing skill (e.g., bed making, taking a pulse) and attempt to teach friends or family members how to perform the procedure correctly. They can identify the factors that have assisted or interfered with the learning process.

STUDENT RESOURCES

Domains of Learning

Domains	Definition	Strategies for Use
Cognitive		
Affective		
Psychomotor		

Principles of Learning

Principles	Description	Role of the Nurse
Motivation		
Ability to learn		
Learning environment		

Instructional Methods

Methods	Description	Specific Examples
One-on-one discussion		
Group instruction		
Preparatory instruction		
Demonstrations		
Analogies		
Role-playing		
Discovery		

Teaching Plan

Learning Need or Topic	Available Resources	Significant Others	Learning Objectives	Teaching Strategies

CROSS-CURRICULUM GUIDE

Client education is another integral part of the nursing process, and it is applicable within all health care settings. Students will be participating in the care of clients of diverse age groups and sociocultural backgrounds, so this content should be integrated throughout the curriculum. They will have to be aware of the learning needs and abilities of these individuals and their significant others in order to assist them to achieve an optimum level of health.

Maternal/Child: The adaptation of teaching approaches will need to be discussed in order to relate to the developmental level of the child. Parent education is also crucial in ensuring that the treatment regimen will be followed.

Medical-Surgical: Clients with medical-surgical health deviations usually require information on the management of their care. This may include knowledge about prescribed medications and their administration, care of dressings or ostomies, prevention of complications, and other similar topics.

Gerontological: Older adults may require information about the aging process in addition to health management of an acute or chronic disease state. Teaching approaches may also need to be adapted to allow for sensory alterations.

Psychosocial Basis for Nursing Practice

CHAPTER 16

Self-Concept and Sexuality

CRITICAL THINKING ACTIVITIES AND ANSWERS

1. Jack Fisher is a 28-year-old manager of a local food store. He comes to his primary care provider for blood work before his upcoming marriage. The nurse working in the HMO office knows Mr. Fisher because he has been coming to the clinic for minor health issues for the past 4 years. In talking with Mr. Fisher, the nurse learns that this is his first marriage, that his fiancee has a 3-year-old son, and that although he has spent a good deal of time with this boy, he has not lived in a household with young children since his own childhood. The nurse understands that Mr. Fisher will be undergoing several role changes related to his upcoming marriage. What new roles will he be tak-

ing on? How might the nurse explore with Mr. Fisher his readiness to assume these new roles and his awareness of the possible stress of taking them on?

Answer: New roles will include husband and stepfather. Marriage will also affect his relationships with both his and her significant others (e.g., parents, friends). There are numerous ways in which the nurse could explore Mr. Fisher's awareness of the new roles and the possible stressors related to assuming them. Possible approaches would include the following:

a. Explore if he and his fiancee have discussed how getting married may affect their relationship.
b. Explore how he sees the responsibilities of a husband and father.
c. Ask about any concerns he has about his upcoming marriage and how his life will change.
d. Explore expectations of what marriage and relating to a young child will bring into his life.

A referral may be made for more in-depth counseling.

2. Mrs. Smith, a 48-year-old, is scheduled for a hysterectomy tomorrow. She expresses concern about whether this is the right choice. What issues may be influencing Mrs. Smith? How do you proceed with care for her?

Answer: Issues that may be influencing Mrs. Smith include the following: concern about the surgery or anesthesia; grief over loss of her childbearing capacity; impact of the hysterectomy on her femininity; concern about functioning, both general physical functioning and sexuality, following the hysterectomy; concern about how her husband may respond to the loss of her uterus and perhaps ovaries; and experiences of women she knows who have had hysterectomies.

3. Mr. Jackson is 65 years old and admitted post-diabetic ketoacidosis. During his stay you notice great intimacy (hand holding, kissing, massage, affectionate names) expressed between Mr. and Mrs. Jackson. How might you approach the topic of sexuality? What information is relevant to provide regarding age and disease state?

Answer: Mr. Jackson should initially be approached when his wife is not present so he can be free to bring up any issues. Begin with a statement such as "I notice you have a very close relationship with your wife. Have you noticed any changes in your relationship in the past several years?" or "Sometimes people with diabetes notice some changes in sexual response. Have you noticed any changes?" Prompt him with additional questions about his ability to attain and sustain an erection or achieve orgasm.

Educate Mr. Jackson about potential changes in sexual response related to age (delayed erection, shorter durations of erection, less force to ejaculation). Explain potential changes with diabetes related to vascular and neurological aspects of the disease: decreased sensitivity, further diminished or loss of ability to achieve erection and ejaculation. Discuss other methods of expressing intimacy, including hugging and oral sex. You might also choose do discuss penile implants and other medical treatment to increase his awareness of various options. A referral for more in-depth counseling may be indicated.

4. Mrs. Jones has given birth to her third child. In assisting her with activities of daily living (ADLs) you notice bruises on her neck and both arms. Mr. Jones seem to be in constant attendance and very resistant to leaving the room. You suspect that some form of domestic abuse may be occurring. How do you approach validating this suspicion without putting Mrs. Jones at risk? What referrals, education, and support materials can you provide Mrs. Jones during this brief 24-hour stay? What are your further obligations?

Answer: You need to be alone with Mrs. Jones to ask additional questions. You may need to ask Mr. Jones to go to the admitting office for information, or you might accompany Mrs. Jones to the bathroom to obtain a specimen. There are several ways that you might approach Mrs. Jones. Two of these would be asking the following: "I noticed the bruises you have; are you in a relationship where someone is hurting you?" or "Because it is very common, we think it is important to ask all women: Are you in a relationship in which someone is hurting you?" If the answer is no, provide her with a single resource number (e.g., hot line, self-help center, shelter) and explain that this is given to all women for personal use or to share with a friend who may need it. If the answer is yes, further assessment is needed. Ask questions such as "Do you believe that you or your children are presently in danger?", "Is there a gun in the house?", and "Have you ever considered leaving or working out an escape plan should that be necessary?" Inform her that usually in the course of such a relationship the violence escalates over time. Provide her with a referral or phone number if referral is refused. Numbers may include shelters, a hot line, and/or abuse services.

You are obligated to report suspected abuse; know your state law and contact the head nurse or administration about how to proceed with reporting and documentation in the medical record. Communicate with the physician about the information. Be extremely discreet so as to prevent information from getting to the husband or raising his suspicion, as this will simply increase the violence against Mrs. Jones.

EDUCATIONAL STRATEGIES

1. Discuss self-concept and its development throughout the lifespan. Review Erik Erikson's stages and gender differences in the development of self-concept.

2. Identify and explain the components of self-concept: body image, self-esteem, roles, and identity. Ask students to provide examples of how each of these components might be influenced by life experiences and stressors.

3. Discuss the nurse's role in promoting self-concept for clients in various health care settings. Have students provide examples of situations where the nurse can be a positive or negative influence on the client's self-concept.

4. Review the role of communication in both determining and promoting a client's self-concept. Have students role play client scenarios where they, as nurses, must respond to a client's actual or perceived alteration in self-concept.

5. Apply the critical thinking process to an actual or simulated client situation where the presence of a health deviation has altered the client's self-concept. For example:
   a. A middle-age man who has experienced a myocardial infarction and may not be able to return to a job that requires extensive physical labor
   b. A young woman who has had a mastectomy
   c. A teenage basketball player who required an amputation following injuries suffered in an automobile accident
   d. An older woman who has severe arthritic pain that limits her ability to perform activities of daily living

6. Discuss how psychosocial and cultural factors might influence an individual's self-concept.

7. Apply the nursing process to an actual or simulated client case study where there is an alteration in self-concept. Have students identify nursing diagnoses, goals and outcomes, nursing interventions, and evaluation criteria.

8. Review specific assessment areas related to determination of a client's self-concept and nursing interventions in health promotion, acute care, and restorative care settings for promotion of self-concept.

9. Discuss concepts of sexuality and sexual health.

10. Ask students to provide examples of how the media influence society's perception of self-concept and sexuality.

11. Review the development of sexuality throughout the lifespan, from infancy through older adulthood. Provide students with, or ask them to provide, examples of how individuals in each age group might respond to their sexuality.

12. Define sexual health. Ask students what the concept might mean to individuals, clients, and health care providers. Ask students to share their own feelings about sexuality and sexual health and have them discuss the issues that they might face as health care providers.

13. Review the normal anatomy and physiology of the male and female reproduction systems. Discuss the sexual response cycle.

14. Discuss issues related to sexual health, including contraception, abortion, and sexually transmitted diseases. Assign students to bring in media examples of how these issues can influence or be influenced by the health care system.

15. Identify the nurse's role in assisting the client to achieve optimal sexual health, including providing accurate information and supporting client decision making.

16. Review alterations in sexual health and how the nurse might assess and intervene in instances of infertility, sexual abuse, sexual dysfunction, and personal/emotional conflict with sexuality.

17. Have students discuss the relationship between self-concept and sexuality.

18. Apply the critical thinking and nursing processes to an actual or simulated client situation where there is an alteration in sexual health.

19. Have students formulate questions to ask clients, adapting them to different age-groups, in order to assess the individual's sexual health. Ask students to identify specific nursing interventions that can be implemented to assist the client to achieve optimal sexual health.

20. Have students identify different client situations where a health care deviation and/or treatment regimen (e.g. antihypertensive medication) may influence a client's sexual health.

21. Ask students to identify nursing considerations related to sexual health for clients in different age-groups and health care settings. Have them formulate an age-specific teaching plan related to sexuality and sexual health for an individual or group.

22. Assign students to observe or participate in the care of clients in a variety of health care settings, specifically focusing on the assessment and promotion of self-concept and sexuality. In pre- and post-care discussions, have students relate actual or potential alterations in their clients' self-concept and sexual health. Have students share their ideas for nursing interventions and client education.

23. Use the following, or similar, client situations to have students identify how the client's self-concept and/or sexuality may be influenced:
    a. A 42-year-old married woman who has had a cerebrovascular accident (CVA)
    b. A 22-year-old male paraplegic
    c. An 86-year-old woman, oriented and active, but confined to a wheelchair in a nursing home
    d. A 35-year-old woman, with a diagnosis of cancer who has had a hysterectomy and will require chemotherapy
    e. A 14-year-old girl with scoliosis who is in a full brace
    f. A 6-year-old who is hearing impaired

INDEPENDENT LEARNING

1. Students should review the normal anatomy and physiology of the male and female reproductive systems.

2. Students can look at their perceptions of their own self-concept and sexuality.

3. Students can investigate the available health care agency and community resources that support an individual's or family's self-concept or sexual health.

4. Students can research an article in a nursing journal related to specific nursing measures for the promotion of self-concept and/or sexuality.

STUDENT RESOURCES

Components of Self-Concept

Components	Description	Measures to Promote
Body image		
Self-esteem		
Roles		
Identity		

Stressors Affecting Self-Concept

Stressors	Description	Nursing Interventions to Promote Self-Concept
Body image		
Self-esteem		
Role		
Identity		

Sexual Development Across the Life Span

Life Span	Sexual Development (Physical/Psychosocial)	Health Promotion Strategies
Infancy		
Preschool		
Childhood		
Puberty/adolescence		
Adulthood		
Older adulthood		

CROSS-CURRICULUM GUIDE

Self-concept and sexuality may be influenced by a wide variety of life experiences and health deviations. These concepts may be integrated into discussions of clients of all ages, psychosocial backgrounds, and levels of health. Disease processes, trauma, hospitalization, or institutionalization may have a profound impact upon an individual's perception of self-concept and sexual health. Students may be encouraged throughout the educational program to incorporate actual or perceived client concerns related to self-concept and sexuality into the plan of care.

CRITICAL THINKING ACTIVITIES AND ANSWERS

1. Mr. Bruns is a terminally ill client suffering from AIDS. He has sensed an abandonment of friends and even family as his disease has progressed. The nurse finds him crying, "Oh, I feel that God has left my life." How might the nurse offer him spiritual support?

Answer: Establishing a presence during client care can contribute to the client's sense of well-being. The nurse should be attentive, answer any questions that Mr. Bruns might have, and show caring and competence in any nursing actions. The nurse should provide Mr. Bruns the chance to talk further about his feelings of abandonment. The nurse can respond with a reflective comment such as "Tell me more about your feelings of abandonment" or "What are you thinking when you feel that way?" Listening can be an important therapy. The nurse must take time to listen and be willing to understand Mr. Bruns' feelings and beliefs. He should be referred to an appropriate spiritual support person.

2.	Norma Lee is a 72-year-old woman with advanced glaucoma. Recently her close friend and neighbor, who assisted in administering her eyedrops, died. The friend also regularly attended church with Ms. Lee. The nurse from the home health agency is visiting to evaluate Ms. Lee for home health aid services. How might the nurse help Ms. Lee continue to practice her religious rituals?

Answer: The nurse should explore further those rituals that are important to Ms. Lee. The nurse can suggest calling the church to locate a volunteer willing to transport Ms. Lee to services or participate in prayer sessions with her at home. If that is not an option, the client might enjoy listening to audiotapes or services at home.

3.	Jim Tenant is a 30-year-old construction worker. The company physician explains that he wants Jim to receive a tetanus injection to guard against infection that could be acquired during an industrial accident. Jim is a member of the Christian Science faith and refuses the immunization. What would be your course of action?

Answer: As the nurse, you must respect Jim's choice. However, you want to be sure that he is well educated about the tetanus toxoid and the potential implications of acquiring a tetanus infection so that he can make an informed decision. Many members of the Christian Science faith believe that faith alone will heal any medical problem. The nurse has to respect a client's decision and remain nonjudgmental.

EDUCATIONAL STRATEGIES

1.	Define spirituality and spiritual well-being.

2.	Review the historical relationship of healing, the healing arts, and spirituality.

3.	Discuss the concepts of faith, hope, religion, and spiritual well-being. Identify the difference between spirituality and religion and how talk about spiritual needs can be addressed outside a religious viewpoint.

4.	Discuss spirituality in relation to intrapersonal, interpersonal, and transpersonal "connectedness."

5.	Ask students to provide their own definitions of faith, hope, and spirituality and to explain how they can be applied to the practice of nursing.

6.	Discuss spiritual health and the role of the nurse in assisting clients throughout the lifespan, to fulfill their spiritual needs. Review the use of a holistic approach in client care.

7.	Discuss how spiritual and religious problems can influence the health status of an individual within different health care settings.

8.	Apply the nursing process to an actual or simulated case study where the client is experiencing spiritual distress. Have students identify how the nurse can incorporate spirituality into the plan of care.

9.	Have students formulate questions that can be included in an assessment of a client's spirituality and spiritual health. Review the JAREL Spiritual Well-Being Scale (refer to text).

10.	Discuss different spiritual and religious groups, their beliefs, and the influence of their beliefs on health care practices. Have students provide examples of situations where medical and nursing care might have to be adapted to recognize and respect a client's spirituality.

11.	Given an actual or simulated client case study, have students complete a care plan or clinical pathway for an individual experiencing spiritual distress.

12.	Invite a pastoral care representative to speak to the students about his or her role in promoting clients' spiritual health.

13.	Assign students to investigate and share examples of alternative therapies that can be used by clients instead of, or in addition to, standard medical treatment. Have them identify how cultural and spiritual or religious beliefs are integrated.

14. For the following, or similar, situations ask students to identify how the client's spiritual health can be affected:
    a. A 52-year-old man who has had a myocardial infarction
    b. An adolescent who has been revived after drowning
    c. An 82-year-old woman with severe arthritis
    d. A 36-year-old woman who has been diagnosed with leukemia

INDEPENDENT LEARNING

1. The student can explore his or her own spiritual beliefs and how the recognition and acceptance of clients' beliefs is necessary in nursing practice.

2. Students should investigate available resources in a health care agency and the community to assist clients in meeting their spiritual needs.

3. Students can research an article in a nursing journal on nursing assessment and implementation of strategies to promote spirituality.

STUDENT RESOURCES

Spiritual and Religious Problems

Problems	Description	Nursing Interventions
Spiritual		
Religious		

Role of the Nurse in Promoting Spiritual Well-Being

Nurse's Role	Examples of Nursing Interventions
Establishing presence	
Supporting a healing relationship	
Prayer	
Support systems	
Diet therapies	
Supporting rituals	

CROSS-CURRICULUM GUIDE

Spirituality, like self-concept and sexuality, develops throughout life and is incorporated in some way, into an individual's well-being. As part of a holistic approach to client care, spiritual needs should be integrated into the nursing assessment of the client in different health settings. Students may be uncomfortable with, or unsure about assisting clients in achieving spiritual health, and they may need guidance in determining their role and the use of appropriate resources.

CHAPTER 18

Cultural Care in Nursing

CRITICAL THINKING ACTIVITIES AND ANSWERS

1. Discuss the problems that ethnic stereotyping and ethnocentrism may cause for the nurse. Suggest some ways that nurses can learn to recognize such tendencies in themselves.

Answer: The student or novice nurse may find it difficult to understand that the client may have health beliefs and practices that differ from the model that exists in nursing education. The student ought to be encouraged to learn as much as possible about different cultural health traditions and beliefs. Because it may be difficult for the nurse to understand the client's point of view, he or she may readily stereotype or demean the client in other ways. The nurse must discover how to be open to cultural differences and how to adequately assess the client's health traditions.

2. Discuss practices in the health care system that can discourage members of ethnic and cultural groups to access and continue with health care programs.

Answer: The health care system may be difficult to manage because of the following:

    a. Use of medical terminology and other unfamiliar language

    b. Routines that inhibit the use of alternative health remedies

    c. Forms, rules, and rituals (e.g., limited visiting hours)

Members of the health care system must open their minds to other ways of health care and respect the ancient traditions that many people continue to practice. Nurses must be instrumental in directing this change.

3. Discuss different illnesses and the susceptibility of different ethnic and cultural groups to them.

Answer: There are countless diseases that plague particular groups of people. The information in Box 18-2 should alert the nurse to many of these problems. There should be screening for early detection and practical diagnostic procedures available to those who are high risk.

EDUCATIONAL STRATEGIES

1. Discuss issues related to culture, including demographics, immigration, and heritage consistency.

2. Review culture, ethnicity, religion, and socialization in relation to heritage consistency.

3. Explore in depth the commonalities and differences and among the major ethnocultural groups in the community and/or geographic region.

4. Ask students to share their own cultural beliefs and practices and to identify how they might influence their health care.

5. Assign students to investigate a culture other than their own and prepare and present a brief overview of cultural health care practices. The presentation can be enhanced through the use of videos, photos, and traditional clothing or food.

6. Discuss how traditional cultural remedies can be used instead of, or in addition to, standard medical treatment. Have students investigate where traditional preventive items or remedies can be obtained in the community.

7. Review the role of the healer or traditional medicine person versus the modern physician role. Ask students to determine how these roles differ, where they might conflict, and how they can be integrated into the overall care of the client and family.

8. Discuss the cultural phenomena affecting health, including time orientation, space and territoriality, communication, social organization, physiological and psychological differences, and environmental control. Have students provide examples of each phenomenon, based on personal or professional experience, and identify how the health care system can be adapted to address these phenomena.

9. Review the health traditions model for maintenance, protection, and restoration of health within the context of a cultural approach.

10. Apply the nursing process to an actual or simulated client situation where cultural beliefs and practices must be recognized. Have students identify specific assessment information that should be obtained in order to accurately determine a client's ethnocultural beliefs and practices.

11. Assign students to observe or participate in the care of clients from diverse cultural backgrounds. In clinical discussions, ask students to identify any traditional health practices that the clients and their families might be using and to share how nursing care can be adapted to meet the clients' specific cultural needs.

12. Organize a role-playing experience where students interview multicultural clients and their families. Have the class critique the interview and provide constructive suggestions for improving communication. If possible, videotape the interviews for students to review at a later time.

13. Assign students to complete a care plan/clinical pathway for an actual or simulated client who has a strong reliance on culturally based health care beliefs and practices in addition to standard medical care.

14. Use the following, or similar, situations to have students specify how they might approach the clients and families involved:
    a. A client who speaks a different language requires information about dietary restrictions
    b. Home remedies that the client is taking are interacting with prescribed medications
    c. The entire extended family is always in the room with the client
    d. The client always wears a protective amulet and must be prepared for a diagnostic procedure or surgery

INDEPENDENT LEARNING

1. Students can investigate the population demographics in their community and identify ethnocultural trends.

2. Students can look at their own cultural practices and health beliefs. They can complete the Heritage Assessment for themselves and their family.

3. Students can research an article in a nursing journal on cultural assessment and nursing strategies for clients from different cultural backgrounds.

STUDENT RESOURCES

Issues Related To Culture

Cultural Issues	Explanation
Demographics	
Immigration	
Heritage consistency	

Cultural Phenomena That Affect Health

Phenomena	Examples	Nursing Interventions
Time orientation		
Personal space/territoriality		
Communication/language		
Social organization		
Physiological differences		
Psychological differences		
Environmental control		

Heritage Assessment

Childhood development occurred in the country of origin or in an immigrant neighborhood of like ethnic group.

Where were you born?

Where did you grow up?

What was your neighborhood like?

Are your parents from the same or different ethnic and religious or racial background?

Entended family members encourage participation in traditional religious or cultural activities.

Do you and your family celebrate holidays and festivals together at home and in the community?

Do you participate in other religious or fraternal events with family members?

Client and family members frequently visit the country of origin or the "old neighborhood."

How often do you return to the neighborhood in which you grew up?

Client's and family members' homes are within an "ethnic" community.

What ethnic group or groups live in your neighborhood?

Client and family members participate in ethnic cultural events such as religious festivals or holidays, sometimes with singing, dancing, and national costumes.

Do you now participate in ethnic or religious events?

Client was reared in an extended family setting.

Who lived in your home when you were young?

Did you live with grandparents, aunts, uncles, and cousins?

What are the present circumstances?

Client and family members maintain regular contact with the extended family.

How often do you visit family members?

Do you keep in close contact with those at a distance?

Family name has not been "Americanized."

What was your family's name when it immigrated?

Have the members kept or changed their name?

Client was educated in a parochial (nonpublic) school with a religious or ethnic philosophy similar to the family's background.

Where did you go to school?

What kind of a school is it?

Client and family members engage primarily in social activities with others of the same ethnic or religious background.

What are the ethnic and religious backgrounds of your friends?

Are they from your same ethnic or religious background?

Client and family members have a knowledge of the culture and language or origin.

Have you studied the history of the people from the nation from which you come?

Do you speak your native language?

What language did you learn first?

What language do you speak at home?

Client and family members possess elements of personal pride about their heritage.

How do you identify yourself?

With which group do you identify, if parents are from different groups?

Client and family members incorporate elements of historical beliefs and practices into the present philosophy.

What is your history?

What can you tell me about your specific health and illness beliefs?

CROSS-CURRICULUM GUIDE

Students should be aware of a client's cultural beliefs and practices, particularly as they relate to health care. Developing an awareness of these beliefs and practices will assist the student in working with the client toward optimal health. Recognizing one's own, as well as the health care system's, cultural values is also important so that they are not imposed on the client. Discussions about and interactions with clients from different cultural groups should promote better recognition of their health care needs and facilitate adaptation (as appropriate) of standard interventions to meet these needs.

MULTIMEDIA RESOURCES

Mosby's Community Health Nursing Video Series:
Set II: Culture in the Community

CHAPTER 19

Family Context in Nursing

CRITICAL THINKING ACTIVITIES AND ANSWERS

1. Imagine one of your clients is a young child with a contagious illness. List some suggestions you might give the parents to deal with the care of the child and to provide a positive family life for the client's siblings. How would your approach differ if the child were from a single-parent family?

Answer: The parents should consider how other members of the family might help with other tasks around the home, and they should think about how to discuss the illness with friends of the children. Determine who can help with the care of the child without becoming ill. A single parent will need more assistance with care of the child, finances, or respite care resources. Adaptation of the home environment to prevent the spread of infection should also be discussed with the family.

2. Think about the family in which you grew up. Describe the values and attitudes you learned in this environment and the influence they might have on how you view your client's family and health practices.

Answer: Use open discussion and identify various types of families of the class or group.

EDUCATIONAL STRATEGIES

1. Discuss the attributes of a family, including durability, resiliency, and diversity.

2. Discuss the meaning of family and current family forms.

3. Have students identify current pressures or problems encountered by today's family. Assign students to investigate and present examples of family stress reported in the media.

4. Review the major concerns of families, including changes in economic status, family violence, and AIDS.

5. Discuss the basic structure and function of the family, its organization, roles, relationships, and communication patterns. Ask students to share personal experiences, as appropriate, of common functioning within their families (e.g., who maintains financial and decision-making responsibilities).

6. Discuss the life-cycle stages of family development.

7. Ask students what constitutes strength or "family hardiness." Have them relate family strengths to level of wellness and health care.

8. Discuss family nursing and the approach to the family as context or client. Provide actual or simulated client/family situations and ask students to identify which approach(es) may be used by the nurse.

9. Apply the nursing process to an actual or simulated client/family situation and have students identify nursing diagnoses, goals, and nursing interventions specific to the client within a family or the family as a client.

10. Have students practice completing a family assessment for a peer, a friend, or their own family member. Ask them to share their information and identify any areas where intervention might be indicated.

11. Discuss general nursing interventions for the promotion of family functioning. Ask students to provide specific examples of nursing care that will support the family and the client within the family.

12. Invite a family therapist to speak to the class about his or her role in assisting clients and families.

13. Discuss specific topics in greater depth, such as caregiver strain or single parent families, that are evident within the immediate community.

14. Assign students to investigate available community resources for families, including any eligibility criteria for access. If possible, have students attend an Al-Anon or similar support group for families with ill or impaired members.

15. Assign students to prepare and present, if possible, teaching plans for the following clients/families:
    a. New parents with their first child
    b. A juvenile diabetic with his single dad
    c. A middle-aged couple with an older parent living with them who has Alzheimer's disease
    d. A married middle-age woman who requires ambulatory peritoneal dialysis

16. Assign students to observe or participate in the care of clients in various settings, particularly focusing on the assessment of family structure and function and the selection of interventions that support the client within the family.

INDEPENDENT LEARNING

1. Students can look at their own family dynamics, including the roles, relationships, and communication patterns of the family members.

2. Students can investigate available community resources that support family functioning.

3. Students can practice using the family assessment tool to become familiar with the areas to focus on and the type of information that can be obtained.

STUDENT RESOURCES

Nursing Process for the Family

Assessment	Nursing Diagnosis	Planning	Implementation	Evaluation

Family Assessment Tool

The family assessment tool is used when the beginning student interviews family members and observes family interaction. It is a guideline only and is not meant to be all inclusive. The student must also ensure that individual health histories accompany this assessment.

FAMILY FORM AND STRUCTURE

Names of adults   Ages

Relationship _____

                          (Single, married, divorced, separated, cohabiting)

Names of children   Ages

Others living in home (include age, sex, relationship)

Cultural background (include pertinent health beliefs, child-rearing practices, related health concerns)

Developmental stage _____
Progress toward accomplishment of developmental tasks _____
Concerns related to developmental stage _____

RESOURCES
Significant relatives and friends not occupying immediate residence _____
Strengths and coping skills _____
How does the family obtain health services? _____
Membership in community groups (e.g., church affiliation) _____
Education (formal and informal) _____
Finances (ability to meet current and future needs) _____

FAMILY PATTERNS
Persons working outside the home _____
Type of work _____Number of hours _____
Satisfaction with work _____
How are the housekeeping tasks accomplished? _____
Are family members satisfied with the way tasks are divided? _____
How are child-rearing responsibilities divided? _____
Who makes the major decisions in the family? _____
Who makes day-to-day decisions? _____
Are family members satisfied with the way decisions are made? _____

FAMILY FUNCTION
Goals
Long-term _____
Short-term _____
Individual family member's goals _____
Are individual and family goals appropriate, considering their current health problem and status? _____
How are individual family members and the family as a whole coping with their current helath problem and status? _____
Communication
Do husband and wife communicate regularly and effectively with each other? _____
Are family members able to communicate openly and honestly with each other?_____
Is conflict openly expressed and discussed? _____
Do family members respect one another's point of view? _____
Do family members offer emotional support to each other? _____

CROSS-CURRICULUM GUIDE

Clients and their families will be encountered by students throughout their educational experience. Although many clients may be viewed independently in the health care environment, the majority of them will return to some type of family unit where their needs and goals will or will not be supported. Families who have an inability to function will have an impact on the overall wellness of the individual members regardless of their age or health status. Students should be involved in experiences that will increase their awareness of client and family relationships, particularly in pediatric, gerontologic, and home care settings.

CHAPTER 20

Growth and Development

CRITICAL THINKING ACTIVITIES AND ANSWERS

1. Zachary, at 2 1/2 years old, is admitted to the hospital with a second-degree burn on the palm of his right hand. He grabbed hold of the barrel of his mother's curling iron, which was plugged in and sitting on the bathroom counter. What measures can the nursing staff take to increase his sense of security and promote his sense of autonomy?

Answer: The nursing staff should incorporate Zachary's parents into his care and encourage one of them to remain with him at all times. They can help feed and bathe him and even participate in his whirlpool treatment and dressing changes. Zachary's sense of autonomy will be promoted by allowing and encouraging him to do those things that will not result in physical or psychological harm to himself or others (e.g., feeding himself, dressing himself, or choosing toys).

2 . Monica, a 5 1/2-year-old, is having a checkup in preparation for beginning school. The nurse needs to do a number of procedures that Monica may perceive as threatening due to their intrusive or invasive nature (e.g., measure her blood pressure, check her throat, and look in her ears). What nursing approaches will be most likely to gain her cooperation?

Answer: Preschoolers often have a fear of bodily harm, and they have a great sense of initiative and imagination and enjoy dramatic play. Demonstrating these procedures on a doll, another child, or a parent, allowing Monica to handle the equipment, and giving her some sense of control are approaches that will encourage her cooperation.

3. Ms. Smith is concerned that her 15-year-old son may soon become sexually active and wants to be sure that he knows the risks involved and how to protect himself from sexually transmitted diseases (STDs) (including AIDS) and from becoming a father before he is ready for the responsibility. As a nurse, how would you advise her?

Answer: If her son does not ask questions, she might use the technique known as "therapeutic seeding." An example is "Some kids aren't sure what safe sex means. Do you have any questions about that?" She might also encourage him to talk to the nurse at school or at the community center and to bring printed materials home from the clinic about safe sex, STDs, and AIDS.

4. Crystal's mother, a 44-year-old woman, began having very short, minimal-flow menstrual periods several months ago and has not had a period for 2 months. She tells the nurse during her checkup that she thinks she's experiencing an early menopause and doesn't need to use birth control any longer. What information should the nurse give her?

Answer: Menopause occurs over a period of several years before it is complete. Not until a woman has gone 12 months without a menstrual period is menopause considered complete and it is no longer necessary to use birth control.

5. Crystal's 40-year-old uncle has felt healthy and has not been to the neighborhood clinic for a number of years. Since he has entered middle age, his wife has convinced him to go to the clinic for a checkup. What should the assessment of a middle-age male include?

Answer: Assessment should include an annual digital exam of the rectum after the age of 40 to assess for colorectal and prostate cancer, and there should also be an annual stool guaiac test and a proctosigmoidoscopic examination after the age of 50. Assessments for stress-related illnesses such as heart attacks, hypertension, migraine headaches, ulcers, backache, arthritis, colitis, and autoimmune diseases should also be done. Discuss the seven recommended health practices outlined in the young adult section of this chapter.

EDUCATIONAL STRATEGIES

1. Ask students to identify internal and external factors that can influence growth and development.

2. Compare and contrast the major developmental theories for childhood and adulthood.

3. Review, using available educational media (e.g., videos, illustrations), the stages of life from conception through older adulthood, including the following:
   a. Physical development
   b. Psychosocial and cognitive activities
   c. Specific health promotion and acute care needs

4. Ask students to identify how the approach of the nurse is adapted for the different developmental stages.

5. Assign students to prepare a diabetic teaching plan for a school-age child, an adolescent, a young adult, and an older adult. Have students compare the similarities and differences in the plans depending on the age of the client.

6. Have students bring in toys and activities for children of different ages and ask them to explain why they are appropriate for that particular age-group.

7. Review the changes in dietary needs that occur throughout the lifespan. Have students prepare sample daily menus for clients of different ages.

8. Assign students to observe or participate in the care of clients of different age groups in a variety of health care settings. Ask students how their nursing activities can be age-adapted for the specific client population. Discuss specific health and safety concerns for the clients.

9. Arrange for students to observe or participate in community activities geared toward specific age-groups at a senior center, the YMCA/YWCA, or child day care center. Have students present orally or in writing their observations of the behaviors and interactions of the individuals at these sites, comparing them to the expectations of that developmental level.

10. Assign students to prepare an oral and/or written presentation on a health problem specific to a particular age group. Have them write a nursing care plan/pathway for an actual or simulated client situation.

11. Have students bring in media examples (e.g., advertisements, TV programs) that are focused on particular age-groups. Discuss how media presentations stereotype individuals of different ages.

12. Discuss the effect that hospitalization has on individuals of different ages.

13. Invite a mother/child, adult, and/or gerontological nurse practitioner to speak to the class about his or her role, educational background, and experiences.

14. Ask students to identify possible subjects for health promotion/maintenance to teach clients from each age-group.

15. Organize a role-playing activity and have students simulate their responses and interactions with the following clients:
    a. A 6-month-old infant requiring numerous injections
    b. A 3-year-old child having surgery
    c. An 8-year-old child with heart disease
    d. A 16-year-old who has been severely burned
    e. A 24-year-old who admits to illegal drug use
    f. A 52-year-old who has lost his or her job
    g. An 81-year-old with a fractured hip

16. Ask students to share their own experiences in dealing with children, families, employment, school, and other lifestyle decisions and responsibilities.

INDEPENDENT LEARNING

1. Students can observe individuals of different ages in the community in order to identify the differences in behavior.

2. Students can research an article in a nursing journal on how nursing care may be adapted to meet a client's growth and development needs.

3. Students can review the theories of growth and development and select one that best fits their style and beliefs.

STUDENT RESOURCES
Comparison of Developmental Theories

	Freud	Erikson	Piaget	Kohlberg
Infancy				
Toddlerhood				
Preschool				
School age				
Adolescence				
Adult				
Older adult				

Growth and Development Overview

	Physical Abilities	Psychosocial/ Cognitive Activities	Health Promotion Activities
Neonate			
Infant			
Toddler			

Growth and Development Overview (continued)

	Physical Abilities	Psychosocial/ Cognitive Activities	Health Promotion Activities
Preschool child			
School-age child			
Adolescent			

Growth and Development Overview (continued)

	Physical Abilities	Psychosocial/ Cognitive Activities	Health Promotion Activities
Young adult			
Middle adult			
Older adult			

CROSS-CURRICULUM GUIDE

Concepts of growth and development should be integrated throughout the nursing curriculum, and they should be reviewed or presented before discussions about health deviations and nursing interventions. Students participating in client care activities must be aware of the basic physical changes and psychosocial and cognitive abilities of the client population. The adaptation of nursing skills (e.g., medication administration) may be demonstrated for clients of different ages. Differences in learning needs across the lifespan should also be highlighted in discussions of health promotion and maintenance.

MULTIMEDIA RESOURCES

Whaley and Wong's Pediatric Nursing Video Series:
Growth and Development

CHAPTER 21

Loss and Grief

CRITICAL THINKING ACTIVITIES AND ANSWERS

1. Kim Harbor, a 29-year-old diagnosed with breast cancer following what was anticipated to be a benign cyst removal, has become very withdrawn and threatens to sign herself out of the hospital against medical advice (AMA). She refuses to have any further surgery, stating that to lose a breast would be the "end of life anyway, so why bother?" Describe how you would approach Kim and what you think you need to assess.

Answer: The nurse should assess Kim's individual perceptions of the event. Include her past experience with illness, any knowledge that she might have about breast cancer, treatments for breast cancer, or prosthetic devices and/or breast reconstruction. Evaluate the nature of her social supports, including the presence and attitudes of a spouse or significant other. What is her family situation? Does she have children or plan to have children? What is her past history with depression? Is she suicidal?

2. Mr. Hightower, an 84-year-old single (never married) man, has been admitted for the third time for complaints of dizziness, numbness and tingling in his fingers, and difficulty breathing. He tells the emergency department physician that he thinks he has a brain tumor. His tests continue to reveal no physical cause for the symptoms, and once he is admitted to

the hospital his symptoms resolve within a matter of hours. A review of the chart indicates that he lost his 17-year-old cat to bone cancer 2 months ago. What do you think is happening, and how would you approach Mr. Hightower?

Answer: Mr. Hightower is likely to be experiencing complicated bereavement due to the loss of his cat. His symptoms might be similar to those that he imagines his cat endured, or they might reflect symptoms of an acute anxiety or panic reaction to his social isolation. The nurse should discuss this loss with him and possibly refer him to a counselor with whom he could discuss his feelings.

3. Harvey is in the final phase of his terminal illness. It is clear he will die soon. He has no family in this state but is very involved with his church, and his minister visits often. His minister asks if it would be appropriate for members of the church to keep a vigil at the bedside until Harvey dies. The medical resident who is following the case has written an order that reads, "Family visitors only." Identify three needs that Harvey is likely to be experiencing as he approaches the end of life. Discuss what nursing interventions would be the most appropriate.

Answer: Harvey might need to make contact with at least some members of his family, and the nurse should facilitate this contact if possible. He needs companionship and comfort in his final days. This likely means that he needs approval to have members of his church stay with him. Since they are his primary support at this time, they should be considered "family." He might need increased nursing involvement, both for comfort care that will not be provided by his attendant or family members and to supplement the care provided by these persons. He will also need vigilant observation for pain management.

EDUCATIONAL STRATEGIES

1. Discuss the concept of loss, including actual and perceived loss and maturational and situational loss.

2. Review the different types of loss, the grief experience, and responses.

3. Ask students to share personal experiences with loss and grieving.

4. Identify the differences between bereavement, grief, and mourning.

5. Compare and contrast the theories of loss and grief, including those of Kübler-Ross, Bowlby, and Worden. Ask students to identify examples of different behaviors that can be demonstrated in the stages specified by each theorist.

6. Discuss anticipatory grief and the circumstances that can lead to this process.

7. Present situations that can affect grief and lead to complicated bereavement. Have students identify examples of special circumstances that might affect the grieving process.

8. Review possible responses of individuals across the lifespan to loss and grief. Ask students to provide specific examples of responses that might be expected from individuals of different ages.

9. Discuss the relationship of hope, spirituality, and self-concept to loss and the grieving process.

10. Guide students in the application of the critical thinking process to situations of loss and grief.

11. Apply the nursing process to an actual and/or simulated client situation where the individual has experienced loss. Assign students to prepare a nursing care plan/pathway for this individual, identifying specific interventions to assist the client in the grieving process.

12. Invite a hospice and/or oncology nurse to speak to the class about his or her role in assisting clients through loss, about the stages of death and dying, and about the available support for the nurse in these situations.

13. Ask students to discuss how nurses might respond to the death of a client, and identify the resources that the nurse can use for emotional support.

14. Assign students to investigate the resources available in the community for clients and families to work through loss and grief.

15. Review the Dying Person's Bill of Rights, living wills, and advance directives.

16. Discuss how therapeutic communication is utilized to assist clients and families through loss and grief.

17. Use the following, or similar, situations to have students identify how the clients might react to loss and how the nurse should respond:
    a. A 32-year-old unmarried woman who has had a mastectomy
    b. A 26-year-old woman who has been diagnosed with multiple sclerosis
    c. A 16-year-old adolescent male with diabetes
    d. A 62-year-old man going through the process of aging
    e. A 45-year-old with a terminal disease
    f. Parents of a 7-year-old child with leukemia

18. Discuss the role of the nurse with clients who are experiencing a loss in health promotion and acute care settings. Ask students to identify specific interventions that might help the client and family to cope with loss and the process of death and dying.

19. Review how religious and cultural beliefs can influence an individual's response to loss and death and dying.

20. Explain and demonstrate postmortem care. Review the religious and cultural beliefs and practices that can influence the preparation of the deceased. Arrange, if possible, for students to observe or participate in the performance of postmortem care.

21. Assign students to observe or participate in the care of clients experiencing loss or terminal illness. Discuss student feelings before the experience and have the group identify specific plans for communication with the clients and their families or significant others.

INDEPENDENT LEARNING

1. Students should review the Dying Person's Bill of Rights to determine expectations of the health care provider.

2. Students can reflect on their own experiences with loss and grief in order to see how past responses might help them to work with their clients.

3. Students can investigate available resources in the community for assisting clients and families to work through loss and grief.

4. Students should review the procedure for postmortem care, including cultural and religious practices that can influence the preparation of the deceased.

STUDENT RESOURCES

Comparison of Theories on Loss and Grief

	Kübler-Ross	Bowlby	Worden
Identification of stages and behaviors of clients and significant others			

Care of the Client and Family Experiencing Loss or Grief

Nursing Interventions for Health Promotion	Nursing Interventions in Acute Care

CROSS-CURRICULUM GUIDE

Students might be interacting with clients who will experience loss and go through the process of grieving. Some clients might respond to a loss of appearance or function, whereas others will need to cope with death and dying. Clients who have been diagnosed with a terminal disease, along with their families, are especially in need of supportive nursing interventions. In addition, students should be aware of other disease processes, traumatic injuries, and sudden events that will result in the client and family experiencing loss and grief. For example, heart and lung disease, sensory impairments, suicide, and sudden death from accidents or violence will necessitate assessment of grief behaviors.

CHAPTER 22

Stress and Adaptation

CRITICAL THINKING ACTIVITIES AND ANSWERS

1. You are caring for a 30-year-old single mother who has recently received a diagnosis of metastatic breast cancer. She is the sole provider for three young children (all under 7 years of age). Discuss the various stressors that will need to be considered when writing an appropriate discharge plan.

Answer: The stressors that need to be considered are as follows:
   a. Family support and extended social support availability
   b. Financial considerations
   c. The developmental stages of the children and their ability to understand what is happening to their mother
   d. The mother's consideration for child care
   e. The mother's ability and resources to keep doctor's appointments, including such factors as transportation and coordination of appointments with children's schedules
   f. The mother's physical ability and endurance for child care (does she need some form of home health care?)
   g. The mother's concerns for discussing death and dying issues with children
   h. The need for legal assistance in the development of a will
   i. The possible need for spiritual assistance and support

2. A client comes to the emergency room with complaints of dizziness, which are not related to any physical finding on examination. During the health history the client reports that her life is very stressful, and she is barely coping. She finalized her divorce 3 months ago, is working 32 hours per week, and is attending college. Her ex-husband recently lost his job and can no longer pay child support. Finally, she tearfully confesses that she thinks she might be pregnant but does not want her ex-husband to know. Develop nursing diagnoses related to this situation.

Answer: Nursing diagnoses include:
   a. Ineffective personal coping related to financial, marital, and school stressors
   b. Anxiety related to the possibility of pregnancy
   c. Fear related to the uncertainty of her future and possible reaction of her husband to pregnancy
   d. Fatigue resulting from excessive demands of work, school, and home responsibilities

3. An older adult woman is admitted to the hospital with a fractured hip. Before her injury she lived with her husband, who suffers from advancing Alzheimer's disease. While she is hospitalized, he is staying with a niece who lives 100 miles away, but this cannot be a permanent situation because her niece is also in frail health. The client has no children who can help her when she returns home. She is concerned not only about who will care for her after she is discharged but also about her husband. What approach would be the best to take in establishing goals for her treatment?

Answer: Speak with the patient to help identify her primary concerns and prioritize her health care needs. Take into consideration the following: her own health status, which demands immediate nursing care, and the health status of her husband. Nursing planning would be directed toward developing short-term goals, focused on healing her hip fracture and returning to independent functioning, and long-term goals, including planning care for her husband. Outside resources and collaboration with professionals in other disciplines, such as social service, will help in achieving the stated goals.

EDUCATIONAL STRATEGIES

1. Discuss what stress is, including its positive and negative aspects.

2. Provide an overview of stress and adaptation theories and their relation to health care delivery.

3. Describe the stress response. Compare and contrast the local and general adaptation syndromes. Ask students for examples of situations that might elicit a stress response.

4. Discuss nursing theories on stress and stressors and their application to client care. Assign students to apply one of the theories to an actual or simulated client situation.

5. Discuss factors related to stress and the response to stress, including developmental, psychological, sociocultural, and spiritual considerations.

6. Review defense and coping mechanisms. Have students provide examples of how each mechanism might be used.

7. Describe the relationship of stress and illness, using the mind-body interaction framework. Ask students to give examples of stress-related illnesses.

8. Apply the critical thinking process to situations with clients experiencing stress.

9. Organize a role-playing experience with students interviewing their peers about stressors and stress-related symptoms and behaviors. Have students use the sample questions (box in text) or develop their own questionnaire.

10. Guide students in the application of the nursing process for an actual or simulated situation where a client is experiencing stress. Assign students to develop a care plan/pathway based on the situation, specifically identifying assessment measures to determine the level of stress and interventions focused on stress management.

11. Discuss crisis, the types of crises, and crisis intervention. Identify the steps of crisis intervention and the role of the nurse.

12. Invite a nurse working in a crisis intervention center to speak to the class about his or her responsibilities and specific interventions for clients in crisis.

13. Ask students to share their own feelings and reactions to stress, including coping mechanisms that they have used to deal with stress.

14. Describe specific nursing interventions for stress management, including promotion of nutrition, exercise, rest, support systems, relaxation techniques, and time management.

15. Explain and demonstrate a variety of relaxation techniques. Have students practice the techniques in class and determine how they will instruct clients in the use of the techniques.

16. Ask students to complete a usual weekly schedule of their activities, then have them critique the schedule for best use of time. Have students re-do their schedules using time management concepts.

17. Stimulate a discussion on nursing "burnout." Ask students what they think about this phenomenon and how it may be prevented.

INDEPENDENT LEARNING

1. Students can review their own experiences with and responses to stress. They can focus on how or if they identified stressors and whether or not their responses were helpful.

2. Students should practice relaxation techniques for use in school, at home, or at work.

3. Students should develop a time management plan that includes school, home, work, and other regular responsibilities.

STUDENT RESOURCES

Stress Response

Stress Response	Description
Local Adaptation Syndrome Reflex pain response	
Inflammatory response	
General Adaptation Syndrome Alarm reaction	
Resistance stage	
Exhaustion stage	

Factors Related to Stress Response

Factors	Description
Developmental	
Psychological	
Sociocultural	
Spiritual	

Crisis Intervention

Steps	Nursing Interventions
Assessment of client problem	
Planning the intervention	
Implementing the intervention	
Reflecting on the resolution	

Sample Interview Questions for Gathering Subjective Data

1. In your own words, what has been the most-stressful thing for you during this hospitalization?

2. When you have experienced stress in the past, how did you resolve it?
   a. Sought out reasons for those feelings
   b. Blamed others
   c. Withdrew from family, friends, or co-workers
   d. Talked with others (spouse, clergy, friends, suppport groups)
   e. Used distraction
      (1) Examples of positive distractors (music, exercise, relaxation techniques)
      (2) Examples of negative distractors (alcohol and drug use, smoking, changes in eating habits)

3. Describe any stress–related problems for which you have been treated in the past.

4. Describe any recent major life changes (within the last year) related to any of the following:
   a. Health (physical and mental)
   b. Family
   c. Lifestyle habits
   d. Changes in daily activities (eating, sleeping, getting up to go to work)
   e. Supportive network
   f. Work (Do yo enjoy your work?)
   g. Financial and legal problems
   h. Recent losses or trauma

5. Can you rate how stressful these major life changes have been on a scale of 1 to 10 (from least stressful to most stressful)?

6. How many people are you responsible for (older adult parents, children, other dependents)?

7. Tell me how you spend your leisure time. Are these activities done alone or with a group of friends?

8. How often do you take vacations or mental health days?

Select Components of Assessment of Mental Status

Mental Status Examination

Appearance
Dress, grooming, hygiene, apparent age, posture, facial expression

Behavior and Activity
Hypoactivity or hyperactivity, rigid, relaxed, restless or agitated motor movements, gait and coordination, facial grimacing, gestures, mannerisms, passive, combative, bizarre

Attitude
Interactions with the interviewer: cooperative, resistive, friendly, hostile, ingratiating

Mood and Affect
Mood (intensity, depth, duration): sad, fearful, depressed, angry, anxious, ambivalent, happy, ecstatic, grandiose
Affect (intensity, depth, duration): appropriate, apathetic, constricted, blunted, flat, labile, euphoric, bizarre

Perceptions
Hallucinations, illusions, depersonalization

Thoughts
Form and content: logical vs. illogical, loose associations, flight of ideas, autistic, blocking, broadcasting, delusions, abstract vs. concrete

Sensorium and Cognition
Levels of consciousness, orientation, attention span, recent and remote memory, concentration; ability to comprehend and process information; intelligence

Judgment
Ability to assess and evaluate situations, make rational decisions, understand consequences of behavior and take responsibility for actions

Insight
Ability to perceive and understand the cause and nature of own and others' situations

Reliability
Interviewer's impression that individual reported information accurately and completely

Psychosocial Criteria

Stressors
Internal: psychiatric or medical illness, perceived loss, such as loss of self-concept or self-esteem
External: actual loss, such as death of a loved one, divorce, lack of support systems, job or financial loss, retirement, dysfunctional family system

Coping Skills
Use of functional adaptive coping mechanisms and techniques, management of activities of daily living

Relationships
Attainment and maintenance of satisfying, interpersonal relationships congruent with developmental state

CROSS-CURRICULUM GUIDE

Accessing the health care delivery system, whether a client is demonstrating signs and symptoms of an illness or not, can be a stressful experience in itself. Individuals awaiting the results of diagnostic tests, anticipating surgery, or responding to the illness of a family member are likely to evidence a stress response. Students can have a preliminary discussion on stress and adaptation early in their program so that they can apply the concepts and be alert to indications that clients and significant others are experiencing stress. Early intervention can offset severe stress reactions, promote a sense of well-being, and improve clients' overall ability to deal with health-related concerns.

Scientific Basis for
Nursing Practice

CHAPTER 23

Vital Signs

CRITICAL THINKING ACTIVITIES AND ANSWERS

1. A 68-year-old widowed woman has been referred to the hypertension clinic held by the Visiting Nurses Association. During her visit, you are assigned to do an admission assessment. She reports that her primary care physician told her that her blood pressure was 164/94. You obtain a blood pressure of 148/86. What further data are required to analyze the discrepancy of blood pressure findings? How would you explain the difference to the client? Develop a plan for the health promotion of this new client.

Answer: Time of day, stress level, and activity all contribute to the elevation of blood pressure in the physician's office. Technical differences can also be a factor, such as type of sphygmomanometer, the arm being assessed, and the technique of the health care provider who is measuring blood pressure. The nurse should assess the blood pressure in both arms and perhaps reassess at the end of the visit. The nurse should educate the client on the effects of stress and activity on blood pressure. Health promotion includes evaluating and modifying risk factors.

2. A 23-year-old college athlete is brought to the emergency room after collapsing during a basketball game. He is awake and oriented but complains of being dizzy and sweaty. He is 6 feet 6 inches tall and weighs 105 kg. He states that just before he passed out he felt his "chest beating like a drum." List the vital signs to be obtained from this client in order of priority. What signs and symptoms would indicate orthostatic hypotension?

Answer: The "chest beating like a drum" is a frequent description of palpitations resulting from dysrhythmias. The suggested order of vital sign priority is apical pulse, blood pressure, SpO_2, respiratory rate, and temperature. Additional data to assess pulse deficit should be obtained. Orthostatic blood pressure assessment should be completed after baseline vital signs are obtained. Orthostatic hypotension related to fluid volume depletion could be suspected based on client complaints of dizziness and recent participation in strenuous activity to increase insensible water loss.

3. A 78-year-old retired coal miner, is admitted to the surgical floor after a left pneumonectomy for carcinoma of the lung. An IV is present in his right forearm. He complains of shortness of breath and pain. During the report the PACU nurse states that his preoperative SpO_2 was 95% and in the immediate postoperative period his SpO_2 was 92% on 4 L O_2 via nasal cannula. What are the most effective methods for obtaining this client's vital signs? What is the priority nursing diagnosis for this client? Explain the difference between the SpO_2 readings.

Answer: Pulse should be obtained apically (pain and postanesthetic status could contribute to peripheral vasoconstriction); both radial pulses should be assessed for equality (positioning during surgery can compromise circulation to extremities); blood pressure should be measured in left arm (infusing IV in right arm means that the left surgical thoracic site is not a contraindication): temperature should not be taken orally but via tympanic membrane (client may be mouth breathing or surgical status may have dried oral mucous membranes); SpO_2 is related to effects of anesthesia, splinting from incisional pain, and surgical procedure. Change in position after pneumonectomy may also contribute to difference in SpO_2 readings. Continuous SpO_2 measurement would be indicated.

4. During a home visit, the client requests that you "take a look at" her 4-year-old son. The child has been quietly lying on the couch watching television for the past 30 minutes of your visit. You note flushed skin that is warm and dry to the touch. Skin lesions indicative of chicken pox are present on his face and torso. Vital signs are: apical rate 126, regular; BP RA 90/52; RR 18; tympanic temperature 103° F (39.3° C). Which vital signs are outside acceptable limits? What is the likely cause of the alteration in vital signs? Provide three nursing diagnoses to be included in the plan of care.

Answer: The temperature is the only vital sign outside the range of acceptable values for a 4-year-old child. The fever is the likely result of the varicella pyrogen, and secondary infection of the lesions should be considered. The lethargic nature of the child (4-year-old children don't sit still for 30 minutes) might be related to the fever. Nursing diagnoses include hyperthermia, risk of fluid volume deficit, and knowledge deficit (mother's).

EDUCATIONAL STRATEGIES

1. Review, or have the students review, the anatomy and physiology associated with temperature regulation, circulation, and respiration.

2. Discuss the guidelines and indications for measurement of vital signs. Emphasize the importance of vital sign measurement and the relation of the findings to the client's status.

3. Discuss the mechanisms that regulate body temperature, pulse, respiration, blood pressure, central venous pressure (CVP), and oxygen saturation.

4. Have students identify factors that can influence the client's vital signs.

5. Review how vital signs change throughout the process of growth and development. Have students identify expected findings for individuals of different ages.

6. Discuss alterations in vital signs and the underlying etiology of the alterations. Ask students to identify nursing interventions appropriate for clients with the following alterations:
   a. Hypothermia, hyperthermia, pyrexia
   b. Bradycardia, tachycardia, pulse deficit, general dysrhythmias
   c. Hypotension, orthostatic hypotension, hypertension
   d. Bradypnea, tachypnea, dyspnea
   e. Decreases and increases in CVP
   f. Reduction of oxygen saturation

7. Explain and demonstrate (with educational media, simulation mannequins/models, or volunteers) the procedures for assessment of vital signs, including the sites for measurement and use of equipment for the following:
   a. Temperature–oral, axillary, rectal, and tympanic
   b. Pulse–apical and peripheral
   c. Respiration
   d. Blood pressure–brachial, femoral, auscultated, palpated
   e. CVP
   f. Pulse oximetry

Have students work in small groups to practice the procedures and record the results.

8. Evaluate the students' ability to assess vital signs through return demonstration/skill testing before clinical experiences. Identify areas that require additional practice for refinement of technique.

9. Have students identify how the environment can affect vital signs and how the nurse can manipulate the environment to reduce or eliminate distractions or influences.

10. Guide students in the application of the nursing process for clients with alterations in vital signs. Ask students how the assessment of vital signs can be integrated into the plan of care/pathway.

11. Assign students to prepare teaching plans for clients and family members on the assessment of vital signs. Have students identify how the procedure may be adapted for clients with special needs (e.g., right-sided weakness).

12. Assign students to assess clients' vital signs in a variety of health care settings. Have students monitor, report, and record the results. Discuss client findings in post-care conferences and ask students to identify alterations and possible indications for these alterations.

13. Have students identify how measurement of vital signs should be altered or adapted for the following, or similar, situations where the client
    a. has just finished eating or drinking
    b. is awaiting outpatient surgery in 20 minutes
    c. has a history of a heart murmur or dysrhythmia
    d. had a right-side mastectomy
    e. is taking anticoagulants, bronchodilators, or muscle relaxants
    f. had oral or rectal surgery
    g. has bilateral arm casts
    h. is obese or extremely thin
    i. has an IV or A/V shunt in the left arm
    j. is 6 months old, 2 years old, or 10 years old

14. Provide students with examples of clients experiencing different health deviations and ask them to identify how the vital signs may be affected.

INDEPENDENT LEARNING

1. Students should review the normal anatomy and physiology associated with the body's temperature-regulating mechanisms and circulatory and respiratory systems.

2. Students should practice taking vital signs with peers, family members, or friends. A skills practice laboratory should be used, if available.

3. Students can investigate strategies for adaptation of vital sign measurement for clients with different health problems (e.g., casts, contractures).

4. Students can research an article on new developments or guidelines for vital sign measurement.

STUDENT RESOURCES

Obtain samples of flowsheets for vital sign recording from clinical agencies for student practice.

Vital Signs across the Lifespan–Expected Finding

	Temperature	Pulse	Respiration	Blood Pressure
Infant				
Toddler				
Preschool child				
School-age child				
Adolescent				
Adult				
Older adult				

Alterations in Vital Signs and Nursing Interventions

Alterations	Nursing Interventions
Temperature	
Pulse	
Blood pressure	
Respiration	

CROSS-CURRICULUM GUIDE

Alterations in vital signs can be associated with a wide variety of health deviations but should be highlighted in discussions on clients with circulatory and respiratory disorders. Review and accurate implementation of these procedures is critical before client care experiences.

Maternal/Child: Students will have to adapt vital sign measurement techniques for infants and children to obtain accurate readings.

Gerontological: Changes that occur with aging will alter vital signs, and students should be aware of expected results. In addition, physiological and pathological changes might require adaptation of the techniques for measurement (e.g., client might not have the musculature to hold a thermometer in the mouth).

MULTIMEDIA RESOURCES

Applying Critical Thinking to Nursing Skills: An Interactive Videodisc Series
    Shift Assessment

Mosby's Nursing Skills Video Series:
    Set I: Vital Signs

TOPICAL OUTLINE

CRITICAL THINKING ACTIVITIES AND ANSWERS

1. A 32-year-old client entering a neighborhood clinic exhibits the following symptoms: frequent productive cough, fatigue, decreased appetite, and persistent fever. What focused assessment should the nurse conduct?

Answer: The nurse should perform a detailed history, identifying that this client is at risk for lung disease (e.g., tuberculosis, HIV pulmonary disease, pneumonia). All techniques of respiratory assessment should be completed: inspection, palpation (excursion, tactile fremitus), percussion, and auscultation; also take pulse, blood pressure, and temperature.

2. The nurse is performing an abdominal assessment and observes a pulsating midline abdominal mass. What is the nurse's next line of action?

Answer: The nurse must not palpate a pulsating abdominal mass as it may be an abdominal aneurysm. The physician should be notified immediately.

3. What physical examination techniques does the nurse use during the following situations: evaluating a client's oral hygiene, a client with a cast on the lower leg, a client found on the floor, and a client reporting abdominal pain?

Answer: Physical examination measures used for:

Oral hygiene: Client's history, inspection and palpation, also use of smell

Application of cast: Inspection and palpation of skin, also neurovascular assessment

Client found on floor: Neurological, musculoskeletal, and integumentary assessments

Abdominal pain: Client's history, palpation of affected area, auscultation of bowel sounds

4. An elderly woman with reduced visual acuity would have difficulty performing what aspect of breast self-examination?

Answer: An elderly woman with reduced visual acuity would have difficulty with the technique of inspection when performing a breast self-exam.

5. A 75-year-old black male is being visited 1 week postoperatively by the home health nurse to assess peripheral vascular status following a femoral-popliteal bypass graft for arterial insufficiency. What assessment data should be obtained by the nurse?

Answer: Assessment criteria include color, temperature, pulse, edema, and skin changes. Systems to be assessed are skin and neurovascular. The client's history, especially pain, helps to identify occlusion (3 Ps: pain, pallor, pulselessness). Also check pallor in a dark-skinned client: normal brown skin appears yellow brown, and normal black skin looks ashen gray.

6. Explain the different findings the nurse might gather when assessing coordination in a 40-year-old versus an 80-year-old.

Answer: Coordination of a 40-year-old should be smooth and balanced; an 80-year-old might demonstrate slow reaction time with movements that are less rhythmical, depending on the individual's level of physical activity and fitness.

EDUCATIONAL STRATEGIES

1. Discuss the purposes of the physical examination.

2. Ask students to identify how cultural and gender sensitivity should be applied to the performance of the physical examination.

3. Have students review normal anatomy and physiology and the alterations that occur with growth and development.

4. Ask students to provide examples of when and how physical assessment can be integrated into the client's care.

5. Discuss the preparation of the client and the environment before the physical exam. Have students set up an actual or simulated setting in preparation for a physical examination.

6. Explain and demonstrate the following (using educational media, simulation mannequins/ models, and/or volunteers):
   a. Skills of physical assessment: inspection, palpation, percussion, auscultation, and olfaction
   b. Client positioning during the examination
   c. Procedure and sequence for completion of the examination
   d. Special equipment used for the examination

7. Ask students to identify how the skills of physical assessment are applied in the examination and what information is elicited with their use.

8. Have students discuss the rationale for different client positions and the sequence for performance of the physical exam.

9. Discuss precautions that should be implemented for infection control and asepsis.

10. Have students identify how communication and teaching can be integrated into the physical examination.

11. Assign students to prepare and implement, if possible, teaching plans for specific areas of adolescent/adult client self-examination, such as skin and breast exams.

12. Explain and demonstrate (using educational media, simulation mannequins/models, and/or volunteers) the physical examination.

13. Working in small groups, have students practice physical assessment skills for selected elements of the physical exam (e.g., head and neck, thorax). If appropriate, have students complete a supervised, limited physical examination. (Students at this level do not usually perform complete examinations, especially in regard to the visual and genital areas.)

14. Evaluate the students' ability to perform the skills of physical assessment and the components of the examination through return demonstration. For example, accurate use of the stethoscope is important for the student to develop.

15. Discuss the expected and unexpected findings that might be noted for each system during the physical examination. Provide students with examples of possible findings from a physical examination and have them identify which are normally expected or unexpected for a client.

16. Review the reporting and documentation of the findings of the physical assessment/exam. Have students practice recording findings on available agency forms.

17. Invite a nurse practitioner to speak to the class about his or her development, the implementation of physical examination skills, and the application of exam findings to client care.

18. Assign students to integrate learned elements of physical assessment into client care in the clinical setting. Discuss findings with students in post-care conferences. Supervise and evaluate the reporting and documentation of physical assessment findings. Ask students to identify and explain, according to their level of knowledge, any expected and unexpected client findings.

19. Have students identify how the physical exam and its findings can be integrated into the care plan/pathway.

20. Have students discuss how the physical examination might be adapted for the following, or similar, clients:
    a. A 2-year-old child
    b. A 14-year-old boy or girl
    c. A woman with severe abdominal pain
    d. An older adult with arthritis
    e. A client from another culture who speaks a different language
    f. A severely anxious or fearful client

INDEPENDENT LEARNING

1. Students should review normal anatomy and physiology in preparation for discussion and practice of the physical examination.

2. Students should review medical terminology for reporting and documentation of findings.

3. Students can practice physical assessment techniques as appropriate with peers, family, and friends. They can think about expected and unexpected findings and how these findings should be reported and recorded.

STUDENT RESOURCES

Physical Examination: Expected and Unexpected Findings

Body System/Area	Expected Findings	Unexpected Findings
Integument		
Head and neck		
Thorax and lungs		
Heart		
Vascular system		
Breasts		
Abdomen		
Female genitalia		
Male genitalia		
Rectum and anus		
Musculoskeletal system		
Neurological system		

Folsteins Mini–Mental State

"Mini–Mental State"
Maximum
Score

Orientation
5 ( ) What is the (year) (season) (date) (day) (month)?
5 ( ) Where are we (state) (country) (town) (hospital) (floor)?

Registration
3 ( ) Name 3 objects; 1 second to say each. Then ask the client all 3 after you have said them. Give l point for each correct answer. Then repeat them until he or she learns all 3. Count trials are record.

Attention and Calculation
5 ( ) Serial 7's. 1 point for each correct answer. Stop after 5 answers. Alternatively, spell "world" backwards.

Recall
3 ( ) Ask for the 3 objects repeated above. Give 1 point for each correct answer.

Language
9 ( ) Name a pencil and a watch (2 point)
Repeat the following: "No ifs, ands, or buts" (1 point)
Follow a 3–stage command:
"Take a paper in your right hand, fold it in half, and put it on the floor" (3 points)
Read and obey the following:
Close your eyes" (1 point)
Write a sentence (1 point)
Copy a design (1 point)

Total Score
Assess level of consciousness along a continuum

Alert	Drowsy	Stupor	Coma

Instructions for Administration of Mini–Mental State Examination
Orientation
Ask for the date. Then ask specifically for parts omitted, e.g., "Can you also tell me what season it is?" One point for each correct answer.
Ask in turn, "Can you tell me the name of this hospital?" (town, country, etc.). One point for each correct answer.

Registration
Ask the client if you may test his or her memory.
Then say the names of 3 unrelated objects, clearly and slowly, about 1 second for each. After you have said all 3, ask client to repeat them. This first repetition determines the score (0-3), but keep saying them until client can repeat all 3, up to 6 trials. If client does not eventually learn all 3, recall cannot be meaningfully tested.

Attention and Calculation
Ask the client to begin with 100 and count backwards by 7. Stop after 5 subtractions (93, 86, 79, 72, 65). Score the total number of correct answers.
If the client cannot or will not perform this task, ask him or her to spell the word "world" backwards. The score is the number of letters in correct order, e.g., dlrow = 5, dlorw = 3.

Recall
Ask the client to recall the 3 words you previously asked. Score 0-3.

Language
Naming: Show the client a wristwatch and ask what it is. Repeat for a pencil. Score 0-2.
Repetition: Ask the client to repeat the sentence after you. Allow only one trial. Score 0 or 1.
3-stage command: Give the client a piece of plain blank paper and repeat the command. Score 1 point for each part correctly executed.
Reading: On a Blank piece of paper print the sentence "Close your eyes" in letters large enough for the client to see clearly. Ask him or her to read it and do what it says. Score 1 point only if eyes are actually closed.
Writing: Give the client a blank piece of paper and ask him or her to write a sentence for you. Do not dictate a sentence: it is to be written spontaneously. It must contain a subject and verb and be sensible. Correct grammar and punctuation are not necessary.
Copying: On a clean sheet of paper, draw intersecting pentagons, each side about 1 inch, and ask the client to copy it exactly as it is. All 10 angles must be present and 2 must intersect to score 1 point. Tremor and rotation are ignored.
Estimate the client's level of sensorium along a continuum, from alert on the left to coma on the right.

From Folstein MF and others: Mini–Mental State: a practical method for grading the cognitive state of patients for the clinician, *J Psychiatr Res* 12:189, 1975.

CROSS-CURRICULUM GUIDE

Medical/Surgical: Areas of specific assessment, with expected and unexpected findings, can be discussed along with the associated health deviations/disorders. For example, students learning about and working with clients who have gastrointestinal problems should be referred to the assessment procedures particular to the abdomen and gastrointestinal system.

Maternal/child: Students can be referred to specific physical assessment skills and evaluation of findings during discussions on pregnancy, childbirth, and growth and development.

Gerontological: Older adults may demonstrate changes that are associated with the normal aging process or are a result of a pathological condition. Students should be able to use basic physical assessment skills to investigate the status of the older client.

MULTIMEDIA RESOURCES

Mosby's Physical Examination Video Series:
- Set 1: *Overview of the Physical Examination*
  Taking a Health History
  Examination Techniques
  The General Survey
  Skin, Hair, and Nails
  Lymphatic system
- Set 2: *Examining the Head and Neck*
  Examining the Eyes
  Examining the Ears
  Examining the Nose, Mouth, and Pharynx
  Examining the Lungs and Thorax
  Examining the Heart
- Set 3: *Examining the Vascular System*
  Examining the Breast
  Examining the Abdomen
  Examining the Male Genitalia and Rectum
  Examining the Female Genitalia, Reproductive Tract, and Rectum
  Examining the Musculoskeletal System
- Set 4: *Neurologic System: Mental Status, Speech, and Cranial Nerves*
  Neurologic System: Motor and Sensory Functions, Reflexes
  Examining the Child
  Examining the Older Adult

Whaley and Wong's Pediatric Nursing Video Series:
- *Pediatric Assessment*

Mosby's Physical Examination Interactive Videodisc Series:
- *Interviewing and Taking a Health History*
  Physical Examination of the Respiratory System
  Physical Examination of the Cardiovascular System
  Physical Examination of the Neurologic System
  Physical Examination of the Adult
  Physical Examination of the Abdomen
  Physical Examination of the Musculoskeletal System

CHAPTER 25

Infection Control

TOPICAL OUTLINE

CRITICAL THINKING ACTIVITIES AND ANSWERS

1. During a home care visit, it is reported that several members of the family have had diarrhea and vomiting after eating a dinner of turkey and stuffing. After further investigation, it is determined that the turkey was thawed at room temperature instead of following the recommendation to thaw it in the refrigerator and that the stuffing was placed in the turkey's cavity before the turkey was completely thawed. The nurse reports this immediately to the physician, and stool cultures are ordered. Three members of the family are diagnosed as having *Salmonella* food-borne illness. Describe in this case (using the chain of infection) how the infection occurred and how the nurse can assist the clients in preventing further food-borne illness.

Answer: The infectious agent was the *Salmonella*, the reservoir was the improperly thawed and cooked turkey and stuffing, the mode of transmission was the consumption of the turkey through the portal of entry, the GI tract, and all persons consuming the turkey were susceptible hosts. The nurse can assist the family in the prevention of food-borne illness by stressing that meat should be thawed in the refrigerator and should not be consumed until they are properly cooked. The nurse should also instruct the family that the physician should be contacted when several members of a family become ill after eating the same foods.

2. In the following client care situations, select the appropriate personal protective equipment (PPE) and give the rationale: (a) starting an IV catheter, (b) blood pressure checks on a client with hepatitis B, (c) changing the bed linen for an incontinent client, (d) entering the room of a client with meningococcal meningitis, (e) entering the room of a client with *Mycobacterium avium,* (f) emptying a suction bottle containing bloody fluid, and (g) changing an infected wound dressing on a client in a home situation.

Answer: The appropriate PPE for these situations include:

a. When starting an IV, washing one's hands and wearing clean gloves is all that is required.

b. No barrier protection is needed when checking blood pressure on a client with hepatitis B because hepatitis B is transmitted in blood and body fluids, not on dry skin. Standard precautions: gloves should be worn if there is visible blood on the client's arm.

c. When changing the bed of an incontinent client, the nurse should wear gloves and a gown if soiling of the uniform is likely.

d. Unless the nurse is within 3 feet of the patient, no PPE is necessary. Droplet precautions are the category used for care of a client with meningococcal meningitis, and a mask is required when within 3 feet of the client until the client has had an effective treatment of appropriate antibiotics.

e. *Mycobacterium avium* is an acid-fast organism in the same family as tuberculosis, but it is not contagious. Thus a mask or respirator is not required.

f. When emptying a suction bottle containing bloody fluid, the nurse should anticipate that splashing could occur; for this reason, eyewear, mask, gown, and gloves should be worn.

g. When changing a dressing on an infected wound, the nurse should assess the size and location of the wound and the amount and color of drainage. The nurse should always wear gloves, but additional barriers might be necessary to prevent contamination of clothing or uniform. The hands should always be washed after removing the gloves.

3. Mrs. Smith is admitted for a major surgical procedure. During the administration procedure, the nurse notices that Mrs. Smith has a productive cough that she says she has had for about 6 weeks. She further states that she has occasionally seen blood in her sputum and has lost weight over the past 4 weeks. Mrs. Smith also tells the nurse that one of the members of her immediate household has recently been diagnosed with tuberculosis (TB). With this additional history, what should the nurse do?

Answer: The nurse should immediately notify the physician about Mrs. Smith's reported history and ask if any additional tests might be needed to rule out TB (chest x-ray, sputum, or skin test) and if airborne precautions can be ordered. The nurse can instruct other members of the health care team to wear a mask or respirator (according to the agency's policy) until TB is ruled out. The client may also have to be moved to a room that has negative air flow or pressure. The nurse should notify the facility's infection control professional for further instructions.

EDUCATIONAL STRATEGIES

1. Discuss the nature, chain, and course of infection. Have students provide specific examples for each component in the chain of infection.

2. Review the normal body defenses against infection. Ask students to identify how the body defenses can be altered and broken down.

3. Discuss nosocomial infections, clients with the greatest susceptibility, and preventive measures. Ask students to provide specific examples of health care setting activities or procedures that might contribute to the development of nosocomial infections.

4. Compare and contrast medical and surgical asepsis. Provide examples, or ask students to identify situations, where each type of asepsis is applied.

5. Discuss how cultural beliefs might influence a client's or family's response to an infectious process.

6. Identify the diagnostic tests that can be used to determine the presence of an infection. Have students investigate the results of these tests (e.g., WBCs) that will indicate an infectious process.

7. Discuss health promotion strategies for the prevention of infection, including nutrition, immunization, rest/exercise, hygienic measures, and stress reduction. Ask students to provide examples of how individuals can reduce the spread of infection in the home.

8. Review the recommended schedule for immunizations across the lifespan.

9. Discuss how infections can be prevented or controlled in the acute care environment through the use of medical and surgical aseptic techniques, standard precautions, and isolation procedures.

10. Explain and demonstrate (using educational media and available supplies) the procedures for handwashing and surgical handwashing. Ask students to compare and contrast the two procedures. Have students practice both handwashing techniques.

11. Discuss the guidelines and approaches in caring for and transporting a client on airborne, droplet, or contact isolation precautions. Have students set up an actual or simulated isolation room.

12. Explain and demonstrate the procedures associated with isolation precautions, including gowning, gloving, and use of protective eyewear and masks. Have students, working in small groups, practice donning protective apparel, obtaining specimens, and disposing of equipment.

13. Explain and demonstrate the procedures associated with surgical asepsis, including putting on sterile gloves, setting up a sterile field, opening sterile packs, and applying surgical attire. Have students practice opening up actual sterile packs (e.g. towels, catheter or tracheostomy care kits), setting up a sterile field, sterile gloving, and adding or removing materials from the field.

14. Evaluate the students' ability to implement techniques associated with infection control through return demonstration/skill testing before clinical experiences.

15. Discuss how equipment is handled, cleansed, and disposed of in accordance with infection control guidelines.

16. Guide students in the application of the nursing process for a client with a communicable or noncommunicable infectious disease. Have students prepare a care plan/pathway for an actual or simulated client who has a local or systemic infection.

17. Assign clients to observe or participate in the care of clients who have a local or systemic infection. Review standard precautions with students in advance. Ask students how they will be using medical/surgical aseptic techniques with their clients.

18. Have students prepare a teaching plan on prevention or control of infection for the following, or similar, clients and families:
    a. Middle-age man with TB returning home to his large family
    b. Young woman treated for a sexually transmitted disease
    c. Parents with their first child

19. Demonstrate proper and improper aseptic techniques and ask students to identify which techniques are correct and which are incorrect.

20. Invite an infection control nurse and/or risk manager to speak to the class about prevention of infection in a health care setting.

21. Ask students to identify the type of asepsis and precautions that should be used in the following situations where the client has the following:
    a. HIV–hospital and home environments
    b. TB–hospital and home environments
    c. A surgical wound
    d. A draining skin ulcer
    e. A newborn infant–hospital and home environments
    f. A urinary catheter

22. Have students identify whether clean or sterile gloves should be used for the following:
    a. Changing surgical dressings
    b. Taking rectal temperatures
    c. Obtaining arterial blood samples
    d. Performing hygienic care
    e. Inserting a urinary catheter
    f. Administering an injection

INDEPENDENT LEARNING

1. Students should review the processes of the body's immune system.

2. Students should review microbiology concepts, including the chain of infection and common disease-producing microorganisms.

3. Students should practice the skills associated with infection control in the skills laboratory and at home.

4. Students can research an article in a current nursing journal on standard precautions and/or resilient infectious agents.

STUDENT RESOURCES

Chain of Infection

Chain of Infection	Description	Nursing Prevention
Infectious agent		
Reservoir		
Portal of exit		
Mode of transmission		
Portal of entry		
Susceptible host		

Medical and Surgical Asepsis

Nursing Strategy	Medical Asepsis	Surgical Asepsis

CROSS-CURRICULUM GUIDE

Review of infection control and aseptic procedures is essential for students in all clinical settings but especially when they will be working with clients who are experiencing communicable diseases. Students may be interacting with clients who have TB, MRSA (methicillin-resistant *Staphylococcus aureus*), VRE (vancomycin-resistant enterococcus), and other communicable diseases that require strict adherence to standard precautions for client and nurse safety.

Reference to sterile techniques should be made in discussions on perioperative nursing care and implementation of specific invasive procedures (e.g., catheterization, tracheostomy care).

MULTIMEDIA RESOURCES

Mosby's Nursing Skills Video Series:
   Set I: *Medical Asepsis and Infection Prevention*
Mosby's Community Health Nursing Video Series:
   Set II: *Infection Control I: The Epidemiological Process*
          Infection Control II: Communicable Diseases and Specific Problems

CHAPTER 26

Administering Medications

CRITICAL THINKING ACTIVITIES AND ANSWERS

1. You are working with a critical care nurse who has been floated to your unit. You observe this nurse drawing up 0.25 mg of digoxin into a 3-ml syringe. The nurse does not dilute the medication and is preparing to give this medication by IV bolus. You tell her that neither you nor any other nurse has given digoxin by IV bolus. She tells you that she does so almost every day. Would you intervene in this situation? What rationale would you use to justify your position?

Answer: Nurses who work in critical care units may be accustomed to giving cardioactive medications by the IV method frequently. Generally speaking, cardioactive medications for administration by this method may be limited to clients in monitored settings, such as a critical care unit. You may want to suggest to this nurse that the two of you seek assistance from the nurse manager, who may be familiar with the institution's IV medication policies. You should check the nursing department's policy manual, which should identify what medications can and cannot be given by a registered nurse via the IV bolus method. These steps will ensure that medications are administered to clients in a safe manner and will also reduce medication errors.

2. Fifteen minutes after you have hung an IV antibiotic, the client is itching and clawing at the skin and hair. You determine that the client may be having an allergic reaction to the antibiotic. What steps would you take immediately? Why?

Answer: Stop the infusion of the antibiotic immediately. Summon help from other staff members and be certain that someone has alerted the client's physician. Obtain the client's vital signs and remain with the client until out of danger. Provide supportive measures as necessary. Once the client is no longer in danger, review all the events that led up to the time the client received the antibiotic. In particular, did you check the client's allergies?

3. You have prepared an IM injection for your client. You did not assess the client before preparing the medication. You draw the medication up in a syringe with a $1\frac{1}{2}$-inch, 21-gauge needle. When you arrive to give the injection you find that the client is cachectic and has very little muscle mass anywhere. How would you proceed with your assessment and intervention? Give your rationale.

Answer: If the client has some muscle mass, but not enough for a $1\frac{1}{2}$-inch needle, you can change the needle to a shorter length. Don't forget to maintain sterility of the needle during needle changes. If the client does not have enough muscle mass, withhold the medication and notify the client's prescriber. Inform the prescriber of the situation. Suggest that the medication be changed to an alternate form, such as rectal or intravenous.

4. Your client is receiving insulin at home and has run out of syringes. You have some 1-ml tuberculin syringes on hand. The client needs to receive 18 units of NPH and 4 units of regular insulin. How would you draw this up? How many tenths of a milliliter of each insulin would you draw up?

Answer: It is not advisable to use syringes for purposes for which they are not intended. Using tuberculin syringes instead of insulin syringes may confuse the client about the proper procedure for insulin administration. The nurse should call the client's pharmacy or health care provider to obtain a new supply of syringes. In an emergency, 0.1 ml on a tuberculin syringe is equivalent to 10 ml on an insulin syringe.

EDUCATIONAL STRATEGIES

1. Discuss the pharmacological aspects of medication administration, including drug names, classifications, and forms. Have students provide examples of each.

2. Review federal and state legislation and institutional guidelines for medication administration. Ask students to identify the nurse's legal responsibilities in medication administration.

3. Discuss medication abuse and misuse, and the responsibilities of the nurse, especially in reporting professional conduct.

4. Explain pharmacokinetics–drug absorption, distribution, metabolism, and excretion. Have students identify factors that can influence each of these actions.

5. Identify the types of medication actions and have students provide examples of each type.

6. Discuss the routes of medication administration and their advantages and disadvantages. Ask students what circumstances may influence the use or avoidance of a particular route.

7. Review systems of measurement, conversions, and calculations used for dosage prescription and calculation. Provide students with practice problems and have them work individually or in small groups on calculating a variety of drug dosages.

8. Discuss the roles of health care personnel, especially the nurse, in the administration of medications.

9. Describe the types of medication orders and have students provide examples for each type.

10. Stimulate a discussion on how critical thinking can be applied to safe and responsible medication administration by the nurse.

11. Have students identify the five rights of the client regarding medication and identify examples of how each is determined and maintained. Apply the five rights to the components of the medication order.

12. Discuss the assessment data that is critical to obtain in order to administer medications safely. Have students practice assessing each other to determine pertinent data, such as allergies, and current medications.

13. Review the special considerations for administration of medications to clients of different ages. Have students provide suggestions for reducing a child's fear of or reluctance to taking medications.

14. Assign students to complete and present, if possible, a teaching plan for an actual or simulated client who is inconsistent or noncompliant in medication use at home.

15. Review the application of aseptic technique to medication administration. Have students identify when medical and surgical asepsis should be used.

16. Show students the equipment that is used for medication administration by different routes. Have students identify when the equipment should be selected for use and how it is used safely.

17. Explain and demonstrate (using educational media, simulation mannequins/models, and appropriate equipment) the procedures for administration of the following:
    a. Oral medications or medications given through enteral tubes
    b. Topical medications
    c. Inhaled medications
    d. Intraocular medications
    e. Parenteral medications

Have students practice the preparation and administration of medications through the specified routes using mannequins/models, "practice fruits" (e.g., grapefruits, oranges), and/or injection pads. Allow ample time for students to manipulate the equipment.

18. Review special considerations for IV administration of medications (per level of student).

19. Assign students to participate in the care of clients who will be receiving medications by various routes. Determine the students' level of knowledge about the prescribed medications, their actions, effects, and nursing responsibilities. Discuss client considerations and safety measures before administration. Supervise the preparation, administration, and documentation of medications.

20. Guide students in the application of the nursing process for clients requiring information about, or having difficulty complying with, the medication regimen. Have students recommend creative strategies for assisting older adults in the home environment with medication administration.

21. Have students provide examples of circumstances that might contribute to medication errors.

22. Ask students to identify how oral and parenteral medication administration can be adapted for infants, preschool children, and older adults.

23. Have students discuss how the nurse should respond in the following situations where the client:
    a. Has no identification band
    b. Questions or refuses a medication
    c. Needs tablets to be cut or crushed
    d. Requires a very small liquid amount of medication
    e. Is not able to swallow pills
    f. Cannot hold the medication cup or inhaler
    g. Is extremely thin or obese
    h. Is paraplegic and requires IM injections
    i. Has a rash on the chest and arms
    j. Is at physical therapy when medications are to be given

24. Have students identify the responsibility of the nurse for the following situations:
    a. The label on the liquid medication is illegible.
    b. The prescribed dosage is three times the normal amount.
    c. The count for a narcotic to be administered is incorrect.
    d. Another nurse asks you to administer her already prepared medications to her client.
    e. Blood is aspirated back during the IM injection.
    f. The IM site is hard to the touch.
    g. A needlestick occurs after injection of a client.

INDEPENDENT LEARNING

1. Students should practice preparing medications in the skills laboratory. At home, they can practice preparing oral medications for administration by using over-the-counter medications that they have at home. Focus should be on overall safety and asepsis.

2. Students should practice calculation of drug dosages for commonly prescribed medications.

3. Students should review the pharmacological actions and nursing implications of the medications prescribed for their clients.

4. Students can investigate common drug and food interactions.

5. Students can think about the type of information that is necessary to safely administer medications to clients.

6. Students should review abbreviations that are commonly used in medication orders.

7. Students may investigate the costs of common brand name and generic drugs at local pharmacies.

STUDENT RESOURCES
Routes of Administration

Route	Description/Types of Medication
Oral	
Parenteral	
Topical	
Inhalation	
Intraocular	

Parenteral Medication

Route	Equipment	Needle Gauge	Amount of Medication	Sites/ Landmarks	Angle of Injection
Subcutaneous					
Intramuscular					
Intradermal					

CROSS-CURRICULUM GUIDE

Medication administration guidelines and procedures coordinate with discussions on pharmacology, either in a distinct course or integrated with medical/surgical, maternal/child, and gerontological topic areas. This information is essential before clinical experiences where medications will be administered. Students should be aware of how medication administration must be adapted in accordance with the client's age, developmental abilities, health status, and environment.

MULTIMEDIA RESOURCES

Mosby's Nursing Skills Video Series:
    Medication Administration III Set: *General Medication Administration Skills Guideline*
                                         Administering Medication by Injection
                                         Administering Medication by Nonparenteral Routes
                                       Administering Medication by IV
Whaley and Wong's Pediatric Nursing Video Series:
    Medications and Injections

CHAPTER 27

Body Mechanics

CRITICAL THINKING ACTIVITIES AND ANSWERS

1. Jon, who is 82 years old, is being released from the hospital today. He is going home with his daughter, who will be caring for him. He is unable to transfer to a chair without assistance. List and discuss the guidelines to be given to Jon's daughter concerning body mechanics safety for herself and for her father. What transfer techniques would you encourage her to use?

Answer: Guidelines for the daughter include the following: Lift with her legs, not her back; make certain she maintains her body in alignment while assisting her father; get extra help if she is in any doubt that she is able to perform procedures herself; and have her father wear non slip shoes. The daughter could consider a hospital bed to assist with position changes. If Jon has limited weight-bearing, a pivot transfer would be the easiest.

2. You are assisting a client to ambulate to the bathroom. The client is 2 days postoperative from major abdominal surgery. Halfway to the bathroom the client complains of dizziness and begins to fall to the floor. What is your initial response? What would you chart regarding this incident?

Answer: Assist the client easily to the floor, allowing her to "slide gently down" your body. Try to avoid the surrounding furniture and make certain that she does not strike her head on the floor. You should chart exactly what happened, using objective terms:

"Ambulated in hallway with assistance. Halfway from room, client stated she 'felt dizzy and weak' Unable to support her own weight, she was helped to a sitting position on the floor. She did not lose consciousness and had no complaints of pain or injury. No bleeding or bruising noted. Assisted in standing, placed in wheelchair, and returned to room. Transferred to bed with minimal assistance. Has no complaints, resting quietly, call bell in reach."

Vital signs should also be recorded, as well as the condition of the abdominal dressing and surgical site.

3. You are assigned to a client who has a trapeze bar across the bed, trochanter rolls, a footboard, and side rails. Explain the rationale for each of these devices in maintaining proper body alignment.

Answer: The trapeze bar assists clients in changing position in bed. The use of the bar requires upper arm strength by clients to enable them to lift themselves from the bed. Trochanter rolls assist the nurse in positioning clients by maintaining alignment against the pull of gravity. Footboards maintain alignment by keeping the feet in dorsiflexion. Side rails prevent clients from falling. It is important to not employ the use of side rails indiscriminately.

4. Before your client with a full-leg cast can go home, he or she must be taught to ambulate with crutches and a three-point gait. Develop a teaching plan for your client.

Answer: A client who is using crutches should bear weight on the hands and be careful of placing too much pressure in the axilla. Make certain that arm pads and rubber tips are secure. This client will bear weight only on the unaffected leg. The crutches are advanced forward first, with the unaffected leg following.

EDUCATIONAL STRATEGIES

1. Define body mechanics, including body alignment, balance, and coordination.

2. Review the anatomy and physiology of the musculoskeletal and nervous systems in regard to body mechanics.

3. Discuss developmental changes that occur throughout the lifespan and their influence on body mechanics.

4. Identify possible pathological influences on body mechanics and have students provide examples of the effects of specific health deviations. Have students identify how a client's body mechanics can be affected by the following, or similar, health problems:
   a. Left-sided CVA
   b. Surgical repair (pinning or replacement) of fractured right hip
   c. Body cast
   d. Abdominal or back surgery
   e. Unconscious state
   f. Scoliosis or kyphosis
   g. Quadriplegia or paraplegia

5. Describe the assessment of a client's posture, alignment, mobility (ROM, gait, exercise), and activity tolerance. Ask students what and how objective and subjective information can be obtained from the client relevant to body mechanics.

6. Discuss general guidelines for safely lifting and moving clients and objects.

7. Explain and demonstrate (using educational media, simulation mannequins/models or volunteers, and appropriate equipment) the procedures for client positioning and transfers. Have students practice these procedures, using available equipment and safe, appropriate techniques.

8. Evaluate the students' ability to implement these procedures through return demonstration and skill testing before clinical experiences.

9. Provide students with examples of different client scenarios and have them specify how the procedure should be implemented or adapted to meet the client's needs (e.g., client with right-side paralysis or episodes of dizziness).

10. Explain and demonstrate ROM exercises. Have students move their own joints as each exercise is discussed.

11. Describe the correct procedures for helping clients to ambulate with assistive devices, including gait belts, canes, walkers, and crutches (at different gaits).

12. Have students prepare and present, if possible, a teaching plan for a client who will be using an assistive device for ambulation.

13. Assign students to participate in the care of clients who require assistance in maintaining proper body mechanics. Focus on maintenance of client comfort and safety.

14. Guide students in the application of the nursing process and completion of a care plan/pathway for a client who requires assistance with mobility.

15. Have students identify how nurses should apply the principles of body mechanics in providing client care so that they may avoid injury.

16. Invite a physical therapist to speak to the class about his or her role in promoting body mechanics.

INDEPENDENT LEARNING

1. Students should review the anatomy and physiology of the musculoskeletal system.

2. Students should practice the skills associated with body mechanics in the skills laboratory and at home with friends or family members.

3. Students can investigate available community resources where assistive devices, such as canes and crutches, can be borrowed, rented, or purchased.

Developmental Changes in Body
Appearance and Function

Developmental Stage	Body Appearance and Function
Infant	
Toddler	
Preschool or school-age child	
Adolescent	
Adult	
Older adult	

Pathological Influences On
Body Mechanics

Pathological Influence	Effect on Client
Congenital defects	
Bone, joint, and muscle disorders	
Central nervous system damage	
Musculoskeletal trauma	

Assistive Devices for Ambulation–
Safety Precautions and Client Instruction

Assistive Devices	Safety Precautions/Client Instruction
Gait belt	
Cane	
Walker	
Crutches	

CROSS-CURRICULUM GUIDE

The information on and techniques for promoting body mechanics are applicable for clients of all ages who may be experiencing prolonged immobility, neuromuscular impairment, or skeletal abnormalities (e.g., scoliosis).

MULTIMEDIA RESOURCES

Mosby's Nursing Skills Video Series
    Set I: Body Mechanics, Exercise, and Activity
Mosby's Applying Critical Thinking to Nursing Skills: An Interactive Videodisc Series
    Activity and Mobility

Basic Human Needs

Safety

CRITICAL THINKING ACTIVITIES AND ANSWERS

1. The newest admission to the nursing unit is an older adult woman with arthritis and limited mobility. She is legally blind but is mentally alert. What are some nursing interventions that will help protect her safety while in the nursing unit?

Answer: Discuss a plan with the client and ask her how the nursing staff could best help her to remain safe. Place her in a room close to the nursing station if possible. Place her in a bed closest to the bathroom to shorten the walking distance. This will conserve her strength and minimize fatigue from extended walking. If this is not possible, a bedside commode may be a safer alternative. Instruct the client in the use of the call bell, pointing out the button by placing her hand and fingers over it so that she can use her sense of touch to supplement her limited vision. Alert staff members to do the following:
   a. Answer the call bell promptly.
   b. Check frequently on the client and toilet often.

c. Avoid the use of restraints, as they will further immobilize her and increase joint stiffness. Decreased activity places her at risk for complications related to immobility (e.g., impaired skin integrity, ineffective airway clearance, altered tissue perfusion). Increased stiffness will increase the risk for injury.

d. In setting up her meal trays, pay attention to scald hazards from hot liquids. Inform her of the foods on the tray and place items in a pattern that is familiar to her.

2. During your clinical experience in maternal-child health you have the opportunity to teach new parents about safety and the newborn. Your time is limited because your clients will be discharged before you return tomorrow. What will you teach today, and what will you teach in 3 days when you make a follow-up home visit?

Answer: The immediate teaching priorities are:
a. Importance of a safe ride home, with the infant in a federally approved infant restraint in the rear-facing position. The restraint must be properly installed and placed in the rear seat. The infant restraint must never be placed in the front passenger seat of a car equipped with a passenger-side airbag because of the risk of impact injury.
b. Inform parents that placing an infant on its stomach to sleep is not recommended because that position can pose a suffocation risk.

Home visit teaching needs include:
a. Before placing the infant in bath water, check the temperature.
b. Never leave the infant unattended in a bath or in the care of a young child. If the phone rings, let it ring or take the infant out of the water and place in a protected area.
c. Never prop a bottle when feeding the infant.
d. If a pacifier is used, it must be in one piece and never tied to a cord or string around the infant's neck.

3. You enter a client's room to answer the call bell and see the client frantically pointing to the trash can next to the bed. You smell smoke and see small flames. What do you do next?

Answer: The steps to follow are based on the acronym RACE.

R—Rescue the client from the immediate vicinity. If possible, help him to the room doorway and call for assistance. If oxygen is in use in the room, turn it (and any other appliances) off.
A—Alarm should be given to call for the internal agency fire department and, if necessary, the external community fire department.
C—Contain the fire to the trash can if possible by smothering the fire with a tray to cover it like a lid or with a large blanket.
E—Extinguish using a type A (rubbish, wood) fire extinguisher.

EDUCATIONAL STRATEGIES

1. Discuss the basic human needs for safety with respect to oxygen, nutrition, temperature, and humidity. Ask students how these needs can be adversely altered for individuals.

2. Review physical hazards in the environment, including pathogens, inadequate sanitation, and pollution. Have students provide specific examples of these types of hazards.

3. Review changes that occur throughout growth and development that influence an individual's safety needs. Ask students to identify specific safety considerations for individuals of different ages.

4. Discuss how the presence of different risk factors may affect an individual's safety.

5. Ask students to identify safety hazards and risks (especially falls) that may be present in the health care setting and describe nursing measures that can be implemented to eliminate or reduce them (e.g., side rails, client orientation to the unit).

6. Ask students to identify the role of the nurse in promotion of safety in the home. Review measures that can be implemented to reduce fire, electrical, and poisoning hazards. Have students investigate and compare the costs of safety equipment, such as fire and carbon monoxide detectors.

7. Assign students to prepare and present, if possible, a teaching plan for clients on safety in the home. Have students focus on the safety needs of different age-groups.

8. Explain and demonstrate (using educational media, simulation mannequins/models, and appropriate equipment) the use of restraints. Have students identify the situations that indicate need for the use of restraints. Ask students about possible hazards and nursing precautions with restraints and realistic alternatives to their use. Have students practice the application of restraints.

9. Assign students to participate in the care of clients in a variety of available health care settings. Have students complete client assessments, such as the Risk for Falls Assessment Tool, in order to determine client's safety needs.

10. Explain the guidelines for intervention in accidental poisoning. Ask students to identify how accidental poisoning might occur in different age-groups and how the situation can be avoided.

11. Invite a risk-management nurse to speak to the class about measures within a health care agency to reduce the risk of client injury.

12. Invite representatives from the local fire and/or police departments to discuss safety issues.

13. Discuss the types and effects of pollution in the local community and measures that can be implemented to reduce pollutants. Have students investigate any specific anti-pollution organizations (e.g., airline noise reduction group) that may be active in the state or community.

14. Ask students to identify the safety hazards that can be present in the following, or similar, examples:
    a. New parents at home with their first child
    b. An older, visually impaired adult living alone in a third floor apartment with hardwood floors, throw rugs, clutter, and inadequate lighting
    c. A single parent living in an urban area where there is a high rate of crime and drug abuse
    d. New homes constructed around the site of a chemical plant or an airport
    e. A sexual partner who is an IV drug user
    f. A client with TB who is returning home to a large family and tight living quarters
    g. An older adult in an extended-care facility who is disoriented at times and unsteady when moving around
    h. A 3-year-old who is left unsupervised in the kitchen or bathroom

INDEPENDENT LEARNING

1. Students should investigate potential and actual safety hazards that are present in their own homes.

2. Students can investigate resources that are available in the community for the promotion of client and family safety (e.g., poison control center) and compile a listing of emergency phone numbers.

3. Students should review a health care agency's policies and procedures for safety.

STUDENT RESOURCES

Health Care Agency Risks

Health Care Agency Risks	Prevention/Nursing Responsibilities
Falls	
Client-inherent accidents	
Procedure-related accidents	
Equipment-related accidents	

Home Care Safety

Safety Issues	Client/Family Teaching
Falls	
Fire	
Electrical hazards	
Poisoning	
Oxygen/carbon monoxide	
Sanitation/pollution	
Temperature	
Security	

Risk for Falls Assessment Tool

Tool 1: Risk Assessment Tool for Falls

Directions: Place a check mark in front of elements that apply to your client. The decision of whether a client is at risk for falls is based on your nursing judgment. *Guideline:* A client who has a check mark in front of an element with an asterisk (°) or four or more of the other elements would be identified as at risk for falls.

General Data

_____ Age over 60
_____ History of falls before admission°
_____ Postoperative/admitted for operation
_____ Smoker

Physical Condition

_____ Dizziness/imbalance
_____ Unsteady gait
_____ Diseases/other problems affecting weight-bearing joints
_____ Weakness
_____ Paresis
_____ Seizure disorder
_____ Impairment of vision
_____ Impairment of hearing
_____ Diarrhea
_____ Urinary frequency

Mental Status

_____ Confusion/disorientation°
_____ Impaired memory or judgment
_____ Inability to understand or follow directions

Medications

_____ Diuretics or diuretic effects
_____ Hypotensive or CNS suppressants (e.g., narcotic, sedative, psychotropic, hypnotic, tranquilizer, antihypertensive, antidepressant)
_____ Medication that increases GI motility (e.g., laxative)

Ambulatory Devices

_____ Cane
_____ Crutches
_____ Walker
_____ Wheelchair
_____ Geriatric (geri) chair
_____ Braces

Tool 2: Reassessment Is Safe "Kare" (Risk) Tool

Directions: Place a check mark in front of any element that applies to your client. A client who has a check mark in front of any of the first four elements would be identified as at risk for falls. In additon, when a high-risk client has a check mark in front of the element "Use of a wheelchair," the client is considered to be at greater risk for falls.

_____ Unsteady gait, dizziness, imbalance
_____ Impaired memory or judgment
_____ Weakness
_____ History of falls
_____ Use of a wheelchair

Home Hazard Assessment

HOME EXTERIOR
Are sidewalks uneven?
Are steps in good repair?
Do steps have securely fastened handrails?
Is there adequate lighting?
Is outdoor furniture sturdy?

HOME INTERIOR
Do all rooms, stairways, and halls have adequate lighting?
Are night-lights available?
Are area rugs secured?
Are wooden floors nonslippery?
Is furniture placed appropriately to permit mobility?
Is furniture sturdy enough to provide support for getting up and down?
Are temperature and humidity within normal range?
Are there any steps or thresholds that may pose a hazard?
Are all steps in good repair?
Are step edges clearly marked with colored tape?
Are handrails available and secure?

KITCHEN
Are hand-washing facilities available?
Is the pilot light on and the area clean on a gas stove?
Are the dials on the stove readable?
Are storage areas within easy reach?
Are cleaning fluids, bleach, etc., in original containers and stored safely?
Are cleaning fluids stored out of reach of children?
Is the water temperature within normal range (115°F to 145°F)?
Are there clean areas for food storage and preparation?
Is refrigeration adequate?

BATHROOM
Are hand-washing facilities available?
Are there skidproof strips or surfaces in the tub/shower?
Are bath mats secured?
Does the client need grab bars near the bathtub and toilet?
Does the client need an elevated toilet seat?
Is the medicine cabinet well lighted?
Are all medications current and in original containers?
Are medications out of children's reach?
Are two doses of syrup of ipecac available in homes with children?
Is the poison control phone number visible and next to a phone?

BEDROOM
Are beds of adequate height to allow getting on and off easily?
Is day and night lighting adequate?
Are floor coverings nonskid?
Does the client have a telephone nearby?

ELECTRICAL AND FIRE HAZARDS
Are all appliances in good working order?
Is equipment grounded?
Are electrical cords in good condition?
Are extension cords used only when necessary?
Are the correct number of appliances plugged into one outlet?
Are electrical appliances kept away from the sink, tub, or shower?
Are the heating/cooling units and fireplace inspected annually?
Is there a guard or screen in front of the fireplace?
Are combustible materials stored properly?
Are there smoke, fire and carbon monoxide detectors?
Are the emergency numbers for police and fire departments visible near the phone?
Has the family discussed and practiced an escape plan in case of fire?

Modified from Tideiksaar, 1989; Wong, 1995; Top, 1987; Ebersole ad Hess, 1994; and Beck, 1993.

CROSS-CURRICULUM GUIDE

Maternal/Child: Promotion of safety is important for clients throughout the lifespan. Children in particular have an increased risk for accidents related to their increasing exploration of the environment and their inability to understand environmental dangers and consequences. Students should be aware of the value of a home assessment and the anticipation of clients' safety needs.

Medical/Surgical: Clients experiencing neurological, sensory, musculoskeletal, or other health deviations that can alter perception or reaction are very susceptible to injury.

Gerontological: Students should be alert to the needs of older adults in the health care setting and at home. Developmental or pathological changes can occur that result in sensory and musculoskeletal impairment. Safety concerns should be a large focus of discussion with students before their clinical experiences with older adults.

MULTIMEDIA RESOURCES

Mosby's Nursing Skills Video Series:
> *Set I:*   *Applying Restraints*

CHAPTER 29

Hygiene

CRITICAL THINKING ACTIVITIES AND ANSWERS

1. Mr. Roberts, an 80-year-old widower who lives alone, is admitted to the intensive care unit. He is obese and has poor hygiene. His skin is rough and dry with some areas of excoriation. What are the most important assessments to be made in the situation? What appropriate interventions might be used?

Answer: Assess the skin, especially pressure areas, skin folds, perineal area, heels, and occiput. Use interventions designed to reduce the hazards of restricted mobility on the skin, hygiene interventions to keep skin clean, dry, and moisturized, and interventions to promote healing of excoriated areas.

2. Mrs. John, a 30-year-old woman, is admitted to the neurological unit after a spinal cord injury. She is now a quadriplegic. In terms of hygiene needs, what are the issues in taking care of Mrs. John?

Answer: Reduce the effects of immobility and pressure on skin. Promote all aspects of hygiene (e.g., mouth, perineal, hair, skin care). Reduce the effects of impaired circulation on the skin.

3. Mr. Green, a 52-year-old man, has been on long-term therapy for peripheral vascular disease. He has been on coumarin therapy. What home care instructions are essential in his discharge planning in regard to hygiene?

Answer: Because of the risk of shaving when on coumarin therapy, Mr. Green should use an electric shaver. Assess the impact of impaired circulation from peripheral vascular disease on foot and nail care. He will need specific instructions about shoes, socks, and nail care and also about reducing the risks of injuries to the extremities (e.g., thermal, chemical, or friction type of injuries). Finally, he will need specific instructions about what will impede circulation (e.g., crossing his legs, wearing tight elastic) and what will promote circulation (e.g., putting his feet up, exercise).

EDUCATIONAL STRATEGIES

1. Review the anatomy and physiology of the integumentary system.

2. Review the physical assessment skills that can be implemented during hygienic care.

3. Ask students to identify what activities constitute hygienic care.

4. Discuss the variables that may influence hygienic care practices, such as body image, sociocultural background, personal preference, and physical condition.

5. Review the hygienic needs of individuals throughout the lifespan.

6. Discuss the alterations that might be found in an assessment of the skin, mouth, hair, nails, eyes, ears, and nose. Have students identify hygienic care practices and inadequacies or health deviations that might contribute to these common alterations.

7. Ask students to identify what assessment information should be obtained in order to determine the client's self-care ability for hygienic care. Have students provide examples of how different levels of ability might influence the client's hygienic care activities and the degree of nursing intervention.

8. Discuss general guidelines for providing hygienic care to clients of different ages, including the preparation of supplies and the client environment.

9. Explain and demonstrate (using educational media, simulation mannequins/models or volunteers, and appropriate supplies) the following:
   a. Bed bath/shower
   b. Perineal care
   c. Oral hygiene
   d. Denture care
   e. Hair care
   f. Nail and foot care
   g. Care of contact lenses
   h. Unoccupied and occupied bedmaking

Have students practice these procedures with their peers in the skills laboratory.

10. Evaluate students' ability to implement basic hygienic care measures through return demonstration/skill testing before their clinical experiences.

11. Explain and demonstrate the preparation of the client's room, including arrangement and use of equipment (e.g., beds, tables). Have students practice setting up an actual or simulated client environment and orienting the client to it.

12. Assign students to assist clients of various ages with hygienic care. Discuss the type/amount of care to be provided and the related safety concerns. Have students share their experiences and client assessments in post-care conferences.

13. Guide students in the application of the nursing process and the completion of a care plan/pathway for a client with hygienic care needs.

14. Have students prepare and present, if possible, a teaching plan on hygienic care for the following, or similar, clients:
    a. Parents of a 3-day-old newborn
    b. A client with diabetes
    c. An older adult with dry skin
    d. A client on anticoagulant medication

15. Ask students to identify how the provision of hygienic care might be adapted for clients with the following health deviations:
    a. Right-sided CVA
    b. Rheumatoid arthritis
    c. An arm or leg fracture with a plaster cast
    d. Diminished level of consciousness
    e. Severe depression

INDEPENDENT LEARNING

1. Students should review the anatomy and physiology of the integumentary system.

2. Students can investigate commercial products that are available for hygienic care and compare the costs of popular name brands and store brands.

3. Students should practice the techniques of hygienic care in the skills laboratory and at home with family members and friends.

STUDENT RESOURCES
Hygiene Assessment and Nursing Interventions

Body Area	Alterations/Hygiene Needs	Nursing Interventions
Skin		
Feet/nails		
Oral cavity		
Hair		
Eyes, ears, nose		

CROSS-CURRICULUM GUIDE

Hygienic care principles and procedures may be applied to all client situations. Special considerations and adaptations are indicated for infants, children, adolescents, and older adults.

In addition, clients experiencing health deviations such as diabetes, cancer, dermatologic disorders, or neurologic disorders might have specific hygienic needs or alterations in their ability to meet those needs.

MULTIMEDIA RESOURCES

Mosby's Nursing Skills Video Series:
    Set I: *Bathing*
                Bedmaking
                Hygiene/Personal Care

CHAPTER 30

Oxygenation

CRITICAL THINKING ACTIVITIES AND ANSWERS

1. Referring to the advantages and disadvantages of various oxygen delivery devices, make a recommendation for each of the following clients requiring supplemental oxygen:

   a. A 42-year-old client requiring short-term, low-flow oxygen therapy after abdominal surgery.

   b. A 20-year-old client with a fractured nose and multiple chest contusions. The physician has prescribed FiO_2 of 50% to 60%.

Answer:

a. A nasal cannula should be effective for low concentrations of oxygen and short-term therapy.

b. A nonrebreather device would be the only device capable of delivering FiO_2 at the prescribed percentage (90% to 100%). The nonrebreather would be advantageous in this situation because it would not tend to dry the mucus membranes of the nose. However, pain may make it difficult to maintain a tight seal over the nose.

2. How can you determine whether Yankauer or endotracheal suctioning would be most beneficial for a client without an artificial airway?

Answer: The choice of an oral suction approach with a Yankauer suction device versus invasive endotracheal suctioning should be based on the level of secretions. If secretions are primarily confined to the mouth, the Yankauer suction would be adequate. If abnormal lung sounds and symptoms of labored breathing or ineffective cough are present, endotracheal suctioning would be necessary to remove deeper secretions.

3. After entering a client's tracheostomy with a suction catheter, the client begins to cough and his face turns red. What would you do?

Answer: This is an expected response to introduction of the suction catheter. You should proceed with suctioning in a steady, quick manner, making sure to suction no longer than 10 seconds. During the procedure, be sure to provide verbal support and encouragement.

4. While caring for a client with a chest tube to water-seal drainage and 20 cm of wall suction, you note excessive bubbling in the water-seal bottle. The client has had the chest tube for 24 hours, after undergoing lung surgery.

a. What should you do and why?

b. During ambulation you note that the drainage is serous and the volume for the last 8 hours is approximately 500 ml. What should your response be?

Answer:

a. Bubbling is expected in the water-seal compartment. However, excessive bubbling may suggest a leak in the water-seal system. All connections should be checked for possible air leakage. If connections are secure, the integrity of the tubing should be assessed using a systematic manner of brief clamping, beginning at the chest wall and moving down toward the water-seal apparatus.

b. The outside of the drainage system should be marked with the date and time at the fluid level. No further action is necessary because this volume of drainage is expected within the first 24 hours after surgery. The fluid should be serous in appearance.

EDUCATIONAL STRATEGIES

1. Review the normal anatomy and physiology and common pathological changes of the cardiac and respiratory systems.

2. Discuss factors that can affect oxygenation, including physiological, developmental, behavioral, and environmental. Ask students to provide examples of how and why these factors affect oxygenation.

3. Describe the following alterations in cardiac functioning that influence oxygenation, along with their etiology and signs and symptoms: conduction disturbance, altered cardiac output, impaired valvular function, and myocardial ischemia.

4. Describe the following alterations in respiratory functioning that influence oxygenation, along with their etiology and signs and symptoms: hyperventilation, hypoventilation, and hypoxia.

5. Discuss the assessment of the client's oxygenation status, including history, physical examination, and diagnostic/laboratory tests. Have students practice taking histories specific to oxygenation with their peers and then reporting and documenting the results.

6. Identify findings of the client assessment that are relevant to oxygenation, such as fatigue, dyspnea, coughing, wheezing, pain and infections.

7. Review the physical assessment techniques and focus areas that are specific to oxygenation. Demonstrate selected techniques on practice

mannequins/models or student volunteers. Have students practice these techniques on each other in the skill laboratory setting. Use available educational media (especially audiotapes and videotapes) to reinforce the assessment skills and expected/unexpected findings.

8. Identify and describe diagnostic/laboratory test results that are indicative of inadequate oxygenation.

9. Ask students to identify nursing interventions that can be implemented for the promotion and maintenance of a client's oxygenation. Discuss how interventions might be adapted to meet the client's specific developmental needs.

10. Discuss the use of pneumoccocal and influenza vaccines, including target groups and contraindications for use. Have students investigate where and when vaccines may be offered in the community.

11. Discuss which clients are at an increased risk for inadequate oxygenation because of their occupation or geographic location.

12. Describe specific nursing interventions to assist the client with the following:
    a. Dyspnea management
    b. Maintenance of a patent airway
    c. Mobilization of pulmonary secretions
    d. Lung expansion

13. Demonstrate the techniques for coughing, deep breathing, use of the incentive spirometer, positioning, chest physiotherapy, and postural drainage. Have students practice the techniques with their peers in the skills laboratory setting.

14. Ask students to specify the rationale for nursing interventions that promote oxygenation.

15. Explain and demonstrate (using educational media, simulation mannequins/models or volunteers, and appropriate supplies) the following:
    a. Suctioning
    b. Care of chest tubes

Have students practice these procedures with their peers in the skills laboratory.

16. Evaluate students' ability to suction and care for chest tubes through return demonstration/skill testing before their clinical experiences.

17. Discuss oxygen therapy and the responsibilities of the nurse in the health care and home environments. Have students identify the specific safety measures that must be implemented in the presence of oxygen therapy. Provide photos or bring in actual oxygen delivery equipment and have students identify its use, flow rate, and client considerations.

18. Invite a respiratory therapist to speak to the class about the oxygenation needs of clients. Ask the therapist to describe and demonstrate different types of equipment and monitoring requirements.

19. Discuss and demonstrate cardiopulmonary resuscitation (CPR). Assign students to complete a CPR class (preferably at a health care provider level) through an approved provider and verify attendance with a completion card.

20. Assign students to observe or participate in the care of clients experiencing difficulty with oxygenation in a variety of health care settings. Focus on the assessment of the client's oxygen needs and the selection of nursing interventions that promote cardiopulmonary functioning. Supervise the students in the administration of medications and oxygen therapy. Evaluate the students' implementation and documentation of nursing measures for the promotion of oxygenation.

21. Have students design and implement, if possible, a teaching plan for a client who requires portable oxygen in the home.

22. Have students complete a care plan/pathway for a client experiencing alterations in oxygenation.

23. Ask students to identify how the following health deviations could alter a client's oxygenation status:
    a. Kyphosis
    b. Quadriplegia
    c. Emphysema
    d. Premature birth
    e. Hypertension
    f. Anemia
    g. Atherosclerosis
    h. Cardiac arrhythmia
    i. Hyperthyroidism

INDEPENDENT LEARNING

1. Students should review the normal anatomy and physiology of the cardiovascular and respiratory systems.

2. Students should practice the techniques associated with assessment and promotion of oxygenation in the skills laboratory.

3. Students should practice at home the techniques for coughing, deep breathing, and pursed-lip breathing and the positions for postural drainage.

4. Students can investigate actual and/or potential sources of environmental pollution in the community that might influence oxygenation.

STUDENT RESOURCES

Factors That Affect Oxygenation

Factors	Description of Effect on Oxygenation
Physiological	
Developmental	
Behavioral	
Environmental	

Alterations in Cardiac Functioning

Alteration	Effect on Cardiac Functioning
Conduction problems	
Altered cardiac output	
Impaired valvular function	
Myocardial ischemia	

Alterations in Respiratory Functioning

Alteration	Effect on Respiratory Functioning
Hyperventilation	
Hypoventilation	
Hypoxia	

Nursing Assessment

Assessment Areas	Findings Indicating Alteration in Oxygenation

CROSS-CURRICULUM GUIDE

Maternal/Child: Students can be referred to techniques for oxygen promotion during class discussions on or clinical experiences with premature infants or children with respiratory difficulties such as croup, asthma, or cystic fibrosis.

Medical/Surgical: Discussions on nursing interventions for promotion of oxygenation is especially important for clients with respiratory health deviations such as emphysema. Clients in the postoperative phase, or who experience chest trauma or cardiovascular or neurologic disorders, are also subject to inadequate oxygenation.

Gerontological: Changes in the skeletal structure and cardiopulmonary functioning, along with decreased resistance to infections, place the older adult client at a greater risk for insufficient oxygenation.

Clients may also need oxygen therapy in the home, and they and their significant others will require instruction on the purpose and safe use of this therapy.

MULTIMEDIA RESOURCES

Mosby's Nursing Skills Video Series:
    Oxygenation Skills IV Set: *Oropharyngeal, Nasopharyngeal, and Nasotracheal Suctioning*
                                                  Tracheostomy Care
                                                  Equipment and Oxygen Therapy
                                                  Artifical Airways
                                                  Care of Clients with Chest Tubes
                                                  Promoting Adequate Oxygenation

Mosby's Applying Critical Thinking to Nursing Skills: An Interactive Videodisc Series -
    Promoting Oxygenation

CHAPTER 31

Fluid, Electrolyte, and Acid-Base Balances

CRITICAL THINKING ACTIVITIES AND ANSWERS

1. Mary Beth is a 24-year-old healthy adult. While at work she received a phone call that her husband had been involved in a serious accident. When she got to the hospital, Caroline, the ER nurse, noticed that she was pale, breathing rapidly, and complaining of dizziness. What is the cause of her symptoms? Which intervention would you expect the physician to initiate? How will this correct her problem?

Answer: Mary Beth is hyperventilating probably because of an acute anxiety attack. When you hyperventilate, your respiratory rate increases and you blow off CO_2, causing respiratory alkalosis. Increase the CO_2 by having her breath into a paper bag, forcing her to rebreathe her own exhaled CO_2.

2. Mr. St. John is admitted to the hospital after his wife found him confused, with an increase in his breathing and a fever. She states, "He has had a terrible cold for 2 weeks now." His temperature is 102°F, heart rate 110, respirations 30, and blood pressure 128/64. His serum electrolytes are within normal limits, and his ABG reveals pH 7.25, PO_2 88, PCO_2 55, HCO_3 24. What does Mr. St. John's ABG indicate? Why would the physician order a chest x-ray for Mr. St. John? If left untreated, could Mr. St. John's problem be life threatening?

Answer: His ABG indicates acute respiratory acidosis. His pH is decreased, his PCO_2 is increased, and the bicarbonate is normal. The problem is respiratory, and Mr. St. John is demonstrating signs and symptoms of acidosis. Also, his heart rate and respiratory rate are elevated, and he has had periods of confusion, which are all signs and symptoms of acute respiratory acidosis. The physician ordered a chest x-ray because Mr. St. John is febrile, and the physician must determine if Mr. St. John has pneumonia, which could be the cause of the respiratory acidosis. Untreated, this condition could progress to acute respiratory distress syndrome and then death.

3. Justin is receiving IV fluids because he is NPO after surgery earlier today. His IV fluid order is 1000 ml lactated Ringer's with 20 mEq KCl to run over 8 hours. What IV tubing should be used to administer these fluids in terms of drop size? The nurse hangs a new bag of IV fluids at 5 PM. At 8 PM the nurse notes that 375 ml has infused from the bag. Are these fluids on time?

Answer: 1000 ml over 8 hours equals 1000/8 or 125 ml/hr. Since the infusion has potassium added to it, it would be appropriate to use either an electronic infusion device or a microdrip. Both deliver 60 gtts/ml. In 3 hours, 375 ml should have been infused—125 ml/hr for 3 hours equals 375 ml. The IV is on time.

4. While starting an IV, Alexandra begins to advance the ONC and notes that the area immediately around the insertion site is swelling. What should she do?

Answer: Remove the catheter. The IV is infiltrated, meaning it is out of the vascular space and infusing in tissues. The fluid accumulation causes the swelling.

EDUCATIONAL STRATEGIES

1. Using educational media (e.g., illustrations, transparencies, videos), review the distribution, movement, and regulation of body fluids. Provide examples of different types of IV solutions and ask students how they will influence fluid movement in the body.

2. Review the major cations and anions, their functions, regulatory mechanisms, sources, and normal values. Ask students to provide examples of food sources for each major electrolyte.

3. Discuss acid-base balance and the chemical, biological, and physiological regulatory mechanisms within the body.

4. Discuss disturbances in fluid, electrolyte, and acid-base balance, including possible etiology, signs and symptoms, and high-risk clients. Have students give the rationale for the physical manifestations of the imbalances, and explain why certain clients have a greater risk of developing the problems.

5. Describe the nursing assessment and physical examination of clients in order to determine the presence of fluid, electrolyte, or acid-base imbalances. Demonstrate specific assessment techniques (e.g., checking skin turgor) and have students practice on each other.

6. Ask students which imbalances might occur with the following, or similar, health deviations or situations:
   a. Diabetes mellitus or diabetes insipidus
   b. Congestive heart failure
   c. Cirrhosis
   d. Excessive use of steroids
   e. Excessive use of antacids
   f. Head injury
   g. Pneumonia
   h. Pancreatitis
   i. Increase or decrease in aldosterone secretion
   j. Vitamin D deficiency
   k. Paget's disease
   i Diuretic use
   m. Inappropriate mechanical ventilator settings

n. Renal failure
o. Second- or third-degree burns
p. Vomiting or diarrhea
q. Intestinal fistula

7. Explain the role of daily weights and intake and output (I & O) measurements in the monitoring of fluid balance. Provide students with sample client weights and have them calculate fluid volume changes (using 5 lb = 2.5 L). Discuss what is included in I & O, and have students practice calculating and documenting actual or simulated client fluid I & O.

8. Use the following, or a similar, example to have students determine the client's I & O in cc's or ml's:

$\frac{1}{2}$ cup ice cream   Urine—520 ml
1 cup tea   Wound drainage—100 ml
$\frac{1}{2}$ cup milk
2 cups corn flakes
1 ounce cream
2 cups water

IV started with 950 ml—currently 310 ml left

9. Identify laboratory tests that can be used to determine fluid, electrolyte, and acid-base imbalances. Provide students with sample test results and have them analyze the values and decide what imbalances are indicated.

10. Discuss the following measures and the associated nursing interventions that can be implemented to correct fluid and electrolyte imbalances:
a. Enteral replacement
b. Fluid restriction
c. Parenteral replacement

11. Discuss the initiation, monitoring and maintenance, and discontinuation of IV therapy. Review the principles of aseptic technique associated with this treatment.

12. Describe potential complications of IV therapy, including phlebitis, infiltration, infection, circulatory overload, and bleeding. Provide students with photos or illustrations of different IV complications and have them identify each problem.

13. Discuss blood transfusions and nursing responsibilities. Have students identify the assessments to be made prior before and during the administration of blood products.

14. Explain and demonstrate (using educational media, simulation mannequins/models, and appropriate equipment) the following nursing techniques:
a. Initiation of a peripheral IV infusion
b. Regulation of IV flow rate
c. Changing an IV solution, tubing, and dressing

Have students practice these techniques in the skills laboratory.

15. Evaluate the students' abilities to implement and document the techniques for IV infusions through return demonstration/skill testing before their clinical experiences.

16. Discuss medical interventions and nursing actions that can be implemented to correct acid-base imbalances.

17. Explain and demonstrate the procedure for obtaining an arterial blood sample. Have students observe the procedure in an acute care setting.

18. Assign students to observe or participate in the care of clients in a variety of health care settings, focusing on the assessment of fluid, electrolyte, and acid-base balances. Discuss physical assessment and analysis of laboratory results with the group in preclinical conference. Supervise the initiation (if appropriate) and maintenance of IV therapy. Have students design and implement teaching plans to assist clients with the maintenance of restoration of fluid, electrolyte, or acid-base balance.

19. Have students complete a care plan/pathway for an actual or simulated client who is experiencing a fluid, electrolyte, or acid-base imbalance.

INDEPENDENT LEARNING

1. Students should review the basic physiologic principles of fluid, electrolyte, and acid-base regulation in the body.

2. Students should investigate the components of solutions that are regularly used for IV therapy.

3. Students should investigate the equipment that is used for both acute care and home IV therapy.

4. Students should review diagnostic tests and the results that are indicative of imbalances.

5. Students can research an article in a current nursing journal on nursing interventions for fluid, electrolyte, or acid-base imbalances.

6. Students can investigate possible food-drug or drug-drug interactions that may precipitate imbalances.

STUDENT RESOURCES

Fluid Disturbances

Fluid Disturbances	Cause/Etiology	Diagnostic Test Results	Client Assessment	Nursing Interventions
Isotonic				
Osmolar				

Electrolyte Imbalance

Electrolyte Imbalance	Cause/Etiology	Diagnostic Test Results	Client Assessment	Nursing Interventions
Sodium				
Potassium				
Calcium				
Magnesium				

Acid-Base Imbalances

Acid-Base Imbalance	Cause/Etiology	Diagnostic Test Results	Client Assessment	Nursing Interventions
Metabolic aidosis				
Metabolic alkalosis				
Respiratory acidosis				
Respiratory alkalosis				

IV Infusion Problems

Infusion Problem	Client Assessment	Nursing Interventions

CROSS-CURRICULUM GUIDE

All clients in any health care setting can be subject to fluid, electrolyte, or acid-base imbalances. Slight variations in the body from physiologic disorders, trauma, environmental factors or behavioral changes can result in disturbances. The potential for these alterations should be highlighted throughout the curriculum, from the woman in labor who is hyperventilating to the older adult who has an insufficient fluid intake. In addition, IV infusions for fluid and blood replacement, as well as for medication administration, will be maintained by students in all health care settings.

MULTIMEDIA RESOURCES

Mosby's Nursing Skills Video Series:
　　　　Intravenous Therapy Skills V Set:　*IV Fluid Therapy*
　　　　　　　　　　　　　　　　　　　Maintaining the IV System
　　　　　　　　　　　　　　　　　　　Blood Administration
　　　　　　　　　　　　　　　　　　　Use of the Peripheral Access Device
　　　　　　　　　　　　　　　　　　　Central Venous Access Devices

Fluids and Electrolytes: A Computer-Assisted Instruction Program (Included on the CD-ROM that's free with the text)

CHAPTER 32

Sleep

CRITICAL THINKING ACTIVITIES AND ANSWERS

1. Mrs. Riley is a 66-year-old woman who comes to the community health clinic every 6 months for management of her hypertension. During this visit she reports the following to the nurse: "I am having more difficulty falling asleep. During the last month I bet I got up at least twice every night. My husband is convinced something is wrong. I still go to bed about the same time, around 10 PM, and I awaken around 6 AM." What would your analysis be of this client's assessment? How might you proceed further?

Answer: Mrs. Riley is describing a relatively normal sleep pattern for an older adult. Typically, older adults have more difficulty falling asleep. They have less deep sleep and tend to awaken more during the night. The nurse should focus on the difficulty the client has in falling asleep to determine if environmental factors are aggravating this situation. In addition, a review of Mrs. Riley's medication history might reveal factors contributing to her insomnia.

2. Edward Pena is a 34-year-old businessman who comes to the physician's office complaining of being very sleepy during the day. He has noticed the problem for about 3 months. He states, "If I'm lucky I get about 4 or 5 hours of sleep each night." He spends most of the work-week flying to various cities across the country. His day begins at 5 AM and often does not end until 7 PM or later. He admits that his eating habits are erratic, sometimes not having a meal until 8 or 9 at night. He drinks coffee during the day to keep him going. Mr. Pena likes to play golf on weekends but exercises little during the week. Last month his boss had a long talk with Mr. Pena after hearing that he had fallen asleep during a business meeting. This was the second time it had occurred. Mr. Pena is asking if he might be able to try a sleeping pill to help him sleep. What might be Mr. Pena's problem? What recommendations might you make to help him sleep?

Answer: Mr. Pena is likely suffering from excessive daytime sleepiness. Although narcolepsy is a possibility, Mr. Pena has not had a long-term problem with falling asleep during the day. The nurse could recommend several therapies: avoiding coffee in the late afternoon and evening, trying to find a way to exercise after work (perhaps at a hotel pool or gym), trying to not continue working late into the evening, avoiding eating a single large meal at the end of the day, and trying to find a way to relax for at least an hour before going to sleep.

3. Explain the value of having a client complete a visual analog scale that rates the quality of sleep.

Answer: The quality of sleep is a subjective experience. Only the client can report whether sleep is good or poor. A visual analog scale provides a means of measuring a change in client's perceptions about sleep overtime. If the nurse introduces sleep therapies, the visual analog scale can be used to evaluate if sleep improves or not.

4. Miss Steinman is 50 years of age and suffers from chronic bronchitis. She also has a history of congestive heart failure and receives digoxin daily and furosemide twice a day. She comes to the surgery outpatient center for repair of carpal tunnel syndrome effecting her right wrist and hand. If you were Miss Steinman's home health nurse, what factors might you consider that place her at risk for having a sleep disturbance?

Answer: Miss Steinman's chronic lung disease, complicated by congestive heart failure, could possibly cause shortness of breath or dyspnea, making it difficult to lie flat in bed. The furosemide is a diuretic that might cause nocturia, particularly if the second dose is taken late in the day. The surgical repair for carpal tunnel syndrome will probably cause short-term pain.

EDUCATIONAL STRATEGIES

1. Describe the difference between rest and sleep, and discuss how the nurse can promote rest. Have students share what helps them to feel "rested" or relaxed.

2. Review the physiology of sleep, including the sleep-wake cycle, circadian rhythms, regulation of sleep, and stages of sleep. Discuss how sleep is measured with selected instruments.

3. Ask students to identify how sleep may be disrupted in the home and the health care environment.

4. Describe the functions of sleep and the role of dreams.

5. Have students identify the average requirements and patterns of sleep for individuals throughout the lifespan.

6. Identify factors that can affect sleep patterns. Have students provide specific examples of how the following factors might affect sleep:
   a. Physical illness
   b. Drugs/substances
   c. Lifestyle
   d. Unusual sleep patterns/excessive daytime sleepiness
   e. Emotional stress

f. Environment
g. Exercise and fatigue
h. Food and caloric intake

7. Have students identify how the nurse can eliminate or reduce environmental factors that might interfere with the acquisition of sleep or rest in the health care environment.

8. Describe common sleep disorders, including insomnia, sleep apnea, narcolepsy, sleep deprivation, and parasomnias. Ask students to identify assessment findings that are associated with these disorders.

9. Discuss the assessment of sleep patterns and the available sources of data for information.

10. Review the components of a sleep history and discuss how findings may be correlated with the client's medical history, life events, emotional status, and/or alteration in routine or environment.

11. Use the following, or similar, situations to have students identify how sleep patterns can be disturbed and what interventions might be implemented by the nurse to promote sleep:
    a. A nurse who has been rotated from the day to the night shift
    b. A 2-year-old child admitted to the hospital
    c. A middle-age adult who is having diagnostic testing for a possible malignancy
    d. An older adult with chronic arthritic pain
    e. A young adult preparing to go off to college for the first time
    f. An individual with a bed partner who is very restless during the night
    g. A student who is preparing for examinations

12. Have students investigate available resources in the health care setting and community to assist clients experiencing sleep pattern alterations.

13. Identify interventions that can be implemented to promote a client's rest and sleep that are associated with the following: environmental management, promotion of comfort and bedtime routine, scheduling of treatments, stress reduction, and pharmacological management.

14. Assign students to observe or participate in client care experiences, focusing on the assessment and promotion of sleep and rest. Have students complete a care plan/pathway, including a teaching plan, for a client who is experiencing an alteration in sleep patterns. Supervise the implementation and documentation of sleep promotion strategies. Discuss the evaluation of client responses to implemented strategies in post-clinical conferences.

INDEPENDENT LEARNING

1. Students should review the physiological processes of sleep.

2. Students should investigate how the health care environment might alter sleep patterns and how the nurse can adapt the environment to promote sleep and rest.

3. Students can investigate available nonprescription and nontraditional remedies for sleep promotion.

4. Students should complete a sleep questionnaire for themselves, a family member, or a friend. They can then analyze the adequacy of sleep and rest patterns.

STUDENT RESOURCES

Sleep Patterns Across the Lifespan

Age Group	Sleep Pattern/Needs
Neonate/infant	
Toddler	
Preschooler	
School-age child	
Adolescent	
Young adult	
Middle-age adult	
Older adult	

Factors Affecting Sleep

Factors	Effect on Sleep

Promotion of Sleep

Specific Factors	Nursing Interventions
Environment	
Rituals	
Comfort	
Activity level	
Stress reduction	
Food/snacks	
Medication	
Specific disturbance	

The SMH Sleep Questionnaire

This questionnaire refers to your sleep in the past 24 hours.

Please try to answer every question.

Name: _____

Today's date: _____

Age: _____ Yrs.

Sex: Male/Female (delete whichever inapplicable).

At what time did you:	Hrs.	Mins.
1. Settle down for the night?	_____	_____
2. Fall asleep last night?	_____	_____
3. Finally wake this morning?	_____	_____
4. Get up this morning?	_____	_____

5. Was your sleep: (check below)

   1. Very light _____

   2. Light _____

   3. Fairly light _____

   4. Light average _____

   5. Deep average _____

   6. Fairly deep _____

   7. Deep _____

   8. Very deep _____

6. How many times did you wake up? (check below)

   1. Not at all _____

   2. Once _____

   3. Twice _____

   4. Three times _____

   5. Four times _____

   6. Five times _____

   7. Six times _____

   8. More than six times _____

How much sleep did you have:	Hrs.	Mins.
7. Last night?	_____	_____
8. During the day, yesterday?	_____	_____

9. How well did you sleep last night? (check below)

   1. Very badly _____

   2. Badly _____

   3. Fairly badly _____

   4. Fairly well _____

   5. Well _____

   6. Very well _____

If not well, what was the trouble? (e.g. restless)

1. _____

2. _____

3. _____

10. How clear-headed did you feel after getting up this morning? (check below)

   1. Still very drowsy _____

   2. Still moderately drowsy _____

   3. Still slightly drowsy _____

   4. Fairly clear-headed _____

   5. Alert _____

   6. Very alert _____

11. How satisfied were you with last night's sleep? (check below)

   1. Very unsatisfied _____

   2. Moderately unsatisfied _____

   3. Slightly unsatisfied _____

   4. Fairly satisfied _____

   5. Completely satisfied _____

12. Were you troubled by waking early and being unable to get to sleep again? (check below)

   1. No _____

   2. Yes _____

13. How much difficulty did you have in getting to sleep last night? (check below)

   1. None or very little _____

   2. Some _____

   3. A lot _____

   4. Extreme difficulty _____

14. How long did it take you to fall asleep last night? _____ Hrs. _____ Mins.

CROSS-CURRICULUM GUIDE

Attainment of adequate sleep and rest is important for all individuals. Students need to be aware of the effect that physiological and psychological stressors have on sleep and rest patterns. Clients in inpatient health care settings are subject to unfamiliar routines, environments, and people, all of which may have an impact upon their ability to sleep. Nursing interventions for the promotion of sleep and rest should be incorporated into the client's plan of care.

CHAPTER 33

Comfort

TOPICAL OUTLINE

CRITICAL THINKING ACTIVITIES AND ANSWERS

1. Mrs. Wiegand is a 76-year-old married woman who comes to the outpatient clinic with complaints, in her words, of a severe burning pain in her hands and wrists. She has been diagnosed with arthritis for more than 1 year. What type of questions might you ask of Mrs. Wiegand to assess how this pain has affected her lifestyle?

Answer: Does it awaken her during the night? What precipitates the pain? Are there any activities that make the pain worse? Has the pain affected her ability to independently conduct ADLs?

2. Mr. Jasper and Mr. Stern are clients experiencing back pain. Mr. Jasper's pain resulted from a fall from a ladder 48 hours ago. Mr. Stern's pain has been bothering him for more than 8 months with no known causes. As the nurse caring for both clients, how might you anticipate differences in assessment and treatment?

Answer: Mr. Jasper is experiencing acute pain that has a known cause. Treatment will focus on immediate pain relief measures appropriate to the injury and his response. Mr. Stern has chronic pain of unknown origin. The nurse should consider long-term effects on Mr. Stern, including an intense psychological and emotional impact from pain of unknown cause. Treatment should include strategies to cope with chronic pain. The nurse may initiate nonpharmacological measures, such as guided imagery, to help Mr. Stern cope with his discomfort.

3. Consider the previous example of Mr. Stern. What might influence your approach to assessment if Mr. Stern were 39 versus 80 years of age?

Answer: If Mr. Stern were 39, he might be more physically active, employed, and have young children requiring his care. He would probably report his signs as acute in nature. If he were 80, he might consider his pain a symptom of age. He would be more susceptible to complications of immobility that can occur in response to the pain. The types of interventions that Mr. Stern would be comfortable using could be influenced by the pain they cause. The support systems available might be different, depending on the ages of the people.

4. Ms. Rogers is receiving morphine by way of a PCA device following abdominal surgery for a hysterectomy. During your assessment, you note Ms. Rogers to be more drowsy and that her respirations have decreased from 16 a minute to 10. What actions should you take?

Answer: Stop the administration of morphine. Notify her physician and administer Narcan. Discuss a reduction in dosage or change of medication.

5. Mr. Lake is a 45-year-old man who experienced a traumatic injury to his left arm following an industrial accident 24 hours ago. His arm is in a very bulky dressing, and pain is aggravated when he lies on his left side. He has an intravenous line with a continuous infusion of intravenous fluids in his right arm. What nonpharmacological pain-relief measures might be helpful for Mr. Lake?

Answer: Elevation of his arm, back massage, and diversions such as television or reading material would all be helpful. Visitors would also help to distract him from the pain.

EDUCATIONAL STRATEGIES

1. Discuss the concept of comfort and the holistic approach that the nurse can take to assist clients in achieving comfort.

2. Discuss the nature of pain, including its objective and subjective aspects, the sources of pain, and its protective function.

3. Ask students to contribute their ideas about the misconceptions and prejudices that are associated with the pain experience and how nursing care might be influenced.

4. Explain the physiology of pain, including reception, perception, and reaction. Ask students how alterations in the central nervous system can alter the pain experience.

5. Identify the physiological and behavioral responses to pain. Ask students to share personal or clinical experiences where responses to pain have been demonstrated.

6. Compare and contrast acute and chronic pain. Have students identify how ADLs can be influenced by each type of pain. Provide examples of different client situations and ask students to identify whether the client is experiencing acute or chronic pain.

7. Discuss factors that influence the pain experience. Ask students to give examples of how and why each factor influences the client's pain.

8. Assign students to investigate and report on different cultural responses to pain.

9. Describe the assessment guidelines for clients experiencing pain, including the following:
   a. Expression of pain
   b. Classification of pain
   c. Characteristics of pain
   d. Physiological and behavioral effects of pain
   e. Neurological status

10. Have students complete a pain assessment with their peers, family members, friends, and clients. Discuss the assessment findings and their documentation.

11. Discuss the correlation of verbal and nonverbal communication for the pain experience. Ask students how they can determine a client's pain if the individual is not able to understand or speak to them.

12. Discuss the importance of explaining treatments and procedures to the client in order to alter the pain experience. Organize a role-playing situation where students explain uncomfortable procedures and prepare a client for these procedures.

13. Identify and describe specific nonpharmacological pain relief measures that the nurse can implement to promote comfort and reduce or eliminate a client's pain. Ask students to provide additional examples of nursing interventions that can be used in different health care settings.

14. Discuss and demonstrate selected comfort promoting and pain relief measures to the class, such as distraction, relaxation, and guided imagery. Have students practice the strategies with their peers.

15. Discuss pharmacological pain relief therapy, including the use of analgesics, PCA, local/regional anesthetics, and epidural anesthesia. Identify the indications, contraindications, and nursing implications for the use of each therapy.

16. Stimulate a discussion on the philosophy of pain management and control by health care personnel.

17. Identify surgical interventions that can be used to relieve pain.

18. Explain the treatment protocol for client's with intractable pain. Ask students how the nurse can assist the client to obtain the optimal effect from the treatments.

19. Have students design and implement, if possible, a teaching plan for a client who will be using a PCA pump in the acute care or home care setting.

20. Review the evaluation and documentation of the client's responses to pain relief measures.

21. Assign students to attend and report on a nursing staff conference, if available, on pain relief strategies.

22. Invite a nurse working in a hospice or on an oncology unit to discuss pain control and relief strategies.

23. Assign students to observe or participate in the care of clients who are experiencing pain, such as clients in labor or on a postoperative unit. Discuss the assessment process and follow-up interventions. Supervise students in the implementation and documentation of pharmacologic and nonpharmacologic strategies for pain relief.

24. Have students complete a care plan/pathway for a client who is experiencing pain, focusing on the individualization of interventions.

25. Have students work in small groups and plan how they might approach the following clients regarding pain relief:
    a. An older adult client with arthritis
    b. A middle-age adult who has just had abdominal surgery
    c. A young adult with appendicitis
    d. A school-age child with a fractured wrist
    e. A toddler who requires daily injections
    f. An adolescent with migraine headaches
    g. A woman in labor
    h. A child or adult with a toothache
    i. A young adult with a sunburn

INDEPENDENT LEARNING

1. Students should review the physiological processes involved in the reception, perception, and reaction to pain.

2. Students can investigate nonprescription and nontraditional measures that are available in the health care setting and community for pain relief (e.g., acupuncture).

3. Students can investigate available over-the-counter medications for pain relief, including their cost and any contraindications for use. They should compare the costs and similarities of trade name and generic brand analgesics.

4. Students can research an article in a current nursing journal on creative nursing strategies for pain relief.

5. Students can consider their own responses to pain and how they were affected by the experience.

STUDENT RESOURCES
Comparison of Acute and Chronic Pain

Pain	Description	Effect on Client
Acute		
Chronic		

Factors Influencing Pain/Comfort

Factor	Client Response	Nursing Interventions
Age		
Gender		
Culture		
Meaning of pain		
Attention		
Anxiety		
Fatigue		
Previous experience		
Coping style		

Nonpharmacological Measures to Promote Comfort

Measures	Effect on Client Comfort
Environmental	
Cutaneous stimulation	
Distraction	
Relaxation	
Anticipatory guidance	
Biofeedback	
Hypnosis	

CROSS-CURRICULUM GUIDE

Information on and procedures for pain relief can be reviewed in general and in relation to situations where discomfort might be anticipated. Antepartum, postoperative, post-traumatic, emergency, oncology, neurology, and orthopedic clients will most likely encounter varying degrees of pain. Nursing interventions in different health care settings to reduce client pain can be integrated into discussions throughout the educational program.

MULTIMEDIA RESOURCES

Whaley and Wong's Pediatric Nursing Video Series:
Pain Assessment and Management

CHAPTER

34

Nutrition

CRITICAL THINKING ACTIVITIES AND ANSWERS

1. You are completing a nursing history for a 24-year-old client who has diabetes. The client is slightly underweight and tells you that he is vegetarian and eats no animal products, including fish, eggs, and milk. What information about his diet would you need to determine whether it is adequate in calories and protein? What laboratory tests would reflect protein status? What physical assessment findings might suggest inadequate protein intake?

Answer: For his diet history, use either 24- or 72-hour recall or ask the client to keep a diet journal. Prealbumin and albumin would be measures of protein. Findings indicating protein loss include peripheral muscle wasting, edema, hair loss, brittle hair, and bruising.

2. Mrs. Evans is 75 years of age and lives alone. She receives a social security check, which pays for her rent and utilities with about $100 a month left over. She has arthritis and has difficulty ambulating more than about 50 feet at a time. How might Mrs. Evan's situation affect her nutritional status?

Answer: Her decreased finances decrease her purchase power. This can be corrected with the use of food stamps. Her limited mobility decreases her ability to shop. Meals on Wheels or congregate meal sites with transportation can provide one nutritionally solid meal for her each day, free or at a low cost.

3. While giving Mr. Orzo a bath, you notice that his PN solution looks odd. There is a small yellow layer at the top of the bag. Mr. Orzo is receiving lipids, amino acids, and dextrose in a single solution. What could this layer indicate, and what should you do first?

Answer: Lipid infusions should be administered within 12 hours. If an infusion has separated or layered, it should not be given. Discontinue administration, including administration tubing, and maintain IV catheter patency with a dextrose solution.

EDUCATIONAL STRATEGIES

1. Discuss the meaning of food in relation to overall health and sociocultural practices. Ask students to share how the preparation and intake of food might be incorporated into familial, cultural, and spiritual practices.

2. Discuss factors that influence dietary intake.

3. Review the principles of nutrition, including metabolism, digestion, absorption, storage, and elimination.

4. Identify the six categories of nutrients, the role and storage of each in the body, and current recommendations for daily intake: carbohydrates, proteins, lipids, water, vitamins, and minerals. Have students identify food sources for each nutrient.

5. Discuss the role of carbohydrates, lipids, and proteins in energy provision. Explain and demonstrate the calculation of kcal/gm for each nutrient. Provide sample exercises for students to use to calculate total energy output.

6. Using educational media (e.g., photos, illustrations, transparencies), explain the food guide pyramid and how it differs from the four basic food groups.

7. Discuss how the promotion of nutrition follows the Healthy People 2000 objectives, with guidelines for reduced sodium and saturated fat intake and increased intake of fruits, vegetables, and grains.

8. Discuss alternative food patterns (e.g., vegetarianism), and their advantages and disadvantages in meeting nutritional needs. Ask students to share personal or clinical experiences with alternative food patterns.

9. Review the nutritional needs of individuals across the lifespan. Have students provide specific examples of how growth and development influence nutritional requirements.

10. Identify and explain the aspects of a nutritional assessment and the information obtained through the following:
    a. Physical measurements—height, weight, anthropometrics
    b. Laboratory tests
    c. Dietary and health history
    d. Clinical observation

11. Have students complete a food intake record (24 hours to 3 days) on themselves, peers, family members, friends, or client and analyze the total nutrient intake for adequacy. If available, use a commercial computer program for analysis.

12. Have students identify what nutritional information and guidelines (e.g., food labels, media stories) are available to the consumer. Assign students to bring in examples of readily found nutritional information.

13. Identify clients who might be at risk for nutritional deficiencies. Use the following, or similar, situations to ask students to provide the rationale for why nutritional problems could develop and how the nurse can assess the presence of a problem:
    a. A postoperative client
    b. An immobilized client
    c. An older adult living alone
    d. A preschool child living in a poor socioeconomic setting
    e. A client in the terminal stages of cancer
    f. An adolescent experiencing socialization and peer pressure

14. Identify measures that can be implemented to promote nutrition for clients in different health care settings. Have students provide specific

examples of how the nurse can improve clients' appetites, meet nutritional guidelines for disease-related treatment, and counsel/teach clients and families about nutritional needs.

15. Stimulate a discussion on client situations where a referral for nutritional needs might be indicated (e.g., Meals on Wheels).

16. Have students identify the general nutritional needs for clients with the following health deviations: diabetes mellitus, cardiovascular disease, renal disease, gastrointestinal disorders, AIDS, or cancer.

17. Discuss specific concerns for clients of diverse cultural and spiritual backgrounds (e.g., kosher or Hindu dietary requirements).

18. Invite a nutritionist or dietitian to speak to the class about his or her role in helping clients to meet their nutritional needs.

19. Discuss enteral nutrition, including its purpose, uses, complications, and associated nursing responsibilities. Ask students to identify situations where clients might need enteral feedings.

20. Have students design and present, if possible, a teaching plan for one of the following simulated situations or an actual client assignment:
    a. Parents of a newborn, a 2-year-old, and a 15-year-old
    b. An older adult with heart disease
    c. A family member responsible for the client's gastrostomy tube care

21. Discuss parenteral nutrition, including its purpose, use, specific solutions, contraindications, complications, and associated nursing responsibilities. Ask students to identify situations where parenteral nutrition might be used for a client.

22. Explain and demonstrate (using educational media, simulation mannequins/models, and appropriate equipment) the following interventions for promotion of a client's nutrition:
    a. Insertion of a small-bore nasoenteric tube
    b Initiation of enteral tube feedings through nasoenteric tubes
    c. Administration of enteral tube feedings through gastrostomy or jejunostomy tube

Have students work in small groups to practice the performance and documentation of these skills.

23. Evaluate the students' ability to provide enteral nutrition through return demonstration/skill testing before their clinical experiences.

24. Assign students to observe or participate in the care of clients in a variety of health care settings, focusing on the assessment and promotion of nutritional status. Have students prepare the environment and assist in oral hygiene in order to stimulate the client's appetite. Supervise the implementation of oral, enteral, and/or parenteral feedings. Have students work with clients in food selection, meal planning, and food preparation in accordance with the prescribed diet therapy. Discuss students' assessments and nursing interventions in pre- and postclinical conferences.

25. Have students complete a care plan/pathway for an actual or simulated client who is experiencing an alteration in nutritional status.

26. Ask students how they can help clients in the following situations to meet the food pyramid's nutritional guidelines:
    a. Overweight
    b. Underweight
    c. Reduced fat diet
    d. Limited income

INDEPENDENT LEARNING

1. Students should review the physiological processes associated with nutritional intake, including digestion, absorption, metabolism, and elimination.

2. Students can complete a self-assessment of dietary intake for a selected period of time, in intervals of 24 hours, 3 days, or weekly. They can review their intake for the specified time period to evaluate the intake of essential nutrients.

3. Students may investigate available resources in the community (e.g., WIC program, Meals on Wheels) that assist clients and families with nutritional needs.

4. Students can visit community food stores or check advertisements and compare the cost of similar items to determine where clients can get the "best buys." They can inquire if the stores will deliver to clients who are unable to leave their homes.

5. Students should review food labels in order to increase their familiarity with the information that is provided to the consumer.

STUDENT RESOURCES

Nutrients

Nutrients	Use by the Body	Sources
Carbohydrates		
Proteins		
Lipids		
Vitamins		
Minerals		
Water		

Promotion of Nutrition

Strategy	Specific Nursing Interventions
Stimulate appetite	
Provide a comfortable environment	
Assist with Feedings	
Provide Enteral Nutrition	
Provide Parenteral Nutrition	
Implement Diet Therapy	

CROSS-CURRICULUM GUIDE

Maternal/Child: Discussions on growth and development may include the promotion of specific nutritional needs for each age group. Students should be aware of signs in infants and children that indicate a failure to thrive.

Medical/Surgical: Nutritional intake is an essential therapeutic component in the care of perioperative clients and those who are experiencing health deviations. It is a special concern for clients with gastrointestinal disorders, cancer, AIDS, extended immobility, and malnutrition.

Gerontological: Older adults may suffer from nutritional deficiencies related to physiological or psychological changes. Problems with mastication or digestion may limit dietary selection and intake. People who live alone and are confined to their homes might not have any desire to cook or eat regularly.

MULTIMEDIA RESOURCES

Mosby's Nursing Skills Video Series
    Set II: *Nutrition*

Mosby's Applying Critical Thinking to Nursing Skills: An Interactive Videodisc Series
    Nutrition and Elimination

CHAPTER 35

Urinary Elimination

CRITICAL THINKING ACTIVITIES AND ANSWERS

1. Six hours after removal of an indwelling catheter, you are checking on your client and she states her bladder feels full. She says she has only minimal incisional discomfort (1 on a scale of 1 to 5) and demands patient-controlled analgesia of morphine. The patient is 1 day post total abdominal hysterectomy and bilateral salpingo-oophorectomy. This is the second postoperative day. Her I & O balanced in the first 24 hours. She has no intravenous fluids and has had 1000 ml of oral intake this day. At 11 AM when her Foley catheter was removed, there was 700 ml in the bag. She has a midline dressing on her lower abdomen and no drainage tubes. What assessment would you make to determine bladder status? What interventions would you implement to enhance urination?

Answer: *Assessments:* palpate for bladder fullness, obtain vital signs (including temperature), find out how often she is using PCA (narcotic analgesics increase risk of retention), determine her response to previous catheterization, ask if she has attempted to use the bathroom since catheter removal and if she has any known urinary problems. *Interventions:* assist her to the bathroom; once her safety is established, provide privacy, instruct her to use the call light before getting up, and run water in the sink. If she is unable to urinate and is not uncomfortable, encourage her to walk and to try sitting up after the walk. If her bladder is palpable or she becomes uncomfortable, notify the physician to discuss her inability to void, assessment findings, and PCA.

2. You are on a home visit to a client who is using a condom catheter. His wife, who is the caregiver, tells you the "darn thing never stays on." What problems might cause the condom not to stay on? What assessments of the client do you need to make to determine the cause? If the catheter was applied incorrectly by the wife, what steps can be taken to ensure she understands how to do the procedure?

Answer: Problems that might cause a poor fit include the following: urine accumulating at the end of the condom, hair inhibiting adhesion, adhesive strip applied incorrectly, condom too small or too large, or an allergy to latex causing blistering and nonadherence. Assessments to make to determine the cause: Before removing the catheter, look to see if it is draining properly or if the tubing or condom are kinked; assess the penis and scrotum for signs of irritation or breakdown; see if hair is inadvertently caught in adhesive; check size of condom; and check the positioning of the client and if he is manipulating the catheter. If the catheter is incorrectly applied, reapply it and demonstrate the steps to his wife. Leave written instructions for her to refer to in the future.

EDUCATIONAL STRATEGIES

1. Review the anatomy and physiology of the urinary system.

2. Discuss factors that influence urinary elimination.

3. Identify and describe the following alterations in urinary elimination, including possible etiology and client signs and symptoms: urinary retention, urinary tract infection, urinary incontinence, enuresis.

4. Discuss the indications for, surgical treatment of, and resultant client alterations in elimination associated with urinary diversions. Use educational media (e.g., photos, illustrations) to demonstrate the differences between the types of diversions. Assign students to investigate and report back on available resources in the health care setting and community to assist clients requiring dialysis, support groups, and/or special ostomy equipment.

5. Discuss the components of the nursing history that will elicit information on a client's urinary function, including patterns of urination, signs and symptoms, and other related factors. Have students determine the type of questions to ask clients to obtain this information.

6. Review the physical assessment of the client for determination of urinary function. Ask students to identify expected and unexpected findings from the assessment (e.g., distended bladder).

7. Describe the assessment of urinary output, including analysis of I & O, and characteristics of urine. Provide students with a sample urinalysis and have them determine the normal and abnormal constituents.

8. Identify and describe common diagnostic tests used to evaluate urinary function. Discuss the client preparation for, and nursing responsibilities associated with, the testing. Review normal results and the possible meaning of abnormal findings.

9. Explain and demonstrate the procedure for collection of a midstream (clean-voided) specimen. Ask how the procedure can be altered for clients of different ages and self-care abilities.

10. Provide small groups of students with the name of a urinary diagnostic test and have them prepare a teaching plan for a client who will be having the test.

11. Assign students to accompany clients, if possible, to observe urinary diagnostic procedures. Have students share their observations after the experience.

12. Discuss the psychological and emotional factors involved in urinary elimination. Ask students how the nurse can promote client dignity and alleviate anxiety in the health care setting.

13. Using the following or similar situations, ask students to specify how urinary elimination might be affected in:
    a. A quadriplegic client
    b. An older adult with cardiovascular disease
    c. A hospitalized 2-year-old child
    d. An adolescent female with a urinary tract infection
    e. A client diagnosed with bladder cancer
    f. A client with diabetes mellitus

14. Ask students to identify interventions that can be implemented to promote urinary function. Demonstrate how measures to stimulate urination are effective by having students put their hands in warm water or listen to the sound of running water.

15. Discuss how nursing interventions to promote urination can be adapted from the health promotion setting to acute care and restorative care settings.

16. Discuss the types or urinary catheterization, their purposes, complications, nursing interventions, and documentation. Ask students to identify specific nursing measures that will assist in preventing infection.

17. Explain and demonstrate (using educational media, simulation mannequins/models, and appropriate equipment) the following interventions for promotion of urination:
    a. Insertion of a straight or indwelling catheter
    b. Provision of indwelling catheter care
    c. Application of a condom catheter

Have students work in small groups to practice the implementation and documentation of these skills.

18. Evaluate the students' abilities to perform catheterization, catheter care, and the application of a condom catheter through return demonstration/skill testing before their clinical experiences.

19. Discuss the use of medications that will influence urinary elimination.

20. Assign students to observe or participate in the nursing care of clients in different health care settings, focusing on the assessment and promotion of urinary function. Review laboratory and diagnostic test results for assigned clients. Discuss specific measures to be implemented to promote urinary elimination.

21. Assign students to complete a care plan/pathway for an actual or simulated client who is experiencing an alteration in urinary elimination.

22. Invite a nurse who specializes in dialysis/renal care to speak to the class about the specific urinary needs of clients and nursing responsibilities.

INDEPENDENT LEARNING

1. Students should review the normal anatomy and physiology of the urinary system.

2. Students should practice the procedures for promotion of urination in the skill laboratory.

3. Students can research an article on the promotion of urination for clients in the acute, extended, or home care setting.

4. Students may investigate resources for clients in local stores/pharmacies for urinary care in the home (e.g., incontinence pads, catheters, drainage bags). They can compare prices to determine the most cost-effective source for these items in the community.

STUDENT RESOURCES

Common Urinary Elimination Problems

Problem	Cause(s)	Signs/Symptoms	Treatment/Nursing Interventions
Urinary retention			
Urinary tract infection			
Urinary incontinence			
Enuresis			

Influence of Growth and Development on Urinary Function and Patterns

Age-Group	Urinary Function / Patterns
Infants	
Toddlers to School-Age Children	
Adults	
Older adults	

Promotion of Urination

Area of Focus	Specific Nursing Interventions
Micturition reflex	
Elimination habits	
Adequate fluid intake	
Pelvic floor muscles	
Bladder compression	
Drug therapy	
Asepsis	
Comfort	
Skin integrity	

CROSS-CURRICULUM GUIDE

Maternal/Child: Children require specific alterations in interventions for promotion of urinary function. Measurement of I & O is also critical because of their body weight and the related percentage of fluid. Some specific health deviations affecting urinary function in children include nephrotic syndrome, glomerulonephritis, and neurological impairments (e.g., spina bifida).

Medical/Surgical: Assessment, promotion, and evaluation of urinary output is important for all clients. Those experiencing genitourinary, neurological, and oncological disorders or surgical interventions might have impairment of urinary function.

Gerontological: Older adults experience changes as a result of the aging process, such as bladder muscle weakness and decreased renal filtration. In addition, older adults may have a health deviation that places them at greater risk for inadequate urinary function. Careful assessment of urination in these clients should be discussed, especially before clinical experiences in extended care settings.

MULTIMEDIA RESOURCES

Mosby's Nursing Skills Video Series
   Set II: *Catheterization and Urinary Care*

Mosby's Applying Critical Thinking to Nursing Skills: An Interactive Videodisc Series
   Nutrition and Elimination

CHAPTER 36

Bowel Elimination

CRITICAL THINKING ACTIVITIES AND ANSWERS

1. While fulfilling your community service responsibility of taking blood pressures at the senior citizens center, one of the clients tells you that this morning after he had a bowel movement, he noticed bright red blood on the toilet tissue. What further data would you need to gather?

Answer: The nurse should assess the amount of bleeding. Is the client able to estimate (e.g., a spot the size of a dollar or a penny)? Did he strain in having the stool? Does he have a history of hemorrhoids, constipation, colitis, Crohn's disease, or recent surgery? Has this happened before? What was his diet for the past 24 hours? The nurse could also choose to inspect the anal area (if a private room is available) and have the client perform a guaiac test of the next stool specimen.

2. An elderly woman with complaints of constipation tells you high-fiber foods are just too expensive. What would you advise?

Answer: Suggest that she try some high-fiber foods such as brown rice and beans, bran cereal, or whole-grain bread (which are not expensive). These foods are also easily chewed. Include in the discussion information about increasing her fluid intake, especially prune juice or hot tea. Encourage her to begin some form of daily activity if she does not currently exercise.

3. This is your first day of caring for a bedridden, comatose, 87-year-old man. In reviewing his chart you find no entry of a bowel movement for the past 10 days. How would you proceed with your bowel assessment?

Answer: Other staff members who have worked with the client should be asked if he had a bowel movement that was not noted. Assessment would begin with inspection of his abdomen for signs of distention. This would be followed by auscultation for bowel sounds and percussion and palpation of the abdomen. If the client had bowel sounds and there were no contraindications, the nurse should assess his rectum for an impaction.

EDUCATIONAL STRATEGIES

1. Review the anatomy and physiology of the gastrointestinal system.

2. Identify factors that affect bowel elimination. Have students provide specific examples of how bowel elimination can be affected with each factor.

3. Describe the following common bowel elimination problems, including their etiology, client signs and symptoms, and potential complications:
   a. Constipation
   b. Fecal impaction
   c. Diarrhea
   d. Incontinence
   e. Flatulence
   f. Hemorrhoids

4. Discuss the psychological and emotional factors associated with bowel elimination. Ask students how the nurse can recognize and minimize disturbances that are associated specifically with the health care environment.

5. Discuss the indications for, surgical treatment of, and resultant alterations in elimination associated with bowel diversions. Using educational media (e.g., photos, illustrations), demonstrate the difference of continent and incontinent ostomies in location as well as drainage, client and family teaching, and nursing care management.

6. Stimulate a discussion on the potential effect an ostomy has on a client's self-concept and body image.

7. Assign students to investigate resources that are available within the health care agency and community for clients with an ileostomy or colostomy. Have students identify the types and costs of equipment that the client will need to purchase and whether health insurance will cover the expenses.

8. Invite an enterostomal therapy nurse to speak to the class about the specific physical and psychological needs of clients with ostomies.

9. Describe the nursing assessment of a client to determine bowel elimination status, including nursing history, physical assessment, and analysis of laboratory and diagnostic test results.

10. Identify and describe laboratory and diagnostic tests that are used to determine problems with bowel elimination. Discuss the client preparation for, and nursing responsibilities associated with, these tests.

11. Ask students what information should be taught to the client who will be performing a test for occult blood at home.

12. Assign students to accompany clients, if possible, to observe diagnostic tests for digestive or bowel elimination disorders. Have students share their observations after the experience.

13. Have students identify specific nursing interventions that can be implemented to promote bowel elimination in different health care settings.

14. Discuss the use of medications (laxatives, cathartics, stool softeners, antidiarrheal agents) that are used to promote regular bowel elimination. Ask students how these medications might also create bowel elimination problems.

15. Discuss the types, purposes, and administration of enemas.

16. Explain and demonstrate (using educational media, simulation mannequins/models, and appropriate equipment), the following interventions for promotion of bowel elimination:
    a. Assisting the client on and off the bedpan
    b. Digital removal of stool
    c. Measuring occult blood in stool
    d. Administration of a cleansing enema
    e. Pouching of an ostomy

Have students practice the implementation and documentation of these skills in small groups.

17. Evaluate the students' abilities to perform measures to promote bowel elimination through return demonstration/skill testing before their clinical experience.

18. Assign students to design and present a teaching plan based on one of the following situations:
    a. Client/family member care of an ileostomy or colostomy
    b. Maintenance of a regular bowel elimination pattern during pregnancy
    c. Bowel retraining
    d. Hazards of overuse of laxatives, cathartics, and enemas

19. Assign students to observe or participate in the care of clients in a variety of health care settings, focusing on the assessment, promotion, and evaluation of bowel elimination. Discuss with students in preclinical conferences the analysis of information from the nursing history and physical assessment along with laboratory test results. Have students identify specific nursing interventions for promotion of bowel elimination. Evaluate the students' maintenance of client dignity, privacy, and safety.

20. Have students complete a care plan/pathway for an actual or simulated client who is experiencing an alteration in bowel elimination.

21. Ask students to identify how bowel elimination may be altered for the following, or similar, client situations:
    a. A client who has had a myocardial infarction
    b. A client with a new ileostomy or colostomy
    c. A truck driver who is on the road for extended periods of time
    d. An unconscious client
    e An adult client with paraplegia
    f. A 6-year-old hospitalized with cystic fibrosis
    g. A client who has had a cholecystectomy
    h. An older adult with rheumatoid arthritis
    i. An individual taking muscle relaxants
    j. A terminally ill client who is on morphine for pain management

INDEPENDENT LEARNING

1. Students should review the normal anatomy and physiology of the gastrointestinal system.

2. Students should practice the techniques for promotion of bowel elimination in the skill laboratory.

3. Students can investigate the different over-the-counter products that are available to promote or inhibit bowel elimination, including their costs, uses, and hazards.

Bowel Elimination Problems

Problem	Cause(s)	Signs/Symptoms	Nursing Interventions
Constipation			
Diarrhea			
Incontinence			
Flatulence			
Hemorrhoids			
Need for bowel diversions			

Promotion of Bowel Elimination

Strategy	Specific Nursing Interventions
Diet	
Exercise	
Timing and privacy	
Normal defecation	

CROSS-CURRICULUM GUIDE

Individuals of all ages require accurate assessment of bowel elimination. Clients who are experiencing gastrointestinal or neurological disorders or prolonged immobility will need special evaluation and promotion of bowel function.

Gerontological: Older adults may experience the physiological changes that occur with aging, such as diminished muscle tone and peristalsis.

MULTIMEDIA RESOURCES

Mosby's Nursing Skills Video Series
    Set II: Promoting Bowel Elimination

Mosby's Applying Critical Thinking to Nursing Skills: An Interactive Videodisc Series
    Nutrition and Elimination

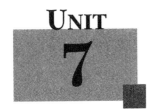

UNIT

7

Clients With Special Needs

TOPICAL OUTLINE

CRITICAL THINKING ACTIVITIES AND ANSWERS

1. You are caring for an 80-year-old female client who is admitted to a nursing home for rehabilitation after a fractured hip. She was in good health and independent until she fell. What evaluative measures should you make to ensure that she is getting proper lung expansion while she is in the nursing home undergoing rehabilitation?

Answer: Evaluative measures for prompting optimal lung expansion include the following:
   a. Inspecting and palpating for symmetrical lung expansion and auscultating lung sounds
   b. Observing her respirations
   c. Monitoring the use of incentive spirometry
   d. Observing her for productive cough and improved coughing ability
   e. Inspecting her sputum for clear, white, watery consistency

2. The client you are caring for is on complete bed rest and has a history of thrombophlebitis. You ask the client during your assessment if she is doing her leg exercises. She replies, "No, I don't need to. I have these fancy stockings." She raises her legs and shows you intermittent compression stockings. What do you reply?

Answer: Explain that the stockings are helping to improve her blood return to the heart but that activity on her part is better than the mechanical help of the stockings alone. Explain that leg exercises will also help to keep her muscles toned, which will help with walking when she can get up again. Ask her to show you how to do the leg exercises and if there are any difficulties when she does them.

3. Mrs. Williams is a client you are seeing in her home after her laparoscopic-assisted vaginal hysterectomy. She has been home 2 hours since she was released from the surgery center. What assessments must you make on this initial visit?

Answer: On the initial visit, a head-to-toe exam is in order and should include the following: level of consciousness and orientation; lung, heart, and abdomen exam; examination of dressing sites and questions about vaginal bleeding; peripheral vascular assessment; posture, gait, and mobility status; and pain assessment.

EDUCATIONAL STRATEGIES

1. Explain the general physiological, developmental, and psychosocial effects of immobility on the client.

2. Ask students what growth and development factors influence mobility status and place an individual at risk for adverse effects of immobility.

3. Have students determine the influences on mobility and the available assistive devices for the following, or similar, health deviations:
   a. Post CVA with left-sided weakness
   b. Lumbar disk herniation
   c. Fractures of the extremities
   d. Rheumatoid arthritis
   e. Quadriplegia
   f. Chronic pulmonary disease
   g. Traumatic knee injury

4. Describe the physical assessment for an immobile client to determine the presence of pathological changes.

5. Have students identify the assessment technique that should be used to determine the presence of the following:
   a. Muscle atrophy
   b. Orthostatic hypotension
   c. Atelectasis
   d. Thrombosis
   e. Fecal impaction

6. Ask students to identify the nursing interventions that should be implemented to prevent or alleviate the negative effects of immobility.

7. Explain and demonstrate (using educational media, simulation mannequins/models, and appropriate equipment) the correct technique for application of elastic stockings. Have students practice the technique in the skill laboratory. Evaluate the student's abilities to apply elastic stockings correctly through return demonstration before their clinical experience.

8. Invite a physical therapist to speak to the class about exercises that can be implemented to prevent or reduce the hazards of immobility.

9. Assign students to observe or participate in the care of clients who are experiencing prolonged periods of immobility. Discuss particular measures that should be implemented frequently during client care, including turning and positioning of clients. Have students complete a care plan/pathway for their clients, with teaching needs of the client/family identified.

INDEPENDENT LEARNING

1. Students should review the normal anatomy and physiology of the body systems that may be effected by immobility.

2. Students should take note of their regular daily activities to get a sense of how immobility would interfere with the ability to complete these activities and interact with others.

3. Students should practice exercises for the immobilized client that promote respiratory, circulatory, and musculoskeletal function.

4. Students can investigate creative diversional activities that may be used for clients with prolonged immobility.

5. Students can research an article in a current nursing journal on new devices that are available to prevent or treat the hazards of immobility.

STUDENT RESOURCE

Nursing Prevention and Treatment
of the Effects of Immobility

Focus Area	Effects of Immobility	Nursing Interventions to Prevent/Treat
Metabolic rate, metabolism		
Fluid, electrolyte balance		
Bone metabolism		
GI system		
Respiratory system		
Cardiovascular system		
Musculoskeletal system		
Integument		
Urinary system		

CROSS-CURRICULUM GUIDE

Clients with orthopedic and neuromuscular disorders—as well as those who have experienced multiple trauma, burns, a diminished level of consciousness or mental orientation, or severe weakness from another pathological condition—may experience prolonged periods of immobility.

Gerontological: Older clients are especially at risk for the adverse effects of immobility. Special emphasis should be placed on careful assessment of older clients, especially in the extended care setting.

CHAPTER 38

Skin Integrity and Wound Care

CRITICAL THINKING ACTIVITIES AND ANSWERS

1. You are teaching a client's family how to irrigate the midabdominal wound that is healing by secondary intention. The spouse states, "I always thought it was best to paint the wound with povidone-iodine to prevent infection." How should you respond? What is the rationale behind your response? What does the spouse need to know about irrigating the wound?

Answer: Current research indicates that povidone-iodine is toxic to fibroblasts and should not be used to clean granulating wounds. Normal saline is the preferred solution to use to clean wounds. It is nontoxic and safe. The spouse needs to know that besides using the correct type of solution, the temperature of the solution is important. Room temperature is recommended. Another point is the system used to clean the wound. Wound-cleaning systems should be of adequate pressure (psi) to effectively cleanse the wound yet not be too high a pressure to injury the healing tissues. A psi range of 4 to 15 is considered safe to use. The spouse will need to learn how to obtain and use the necessary equipment to clean the wound correctly.

2. It is your client's seventh postoperative day. When assessing the wound you note that several sutures remain. What actions do you take?

Answer: Check the MD orders to see if any sutures are to be removed. Assess whether the sutures that you see are whole and intact or just parts of the sutures that were removed previously.

3. A client has two Jackson-Pratt drainage collectors on the right side of the abdomen. What nursing assessments should be made to ensure proper functioning of this system? Can any aspects of care for this type of drain collector be delegated? Explain the rationale for your answer.

Answer: The nurse should assess the location of each of the Jackson-Pratt (JP) containers. They should be numbered or identified so that it is clear which JP the nurse is talking about. The entire JP system should be assessed each shift. Check for patency and presence of clots. Assess whether the JP should be a wall or self-suction. For a wall suction, make sure it's on the proper setting, which is usually low; if a self-suction, make sure that the bulb part of the JP is correctly depressed. Most often the tubing should be pinned to the client's gown. Make sure there is no leakage from any parts in the tubing system, that there are no kinks in the tubing, and that the client is not leaning on any parts of the tubing.

The emptying of the JP can, in most states, be delegated by the nurse to others. Check the nurse practice act in your particular state. The nurse, however, is responsible for the action of the person who is delegated to empty the JP. The nurse retains the responsibility for assessing the characteristics of the drainage and making sure that the amount of drainage is recorded on the client's record.

4. Your 85-year-old black male client is admitted to the hospital with a diagnosis of left cerebral vascular accident. He has right-sided weakness, and he cannot turn or walk without using his walker and another person's assistance. He also has difficulty swallowing, and he is incontinent of urine.
   a. What risk factors, if any, for pressure ulcers does this client have?
   b. What characteristics should the nurse assess to monitor for a stage I pressure ulcer?
   c. How should this be accomplished?

Answer:
   a. Risk factors include paresis, immobilization, malnutrition, incontinence, and age.
      The most common site of pressure ulcers is the sacrum. This client has several risk factors for developing pressure ulcers. These include his decreased sensation and right-sided weakness from the CVA. As a result, his ability to turn, reposition, and ambulate independently are diminished; therefore, pressure can be exerted against his skin without him being able to feel it or change his position. These are major risk factors for developing a sacral or any pressure ulcer. Because he is incontinent of urine, his skin is exposed to a moist environment that contains bacteria. This moisture can cause skin maceration or breakdown. Should an indwelling catheter be inserted to contain his urine, this will also put him a risk for pressure ulcer development from the catheter. The catheter must be properly anchored to his leg, or it can put pressure on the tip of his penis and urethra and cause skin breakdown.
      Because he has difficulty swallowing, he many not be able to consume enough of his prescribed diet. Inadequate intake of his required daily calorie, protein, vitamin, and mineral requirements can lead to malnutrition as evidenced by weight loss, muscle atrophy, and reduced tissue mass. The latter means that there is less tissue that can serve as a "pad" between his bony prominences and his skin. His age also has implications for his skin. Older skin has a flatter epidermal junction. This puts the

client at increased risk for "peeling" away his dermis from shearing that can occur when the head of the bed is higher than 30 degrees and from friction that can occur from improper positioning and transfer that "drags" rather than lifts his skin off the mattress or chair surface.

b. Several characteristics should be assessed to identify a stage I pressure ulcer. For this particular client, the guidelines for assessing clients with darkly pigmented skin should be used. At the minimum, the local characteristics should include color, temperature, hardness, and edema of the skin over the bony prominences.

The following information about the whole person should also be assessed for this client: history and physical, nutritional assessment, pain, psychosocial, comorbid conditions, complications, and risk for additional pressure ulcers.

c. Halogen or natural light sources are best for assessing color changes in darkly pigmented clients. Fluorescent lighting should not be used, as it gives a bluish hue to the skin that can interfere with the accurate assessment of skin color. Wearing clean gloves, the nurse should palpate any areas of skin discoloration. Feel for fluid beneath the skin (fluctuance) and temperature changes—warmer first, then cooler.

EDUCATIONAL STRATEGIES

1. Review the anatomy and physiology of the integument and the physiological processes associated with wound healing.

2. Discuss what pressure ulcers are, their prevalence in health care settings, and the economic consequences of their development.

3. Compare and contrast wound healing by primary and secondary intention. Identify the phases of primary intention healing. Highlight the discussion with photos, illustrations, or models.

4. Review the pathogenesis associated with the development of a pressure ulcer and the staging process, using photos and illustrations.

5. Identify client risk factors associated with the development of pressure ulcers. Have students identify how the following may increase the risk of pressure ulcer development:
   a. Impaired peripheral circulation
   b. Diminished level of consciousness
   c. Impaired sensory or motor function
   d. Use of selected equipment or treatments
   e. Shearing force/friction
   f. Moisture on the skin
   g. Poor nutrition and/or anemia
   h. Cachexia
   i. Advanced age

6. Explain the assessment tools that can be used to predict a client's risk for pressure ulcer development. Have students review the tools and identify their similarities and differences.

7. Provide students with photos/illustrations of pressure ulcers and have them describe and document them, including location, size, and drainage. Use available agency tools for documentation.

8. Review the physical assessment parameters for determination of pressure ulcer development, including condition of the skin, mobility, nutritional status, and pain.

9. Have clients identify how the following clients are at risk for pressure ulcer development:
   a. Unconscious client
   b. Client with restraints in place to the extremities
   c. Client with a spica cast
   d. Client with pelvic traction
   e. An incontinent client
   f. A client with a wasting disease, such as terminal cancer

10. Ask students to identify specific nursing interventions that should be implemented to prevent the development of pressure ulcers.

11. Discuss the assessment information that contributes to the scheduling of turning and positioning and the choice of support surfaces or mattresses.

12. Discuss the newest research on methods used for the prevention and treatment of pressure ulcers and wounds.

13. Have students investigate and report back on the types of treatment, equipment, supplies, and medications that are used in an affiliated agency for the prevention and treatment of pressure ulcers and wounds.

14. Invite a nurse who specializes in the treatment of wounds/pressure ulcers to speak to the class about the nurse's role in prevention and treatment.

15. Describe the complications of wound healing, along with etiology, signs, and symptoms.

16. Identify factors that influence wound healing.

17. Discuss the potential psychological impact of wounds on clients.

18. Explain the process for initial and ongoing assessment of wounds in emergency and stable settings.

19. Describe, using available photos, the potential characteristics of wound drainage.

20. Show students the different types of wound drainage systems.

21. Discuss the use of sutures and staples for wound closure and the nursing care indicated for each type of closure.

22. Identify and describe nursing interventions for wound care, including first aid, dressings, use of bandages and binders, irrigations, and application of heat and cold therapy.

23. Discuss and demonstrate the use of different types of dressings. Ask students to identify the type of dressing that is appropriate for the following:
    a. Small, superficial wound
    b. Necrotic wound
    c. Clean, granulating wound
    d. Clean, surgical wound with a small amount of drainage

24. Explain and demonstrate (using educational media, simulation mannequins/models, and appropriate equipment) the following for pressure ulcers/wounds:
    a. Assessment for risk of pressure ulcer development
    b. Treating pressure ulcers
    c. Applying dry and wet-to-dry moist dressings
    d. Performing wound irrigations
    e. Applying an abdominal, a T, or a breast binder
    f. Applying an elastic bandage
    g. Applying a moist hot compress to an open wound

Have students work in small groups and practice the implementation and documentation of these techniques.

25. Evaluate the students' abilities to implement the techniques associated with pressure ulcer and wound care through return demonstration/skill testing before their clinical experience.

26. Ask students to identify measures that can be implemented to reduce the client's discomfort during wound care.

27. Have students identify the indications for the use of heat and cold therapy, complications from the therapy, and factors that can influence a client's tolerance.

28. Invite an infection control nurse/risk manager to speak to the class about aseptic technique and wound care.

29. Discuss how wound care can be adapted for clients outside the acute care environment.

30. Assign students to develop and implement, if possible, a teaching plan for the following:
    a. A family member who will be caring for an immobile client at home who is at risk of developing pressure ulcers
    b. A client who will be caring for a surgical wound at home

31. Assign students to observe or participate in the care of clients with potential or actual alterations in skin integrity. Discuss client assessment before the experience. Review specific supportive measures and wound treatment, if indicated. Have students identify clients' educational needs for pressure ulcer prevention and/or wound care.

32. Have students complete a care plan/pathway for an actual client with an impairment in skin integrity, or for the following simulated client situation: An 84-year-old man has not regained his prior level of mobility following a right hip replacement. The client has also become progressively more disoriented to his surroundings and unable to participate in activities of daily living without significant support and direction. He is occasionally incontinent of urine and feces. When not in bed, the client spends most of his day in a geriatric chair.

INDEPENDENT LEARNING

1. Students should review the anatomy and physiology of the integumentary system and the physiology of the inflammatory response and wound healing.

2. Students should practice the nursing techniques associated with maintenance of skin integrity and promotion of wound healing in the skill laboratory.

3. Students should investigate resources that are available in the health care setting and community for the prevention and treatment of pressure ulcers.

4. Students can research an article on recent techniques used for prevention of pressure ulcers and wound healing.

STUDENT RESOURCES

Factors Contributing to Pressure Ulcer Development

Factor	How the Factors Contribute to Ulcer Development
Shearing force	
Friction	
Moisture	
Nutrition	
Infection	
Impaired circulation	
Obesity	
Age	

Wound Healing

Wound Healing	Description
Primary intention:	
Inflammatory phase:	
Proliferative reconstruction:	
Maturation phase:	
Secondary intention:	

Pressure Ulcer Prevention

Strategies	Specific Nursing Interventions
Hygiene and skin care	
Positioning	
Therapeutic beds/mattresses	

Wound Care

Strategies	Specific Nursing Interventions
Dressings	
Bandages/binders	
Heat/cold therapy	

CROSS-CURRICULUM GUIDE

Maternal/Child: Application of cold therapy can be used for the postpartum client with an episiotomy. A breast binder can be applied for a non-breast feeding mother. Young children and adolescents might experience traumatic injuries and/or surgery that will result in the need for wound care and dressings. Nursing care for the promotion of wound healing must be adapted to meet the developmental needs of the younger client.

Medical/Surgical: Information on maintenance of skin integrity and promotion of wound healing should be incorporated into discussions on the following: postoperative care, diabetes mellitus, circulatory insufficiency, burns, physical trauma, amputation, and any other client situation where there could be a threat to skin integrity.

Gerontological: Older adults who are immobile and have impaired circulation are especially prone to skin breakdown. They require careful assessment and prompt intervention by the nurse order to avoid further complications.

MULTIMEDIA RESOURCES

Mosby's Nursing Skills Video Series:
    Set II: *Wound Care and Applying Dressings*

CHAPTER 39

Sensory Alterations

CRITICAL THINKING ACTIVITIES AND ANSWERS

1. Mrs. Wilson, 72 years of age, attends the clinic for regular checkups every 6 months. During a routine conversation, she states, "I am not seeing as well these days." Discuss three symptoms clients experience with aging. What strategies can you use to assist Mrs. Wilson to see better?

Answer: Presbyopia is the inability to focus properly. This usually begins to appear around the age of 40. The visual field can also narrow, which makes peripheral vision more difficult. The pupil is less responsive to light because the pupil sphincter hardens and pupil size decreases. Depth perception becomes distorted. Dark and light accommodation takes longer. Reduced lacrimal production can cause dryness of the eyes.

After an eye examination is conducted to identify what problems Mrs. Wilson is experiencing, a nursing plan can be developed. Health promotion is very important. Mrs. Wilson should be encouraged to visit her eye doctor on a regular basis. Keeping her glasses in proper working order, free from scratches, and fitting well is imperative. Other strategies Mrs. Wilson can use include the following:

To minimize glare in the home:
    a. Adjust curtains, use sheers to filter out the light.
    b. Avoid highly waxed or glossy floors.
    c. Avoid facing the sunlight.
    d. Wear sunglasses.
    e. Use only incandescent light bulbs.

To improve vision:
  a. Wear corrective lenses as prescribed.
  b. Use a magnification device.
  c. Read larger-print editions of favorite books or magazines.

To aid with depth perception difficulties:
  a. Differentiate between harder and softer surfaces with the use of colors.
  b. Avoid rearrangement of furniture.

The use of community resources and volunteer agencies may be of assistance to Mrs. Wilson. Service organizations offer transportation, books on tape, and large-print editions of books. When dealing with older adults, encourage independence through health promotion and disease prevention.

2. Mr. Thomas is a 72-year-old client who exhibits a blank, dull affect, a hesitancy to communicate, and a tendency to speak loudly when spoken to. Physical examination should be focused on what potential problem area for this client?

Answer: Mr. Thomas is probably experiencing a hearing disorder. The nurse must perform a bilateral hearing examination to identify his problem. After data is collected, the nurse will be able to formulate a nursing diagnosis and develop a plan of care.

3. Mrs. Tillis lives in a two-room apartment on the second floor. During your home visit you notice there is a single light over the stairwell. The client's apartment is painted in a dull gray, with throw rugs throughout. Mrs. Tillis is 80 years of age and lives alone. What recommendations might you make to improve the safety of Mrs. Tillis' environment?

Answer: Mrs. Tillis' environment requires a few major adjustments to increase her safety and help prevent serious injuries.
  a. Contact the landlord and request lighting improvements in the hallway.
  b. Install an exterior light over the threshold of Mrs. Tillis' door.
  c. Repaint the walls in bright colors, which will add brightness to the living area.
  d. Move any cords, such as extension cords, that can be easily tripped over.
  e. Remove throw rugs.
  f. Use paint to differentiate between walls and floors.
  g. Add incandescent lighting to brighten the environment.

EDUCATIONAL STRATEGIES

1. Review the anatomy and physiology of the nervous system, particularly with respect to the major senses—sight, hearing, touch, smell, taste, and position sense.

2. Discuss common sensory alterations that the nurse might encounter in client situations.

3. Describe sensory deprivation and overload and its recognition in clients. Ask students to provide examples of health care situations that might contribute to these problems.

4. Review the assessment of a client's sensory status, including health promotion behaviors and medical history. Ask students how a clients' sensory abilities can be detected through observation of everyday behavior and interactions.

5. Identify clients who are at risk for sensory alterations.

6. Have students complete a sensory assessment with a peer, family member, friend, or client and report and record the findings.

7. Assign students to observe clients in a health care setting and note the amount and type of stimuli present.

8. Discuss methods of communication that can be used with individuals experiencing sensory deficits. Have students investigate and report on available resources within the health care agency for facilitation of communication with clients.

9. Have students modify an actual or simulated client environment to meet optimum safety and stimulation requirements. Students should consider the scheduling of client care activities to avoid overstimulation.

10. Arrange for students to participate in vision and hearing screenings in a community setting, such as a school, clinic, or pediatrician's office.

11. Invite a speech and/or occupational therapist to speak to the class about promoting the client's self-care abilities and communication.

12. Stimulate a discussion on the importance of promoting sensation/stimulation, especially touch, for the older client in an extended care setting.

13. Organize a role-playing experience for the students based on the following, or similar, scenarios:
    a. Helping a visually impaired individual to maintain independence in activities of daily living and medication administration
    b. Communicating with a hearing-impaired client
    c. Caring for a client on isolation precautions

Supervision of these exercises is recommended if students will be playing sensory-impaired clients.

14. Assign students to observe or participate in the clinical care of clients who have the potential for, or an actual, sensory alteration. Focus on the students' communication techniques and their interventions for promotion of client safety. Review the students' interactions, noting the degree of sensory stimulation provided and the client's responses.

15. Have students complete a care plan/pathway for clients experiencing a sensory alteration.

INDEPENDENT LEARNING

1. Students should review the normal anatomy and physiology of the sensory systems.

2. Students should investigate available community agencies that are specifically designed to assist clients with sensory deficits.

3. Students can think about how they would need to adapt if they experienced a sensory deficit. Students should note areas that must be adapted in the home to better cope with the deficit.

4. Students should complete the Home Care Safety Checklist to determine the safety of their own homes or those of their clients.

STUDENT RESOURCES

Sensory Alterations

Alteration	Description
Sensory deficit	
Sensory deprivation	
Sensory overload	

Promotion of Sensory Function

Strategies	Nursing Intervention
Screening	
Assistive aids	
Meaningful stimulation	
Safe environment	
Communication	

Home Care Safety Checklist

This checklist will guide you in surveying the safety of your home. There may be items you can think of that are missing from the list. Although items are listed for particular areas or rooms, check to see if the safety tip applies for other parts of the house as well.

Front and Back Entrances

Yes No

___ ___ Is your house address easy to see so that your home can be found in case of an emergency?

___ ___ Are walkways to the front and back doors even and free from holes or cracks?

___ ___ Are home entrances well lighted, including walkways?

___ ___ Do you have nonskid strips, safety, treads or rough textured paint on outdoor steps?

___ ___ Are doormats in good repair with a nonskid backing and a tapered edge?

___ ___ Is there a sturdy handrail on both sides of the stairs leading to entrances?

___ ___ Are steps in good condition with even, flat surfaces?

Kitchen

Yes No

___ ___ Do you wear clothing with short or close-fitting sleeves while you are cooking?

___ ___ Do you always stay in the kitchen when cooking?

___ ___ Do you have a loud timer to remind you when food is cooked?

___ ___ Do you keep the stove top and oven clean and grease-free?

___ ___ Do you keep towels, potholders, and curtains away from burners and the oven?

___ ___ Are the stove control dials easy to see and use?

___ ___ Is an easy-to-use fire extinguisher close at hand?

___ ___ Are there emergency numbers for police, fire, and poison control posted on or near the telephone?

___ ___ Do you keep towels, potholders, and curtains away from burners and the oven?

___ ___ Do heat-producing appliances, such as a toaster or iron, have an automatic "off" feature?

___ ___ Can you reach regularly used items in the kitchen cabinets and shelves without climbing to reach them?

___ ___ Is there adequate lighting over the sink, stove, and work areas?

___ ___ Do you wipe up spills on the floor immediately?

___ ___ Are kitchen throw rugs and mats slip-resistant?

Bathrooms

Yes No

___ ___ Can the bathroom door lock be unlocked from both sides of the door?

___ ___ Are the tub and shower equipped with nonskid mats, abrasive strips, or surfaces that are not slippery?

___ ___ Does the bathroom floor have a non-slip surface or a rug with a nonskid backing?

___ ___ Do you avoid use of slippery bath oils when bathing?

___ ___ Do the bathtub and shower have at least one grab bar?

___ ___ Is the grab bar a different color than that of the wall?

___ ___ Are you careful to not place towels on grab bars?

___ ___ Is your bathroom well ventilated to prevent moisture buildup on floors?

___ ___ Are the soap dishes recessed?

___ ___ Are your water faucets clearly marked "cold" and "hot"?

___ ___ Is the water temperature on the water heater 120°F or lower?

Living Room or Family Room

Yes No

___ ___ Are electrical cords removed from under furniture or carpeting?

___ ___ Has the chimney been cleaned within the past year?

___ ___ Can you turn on a light without having to walk into a dark room?

___ ___ Are lamp, extension, or phone cords kept out of the way of traffic?

Home Care Safety Checklist—cont'd

Living Room/Family Room—cont'd

Yes No

___ ___ Are hallways and walkways free from objects and clutter?

___ ___ Are loose area rugs securely attached to the floor and not placed over carpeting?

___ ___ Are your rugs low pile instead of shag?

___ ___ Is furniture arranged in each room so that you are able to walk around easily?

___ ___ Is all furniture steady and without sharp edges?

Around the House

Yes No

___ ___ Are all living areas well lighted?

___ ___ Are windows easy to open and close?

___ ___ Is flooring or carpeting throughout the house in good repair?

___ ___ Are all thresholds level with the floor or no more than $\frac{1}{2}$ inch in height?

___ ___ Are stairways well lighted?

___ ___ Is there a light switch at both the top and bottom of the stairs?

___ ___ Does lighting produce glare or shadows on the stairs?

___ ___ Do handrails run continuously from the top to the bottom on entire flights of stairs?

___ ___ Are sturdy handrails fastened securely on both sides of stairways?

___ ___ Are step coverings in good condition?

___ ___ Are carpet or rubber stair treads securely tacked down?

___ ___ Are all stairs kept free of clutter?

___ ___ Are telephones conveniently located so you don't have to hurry to answer one?

___ ___ Are numbers on the phone large enough to read easily?

General Fire Safety

Yes No

___ ___ Do you have properly working smoke detectors?

___ ___ Do you routinely check detector alarms to be sure batteries are good?

___ ___ Do you have several emergency exit plans in case of fire?

___ ___ Do you practice an exit plan?

___ ___ Is the furnace area free of things that can catch on fire?

___ ___ Do you use portable space heaters?

___ ___ Do you keep any portable space heaters at least 3 feet away from flammable items?

General Electrical Safety

Yes No

___ ___ Do all extension cords carry a proper load, as indicated by the rating labeled on the cord and the appliance to which it is attached?

___ ___ Do you use extention cord or outlet extenders with a built-in circuit breaker or fuse?

___ ___ Are electrical cords kept away from water?

___ ___ Are any electrical cords frayed or damaged?

___ ___ Do all outlets and switches have cover plates?

___ ___ Do you use lightbulbs that are the correct wattage for each lamp?

___ ___ Is your fuse box easy to get to and clearly labeled?

___ ___ Are lamp switches easy to turn so you avoid burns from hot bulbs?

CROSS-CURRICULUM GUIDE

Clients of all ages and experiencing a wide variety of health deviations may be subject to sensory alterations when placed in a health care setting. Awareness of client responses should be incorporated into discussions before clinical experiences.

Medical/Surgical: Certain disease processes, other than those directly related to the senses themselves (e.g., glaucoma), place the client at an increased risk for sensory alterations/deficits. These include diabetes mellitus, tumors, infectious processes, and circulatory insufficiency. Some medication such as aspirin and selected antibiotics and diuretics, can also contribute to the development of sensory problems.

Gerontological: Older clients can be more prone to sensory alterations, especially in circumstances where they are immobilized or isolated.

CHAPTER 40

Surgical Client

CRITICAL THINKING ACTIVITIES AND ANSWERS

1. Mr. Wilson is a 76-year-old client admitted for a fractured hip. He has a history of emphysema. What risk does Mr. Wilson face as a result of surgery and why?

Answer: Mr. Wilson is at increased risk from surgery for the development of respiratory and circulatory complications as a result of his age, emphysema, and fractured hip. Physiological changes occurring with age, such as increased rigidity of the rib cage, reduced movement of the diaphragm, and stiffening of lung tissue, result in decreased vital capacity, reduced oxygenation of blood, and impaired excretion of anesthetic agents. Emphysema also impairs gas exchange, which will further decrease tissue oxygenation. Fractures of large bone increase the risk for development of emobli.

2. Mary is the nurse working in the preadmission center for surgical services. She is interviewing Mrs. Rice, who states that she has been taking one baby aspirin every day to help with her circulation. Why is this important for Mary to document?

Answer: Mrs. Rice has been taking aspirin, which acts to decrease platelet aggregation. Although Mrs. Rice is taking only one baby aspirin per day, there is the potential for a decreased ability of the blood to clot and an increased risk for bleeding and hemorrhage during and after surgery. It would be wise to evaluate Mrs. Rice's prothrombin time (PT), partial thromboplastin time (PTT), and platelet counts to determine if the clotting ability of her blood has been compromised.

3. Angie is a nursing student assigned to Mrs. Lyons, a 45-year-old woman who is recovering from surgery for a colon resection. It is the third day after surgery, and Mrs. Lyons' NG tube was removed yesterday afternoon. During her morning rounds Angie is assessing Mrs. Lyons and finds that her abdomen is distended. What might his indicate?

Answer: General anesthesia and the manipulation of Mrs. Lyons' intestines during the colon resection decreases peristalsis. After removal of the NG tube used for decompression, it is important to assess for adequate bowel motility. Abdominal distention can indicate a paralytic ileus, which is a bowel obstruction that requires the reinsertion of the NG tube.

4. Mr. Pulley had a colon resection yesterday and has a midline incision that extends from the xiphoid process to the symphysis pubis. Carmen has been assigned as his nurse and assesses rales when auscultating his lungs. What information regarding Mr. Pulley's incision must Carmen consider in planning interventions to address the nursing diagnosis of *ineffective airway clearance?*

Answer: Midline abdominal incisions cut through the abdominal muscles, which are used for diaphragmatic breathing. Diaphragmatic breathing promotes full lung expansion, helps to reinflate collapsed alveoli, and mobilizes secretions. Controlled coughing and using an incentive spirometer are other interventions that help to prevent atelectasis and pooling of pulmonary secretions. Clients with midline incisions guard their incisions due to incisional pain and do not fully expand their lungs. Therefore interventions such as timely administration of pain medications, positioning, and splinting the incision help them to accomplish full diaphragmatic excursion.

EDUCATIONAL STRATEGIES

1. Discuss the different classifications (e.g., major, minor, emergency) of surgery and the associated nursing care approaches.

2. Ask students how the nursing assessment and its focus should be altered depending on the location of, and circumstances surrounding, a client's surgery (e.g., same-day or emergency procedures).

3. Describe the components of a comprehensive preoperative nursing assessment of the client, including the following:
   a. Past medical history
   b. Prior surgeries
   c. Medication history
   d. Allergies
   e. Smoking habits
   f. Alcohol/substance abuse
   g. Family support
   h. Occupation
   i. Preoperative pain
   j. Emotional status
   k. Sociocultural background/practices

Ask students how responses from the client to each area can influence the operative experience and determine the nurse's interventions, follow-up, and reporting.

4. Review the preoperative physical assessment. Discuss how findings can influence the client's operative experience and determine the nurse's interventions, follow-up, and reporting (e.g., elevated temperature, decreased respirations).

5. Identify client risk factors that can affect the surgical experience. Have students provide specific examples of how the risk factors might influence the client's experience.

6. Discuss preoperative laboratory and diagnostic tests that can be ordered for client evaluation.

7. Describe general client preparation, education, and nursing responsibilities in the preoperative phase. Ask students how these preoperative interventions might be altered/adapted for the client having ambulatory or same-day surgery.

8. Review the legal parameters and nursing accountability associated with informed consent. Ask students what they should do if the client does not demonstrate an understanding of the surgical procedure and its potential complications or if the client is unconscious and requires emergency surgery.

9. Identify and describe the purposes of preoperative teaching for the client and family.

10. Explain and demonstrate (using educational media, simulation mannequins/models and/or student volunteers, and appropriate equipment) the following perioperative nursing interventions:
    a. Teaching postoperative exercises
    b. Inserting and maintaining a nasogastric tube
    c. Applying antiembolism stockings and sequential compression stockings

Have students practice the implementation and documentation of these techniques with their peers in the skill laboratory.

11. Evaluate students' ability to implement the perioperative techniques through return demonstration/skill testing before their clinical experience.

12. Ask students to share personal or family experiences with surgery. If the experiences were negative, ask if a nurse could have done something to improve the situation.

13. Describe the common physical preparations of the client before surgery, including promotion of fluid and electrolyte balance, skin preparation, bowel and bladder preparation, and promotion of rest and comfort.

14. Review the preparation of the client on the day of surgery, including the following:
    a. Completion of the preoperative checklist
    b. Monitoring of vital signs
    c. Provision of hygienic care
    d. Check of hair and cosmetics
    e. Removal and storage of prostheses
    f. Preparation of bowel and bladder
    g. Application of antiemboli stockings/compression device
    h. Provision of privacy and dignity
    i. Implementation of special procedures (e.g., nasogastric tube)
    j. Storage of valuables
    k. Administration of preoperative medications
    l. Maintenance of client safety

15. Ask students how the preparation for surgery can be adapted for clients of different ages or who speak other languages, have no family support, have specific spiritual or cultural needs, or have a psychiatric history.

16. Have students role-play the preparation of a client and the transport to the operating room.

17. Have students prepare an actual or simulated client room for the acute care postoperative phase.

18. Discuss the intraoperative phase, including the immediate preparation of the client, introduction of anesthesia, client positioning, documentation, and roles of the members of the operating room team.

19. Identify and describe the different types, uses, and risks of anesthesia, and the nursing care that is associated with their use.

20. Discuss the postoperative phase, including transfer to the postanesthesia care unit (PACU), client monitoring, nursing interventions to support vital functions, and critical documentation. Ask students to indicate specific assessments that the nurse in a PACU should conduct to determine overall client status.

21. Have students identify similarities and differences in postoperative/PACU care for clients in an acute care or ambulatory surgery center.

22. Discuss discharge criteria in the PACU for clients returning to an acute care unit or to their homes.

23. Describe postoperative care of clients in the acute care setting.

24. Identify nursing interventions for clients in the postoperative phase for maintenance of respiratory function, prevention of circulation stasis, and promotion of nutrition, elimination, wound healing, rest, comfort, self-concept, and self-care abilities.

25. Discuss postoperative complications and ask students to identify how they can be discovered.

26. Invite a nurse who practices in an operating room or PACU to speak to the class about client assessment and preparation for surgery or discharge.

27. Assign students to accompany clients, if possible, through the intraoperative phase to observe client preparation, surgical asepsis, and nursing roles. Have students share their observations after the experience.

28. Assign students to observe or participate in the care of clients in a PACU. Have students monitor clients' status and provide and document nursing interventions, with supervision. Have students collaborate with the nursing staff on client discharge from the PACU.

29. Assign students to observe or participate in the nursing care of clients on a postoperative unit in an acute care facility. Work with students to prepare and conduct preoperative client teaching. Discuss and supervise the assessment of the client and the appropriate preoperative and postoperative nursing interventions.

30. Have students complete a general care plan/pathway for a surgical client. Have students individualize the care plan for an actual client in an ambulatory or acute care surgical setting.

31. Using the following or similar situations, have students identify interventions that the nurse should implement:
    a. A client, on the day of surgery, who has no blood work or x-rays noted
    b. A client in the PACU who has an erratic breathing pattern or saturated dressings
    c. A client experiencing a significant decrease in urination 2 days postoperatively
    d. A client with an elevated temperature 2 or 5 days after surgery
    e. A client who will not cough or deep breathe because of incisional pain
    f. A client who will be discharged to home following eye surgery

INDEPENDENT LEARNING

1. Students should investigate the types of anesthesia that are commonly used for surgical procedures and the potential adverse reactions and nursing responsibilities for each type.

2. Students should investigate the types of surgery that are usually performed in an outpatient/ambulatory surgery center. They can compare those with procedures that are usually performed in an acute care facility.

3. Students can research an article in a current nursing journal on legal implications and situations that might arise in the perioperative environment.

4. Students can inquire about a family member's or friend's prior surgical experiences to get the client's perspective.

STUDENT RESOURCES
Surgical Risk Factors

Risk Factors	Rationale for Risk
Age	
Nutrition	
Obesity	
Radiotherapy	
Fluid/electrolyte balance	
Medical conditions	
Allergies	
Medications	
Alcohol/controlled substance	
Cognitive function	

Preoperative Nursing History

Focus Area	Implications of Findings
Medical conditions	
Prior surgery	
Medications taken	
Allergies	
Smoking habits	
Alcohol/substance use	
Client expectations	
Family support	
Occupation	
Feelings	
Cultural factors	
Coping resources	
Body image	

Acute Care Nursing Interventions
for the Surgical Client

Focus Area	Nursing Interventions in the PACU	Nursing Interventions on the Postoperative Unit
Respiration		
Circulation		
Temperature control		
Neurological function		
Wound/dressing care		
Gastrointestinal fnction		
Urinary function		
Fluid/electrolyte balance		
Comfort		

CROSS-CURRICULUM GUIDE

Students should be referred to information on and techniques for the care of the surgical client before their clinical experiences in the acute care or ambulatory operative setting or in labor and delivery. Because an increasing number of clients are having ambulatory surgery, preoperative and postoperative client care and education can also be integrated into discussions on home care nursing.

MULTIMEDIA RESOURCES

Mosby's Nursing Skills Video Series
    Set II: *Preoperative Skills*
                  Postoperative Skills

Answers to Case Study Questions and Self-Tests

CHAPTER 1

Case Study

a. This is an individual entering her middle adult years who is experiencing stress in her personal and professional life. Ms. J. has been called upon by her employer and her daughter to meet their expectations, and she believes that this does not allow her the time to meet her health needs. The symptoms of gastrointestinal distress might be a response to the pressures in her life.

b. Initially, the nurse can spend time with Ms. J. to discuss her personal feelings and needs. She might benefit from being taught stress reduction and relaxation techniques, along with a review of time management. The nurse can investigate with Ms. J. if there are support people at work and in the neighborhood to assist her in keeping up with her busy schedule. Ms. J. can also be assisted in making an appointment for medical follow-up to determine her current health status.

Self-Test

1. e

2. d

3. c

4. b

5. a

6. Holistic nursing interventions include music therapy, reminiscence, relaxation therapy, therapeutic touch, and massage therapy. These interventions can be used to provide distraction, reduce pain, relieve anxiety or tension, and promote sleep. Therapeutic touch requires advanced training and is used to decrease pain, increase circulating hemoglobin, decrease headaches, and relieve anxiety and stress.

7. Active strategies for health promotion can include programs for weight reduction, smoking cessation, nutritional guidance, and exercise. Passive strategies for health promotion include fluoridation of drinking water and fortification of foods, such as milk, with vitamins.

8. Genetic and physiological factors include pregnancy, excess weight, and family history of a condition (e.g., diabetes, cancer, or heart disease). Age increases the risk of birth defects and complications in pregnancies of women over age 35, some kinds of cancer (e.g., prostate) in individuals over age 45, and susceptibility to infection in very young and older age.

9. b

10. c

CHAPTER 2

Case Study I

a. You can tell the neighbor that managed care is a type of program where the health needs of the client are funneled through to one party—the case manager. The design of this program is to control the cost of health care services while maintaining quality. Specific guidelines are in place for the type of services covered, length of hospital stay, and access to specialty care. An HMO (health maintenance organization) is a type of managed care program where the focus is on primary care. Usually a comprehensive number of services are provided, either in one location or by different providers specified by the organization.

b. You could review the HMO book with your neighbor in order to clarify some of the terms and conditions of the coverage, which may be confusing for someone without any experience with the health care delivery system. If there are specific questions, the neighbor could be referred to an information telephone number for the program.

Case Study II

a. This client should be eligible for Veteran's Administration benefits and may be referred to the Veterans Affairs Department to receive further information.

b. He could be admitted to a military or Veteran's Administration hospital for ongoing treatment.

Case Study III

a. This client could benefit from the services of a hospice organization for either home care or inpatient care, depending on the program.

Self-Test

1. f

2. h

3. i

4. j

5. g

6. e

7. a

8. b

9. d

10. c

11. Services usually provided by a home care agency include wound care, respiratory care, vital-signs monitoring, promotion of nutrition and elimination, rehabilitative care, medication administration and intravenous therapy, and laboratory study collection and monitoring.

12. Hospice

13. Issues in health care delivery include the following:
   a. Cost control—resulting in staff reduction and limited resources, providing a challenge for the health care professional to continue to offer quality care.
   b. Access to health care—consumers desiring appropriate, cost-effective, quality care within the community.
   c. Accountability—consumers demanding quality and results of interactions.
   d. Professional topics—increased need for diversified nursing competencies, work redesign, and delegation to unlicensed assistive personnel.

14. Patient-focused care involves bringing all care providers and services to the client with the goal of improving the effectiveness of care and client satisfaction. The nurse plays a major part in coordinating client care. Cross-trained personnel can provide multiple services and reduce the number of staff with whom the client will interact in the agency. More emphasis is placed on professional nursing activities (e.g., teaching, client assessment) than on ancillary functions such as bedmaking.

15. b

CHAPTER 3

Case Study

a. The new registered nurse (RN) should consider the clients who are on the unit, with respect to the type of care that they will require regularly. In addition, the backgrounds and experience of the co-workers will determine how each individual will contribute to overall client care.
b. This nurse can use a variety of leadership styles but might find that, as a new staff member with limited experience, democratic and/or situational styles will be most effective.
c. Based on the educational background of the staff and the number of clients on the unit, the new RN may recommend a team nursing model.

Self-Test

1. i

2. j

3. g

4. h

5. f

6. a

7. b

8. c

9. d

10. e

11. The three key elements in decentralized decision making are responsibility, authority, and accountability.

12. Responsibilities of the nurse manager include the following:
    a. Assisting staff in establishing goals and the systems necessary to accomplish the goals
    b. Monitoring professional nursing standards of practice on the unit
    c. Developing an ongoing staff development plan
    d. Recruiting new employees
    e. Conducting routine staff evaluations
    f. Establishing oneself as a role model for positive customer service
    g. Submitting staffing schedules for the unit
    h. Conducting regular client rounds and rounds with physicians
    i. Establishing and implementing a quality improvement plan for the unit
    j. Reviewing and recommending new equipment needs for the unit
    k. Conducting regular staff meetings
    l. Establishing and supporting staff and interdisciplinary committees

13. Time management principles include the following:
    a. Goal setting—reviewing both client and one's own goals, including documentation, treatments, meetings, and conferences.
    b. Time analysis—keeping track of how time is spent accomplishing different activities, including preparation time and actual implementation.
    c. Priority setting—establishing the most important activities, and time frames for those activities, for client and oneself.
    d. Interruption control—focusing on completion of identified activities, with plans for talking to and assisting colleagues.
    e. Evaluation—reflecting on how effectively time was used for client and one's own activities.

14. d

15. b

CHAPTER 4

Case Study

a. The nurse might choose to return to the office to obtain supplies and make a later visit to this client, if there are other visits to make or there is work to be done at the office. This option will, however, take time away from the nurse and extend her visiting hours. She could choose to purchase the necessary items from a local pharmacy but might not have the necessary funds or be able to be reimbursed for this purchase. It might be most appropriate for the nurse to investigate what alternative resources are available in the client's home, such as clean cloths, boiled water, salt, and tongs (all used with client permission).

b. The nurse should determine what resources the client has in the home, including running water, waste disposal, and methods for heating and refrigerating. In addition, a financial screening should be done, if indicated, to determine available funds and/or insurance coverage for supplies and equipment.

Self-Test

1. e

2. d

3. b

4. c

5. a

6. d

7. b

8. d

9. b

10. c

CHAPTER 5

Case Study

a. The nurse should obtain additional data about Mr. B.'s medical history and current health status. Mr. B. might be seeing a physician or other primary care provider and have medication prescribed for hypertension.

b. A community health fair allows for general screening of large numbers of people but does not usually offer the opportunity or space for privacy to complete health histories or physical assessments. Individuals demonstrating alterations from expected norms, such as Mr. B., should be referred to clinics, personal physicians, or other health care delivery agencies, as appropriate.

Self-Test

1. d

2. e

3. c

4. a

5. b

6. Strategies for effective communication include the following:
   a. Being silent—sitting with the client who is crying or dealing with feelings and concerns.
   b. Listening attentively—showing interest in the client who is discussing concerns or sharing family information.
   c. Conveying acceptance—letting the client know that he or she may continue with a subject, saying, "Go on" or "Tell me more."
   d. Asking related questions—asking in language that is understandable to the client how certain events or feelings are associated with his or her current status.
   e. Paraphrasing—taking what the client has stated and putting it in other words for the nurse and the client to hear again.
   f. Clarifying—asking the client to verify that the meaning of the statements is clear.
   g. Focusing—directing the attention of the client to a particular idea in the discussion.
   h. Stating observations—letting the client know what the nurse has observed during the discussion, such as anxiety-related movements or expressions of pain.
   i. Offering information—giving the client information about the health care system, prescribed therapies, available community resources, and so on.
   j. Summarizing—bringing together all the data obtained, highlighting the key points, and allowing the client to validate the information.

7. The three phases of the interview are the orientation phase, working phase, and termination phase.

8. a. Inspection—visual observation of the body's external structure and function, such as the condition of the skin and mucous membranes and the ability to move the muscles and joints.
   b. Palpation—use of the hands to determine temperature, texture, pulsations, and the presence of tenderness or masses.
   c. Percussion—tapping on specific surface areas of the body to produce vibration and sound that indicates the presence of air, fluid, or solid matter.
   d. Auscultation—listening with a stethoscope to sounds produced by the heart, lungs, and gastrointestinal system.

9. d

10. a

CHAPTER 6

Case Study

a. The relevant assessment data obtained from Mr. B. includes the following:
   • Newly diagnosed with hypertension
   • New prescription of an antihypertensive medication
   • Insecurity about the medication regimen
   • Father's death at age 54 from a heart attack
b. Nursing diagnoses for Mr. B. may include the following:
   • Knowledge deficit related to unfamiliarity with the diagnosis and treatment of hypertension
   • Knowledge deficit related to newly prescribed medication
   • Fear related to possible repeat of father's medical history and early death

Self-Test

1. e

2. d

3. c

4. a

5. b

6. The steps of the nursing diagnostic process are analysis and interpretation of data, identification of client needs, and formulation of nursing diagnoses.

7. a

8. b

9. c

10. d

CHAPTER 7

Case Study

a. Sample diagnoses, goals, and outcomes for Mr. B.—see bottom of page.

b. Nursing interventions may include the following:

For knowledge deficit:
- Assess Mr. B.'s willingness and readiness to learn about his diagnosis and medication regimen.
- Identify and present appropriate information about hypertension and the medication regimen.
- Establish an environment and strategy for teaching Mr. B. that is conducive to learning.
- Provide effective learning materials, including pamphlets, videos, photos, and charts.

For fear:
- Assess the degree of Mr. B.'s fear.
- Observe nonverbal and verbal responses.
- Listen to Mr. B.'s concerns and feelings.
- Provide information on coping mechanisms to assist in reducing his level of fear.
- Offer referral to a support program or counseling, as indicated.

Nursing Diagnoses	Goals	Expected Outcomes
Knowledge deficit related to newly prescribed medication (as manifested by his verbalization of uncertainty as to how and when to take his medications)	Mr. B. will recognize the purpose of the hypertensive medication and prepare an administration schedule by the end of the clinic visit.	Mr. B. will restate the use of the antihypertensive medication and scheduling of administration during the visit.
Fear related to possible repeat of father's medical history and early death	Mr. B. will demonstrate effective coping mechanisms within the next month and will identify a reduction or elimination of the feelings of fear.	Mr. B. will discuss his concerns about his father's medical history and early death during this visit. He will acknowledge his fear of repeating this history.
Knowledge deficit related to unfamiliarity with diagnosis of hypertension	Mr. B. will make specific lifestyle alterations and participate in the treatment regimen.	Mr. B. will identify the etiology and therapeutic regimen for hypertension after the next two clinic visits.

1. e

2. d

3. b

4. a

5. c

6. Goals, outcomes, and nursing interventions for the nursing diagnoses are as follows:
   a. Knowledge deficit related to the need for postoperative care at home.
      • Goals: Perform, or obtain assistance in performing, postoperative care at home.
      • Expected outcomes: State the purpose and procedure for postoperative care. Demonstrate postoperative care before discharge.
      • Nursing interventions: Provide appropriate materials for client review of postoperative care before surgery.
      Review and demonstrate the postoperative care to client after surgery
      Observe the client's independent performance of postoperative care before discharge.
   b. Constipation related to lack of physical activity.
      • Goals: Reestablish normal pattern of elimination. Participate in specified daily physical activity to tolerance level.
      • Expected outcomes: Ambulate up and down the hallway 3 times each day. Perform active range of motion twice each day.
      • Nursing interventions: Instruct and assist client in performance of physical activity. Observe tolerance to physical activity. Assess elimination pattern daily. Promote additional measures to improve elimination, such as the intake of fluids and fiber.

7. The steps in the consultation process are the following:
   a. Identification of the general problem area
   b. Direction of the consultant to the appropriate professional
   c. Provision of pertinent information about the problem area to the consultant
   d. Instruction not to bias the consultant
   e. Discussion with the nurse requesting consultation and the consultant
   f. Incorporation of consultant recommendations into the care plan and health system

8. a

9. c

10. d

CHAPTER 8
Case Study

a. In order for his hypertension to be controlled, Mr. B. will have to take his medication on a regular basis. The nurse should focus on the implementation method of teaching. Counseling might also be involved, especially if Mr. B. is experiencing other difficulties at work or home that are interfering with his ability to manage his therapeutic regimen.

b. The nurse will have to look at the original goals, outcomes, and nursing interventions to determine what alterations might be necessary. The strategies for providing the information on Mr. B.'s diagnosis and medication might not have been appropriate. In addition, the client's fear about his father's history could have been blocking his ability to focus or influencing his degree of motivation to participate in the therapeutic plan.

1. d

2. a

3. e

4. b

5. c

6. Examples of how the nurse may use the following skills:
   a. Cognitive—knowledge of the rationale for therapeutic interventions, normal and abnormal physiological and psychological responses, and the needs of the client for health promotion and illness prevention.
   b. Interpersonal—ability to establish a trusting relationship and communicate clearly with, provide instruction and counseling to, and demonstrate sensitivity of the needs of the client, family, and significant others.
   c. Psychomotor—ability to understand the rationale for and demonstrate the physical ability to perform therapeutic skills (e.g., injections, catheter insertion).

7. The nurse must use sound judgment in determining the accuracy and appropriateness of the standing orders for the client. In addition, the nurse should have the knowledge and competency necessary to carry out each order safely.

8. Nursing care may be communicated through written or computerized documentation on the agency care plan or pathway. In addition, end-of-shift reports and nursing rounds provide an opportunity to verbally share nursing interventions with colleagues. Computerization has increased the ability of nurses to communicate interventions quickly and over long distances if necessary.

9. b

10. d

CHAPTER 9

Case Study

a. Mr. B. appears to be achieving the majority of his goals. He states that he is exercising regularly and trying to use the relaxation techniques when he feels stressed. Mr. B. also is expressing his method of coping with his father's medical history.

b. Areas for reassessment can include Mr. B.'s actual medication schedule (because his blood pressure is still slightly elevated) to determine that it is within the prescribed regimen. Determination can also be made to see if Mr. B. could benefit from additional exercise (per review with the physician) and to review the relaxation and stress management techniques.

Self-Test

1. b

2. d

3. e

4. a

5. c

6. FOCUS-PDCA is a model for process improvement that stands for the following:

   Find process to improve
   Organize team that knows process
   Clarify current knowledge of process
   Understand causes of process variation
   Select process improvement
   Plan
   Do
   Check
   Act

7. Examples of quality indicators:
   a. Outcome indicator—change in the client's status after receiving care, such as ability to perform postoperative dressing care or self-catheterization.
   b. Process indicator—manner in which care is delivered, such as the use of a nursing assessment tool or preoperative client education.
   c. Structure indicator—system for delivery of care, such as staffing patterns and compliance with inservice education requirements.

8. Factors involved in the evaluation of nursing interventions include the appropriateness of the interventions selected (per the standards of care) and the correct application of the implementation process (level of care provided, frequency of interventions).

9. c

10. b

CHAPTER 10

Case Study

In order to become a nurse-midwife, this individual will need to complete the Bachelor's degree in nursing that she has begun and progress on to a graduate program in nursing to obtain a Master's degree. Advanced practice nurses, such as nurse-midwifes, require education in advanced physical assessment, pharmacology, and clinical care in addition to expertise in their field. The American College of Nurse-Midwives offers nationwide certification for individuals who have met the criteria for practice.

Self-Test

1. j

2. f

3. g

4. i

5. h

6. b

7. d

8. a

9. c

10. e

11. Henry Street Settlement

12. Diploma program

13. Challenges for nursing in the future include the following:
    a. Ever-expanding need for new skills with new technology
    b. Cross-training
    c. Use of unlicensed assistive personnel, dele-

gation
    d. Increasing need for clinical research
    e. Increasing generalization of practice
    f. Increasing responsibility for coordination of care

14. d

15. a

CHAPTER 11

Case Study

a. The steps are as follows:

Step 1. Is this an ethical dilemma?

Review of scientific data does not resolve Ms. R's situation. Her question is perplexing, and your response and her action will have a profound relevance for human concern.

Step 2. Gather all the information relevant to the case.

Ms. R. is a 38-year-old woman with severe multiple sclerosis who is unable to perform the simplest activities of daily living. She appears to be aware of her situation and is seeking an alternative to her present lifestyle. You are her home care nurse and are aware of the client's situation.

Step 3. Examine and determine one's own values on the issues.

Use of the values clarification process may assist you in determining your own beliefs about assisted suicide and the quality and sanctity of life.

Step 4. Articulate the problem.

Ms. R. has an interest in being "helped to die," and she has involved you in a possible dilemma by asking you to assist her in getting more information about this method.

Step 5. Consider possible courses of action.

You may or may not be able to help the client with her actual pursuit of an assisted suicide because of your beliefs. In addition, the legal view on assisted suicide varies from state to state and will have to be investigated before any action is taken by you or the home care agency. A discussion with your supervisor and colleagues might assist in determining a course of action. (You should inform the client that you will be sharing this information with other members of the health team.) If Ms. R. is intent upon finding out about, and possibly pursuing, an assisted suicide, her family members (if available) might become involved.

Step 6. Negotiate the outcome.

Communicate with the client to determine if there are alternatives to her plan. Work with the client to consider all the possibilities, but respect her wish if she continues to request information and an end to her current existence.

Step 7. Evaluate the action.

The actions taken by the nurse and other members of the home care agency should be documented. Recognize that satisfaction with the outcome by both the client and the nurse might not be possible. There are no inherently right or wrong answers to these types of ethical questions. Evaluation is based on the effectiveness of working through the problem to a reasonable solution.

b. The nurse in this situation should be the client's advocate. The first step is to determine if the client is truly intent on pursuing this alternative measure. If she really is interested, then the nurse may assist her in a number of ways. Information on assisted suicide can be obtained directly or indirectly for the client. The nurse might not be able to become involved but can still be supportive of the client's decision to investigate the procedure. There are legal and ethical considerations that might inhibit the nurse from having *any* involvement, in which case Ms. R. should be referred to others who can assist her.

Self-Test

1. c

2. d

3. e

4. a

5. b

6. The four modes of values transmission are modeling, moralizing, laissez-faire, and responsible choice.

7. The steps in the values clarification process are choosing one's beliefs and behaviors, prizing one's beliefs and behaviors, and acting on one's beliefs.

8. Deontology

9. Examples of how ethical concerns may be involved include the following:
   a. Cost containment—not having enough staff or equipment because of monetary cutbacks, having limitations on coverage and benefits, or providing restricted hours and services.
   b. Cultural sensitivity—accepting a client's refusal of treatment (e.g., Christian Scientist beliefs), recognizing the need for a special diet, or showing concern for the body of the deceased.

10. a

CHAPTER 12
Case Study I

A client who does not appear to understand a procedure should not sign a consent form. The physician should be contacted to provide the information to the client. The nurse's role in this situation is to witness the consent form only if the client demonstrates an understanding of the procedure. Since the nurse will not be performing the procedure, it is not his or her responsibility to describe what will or will not be done during the surgery.

Case Study II

Any question of a written order should be clarified with the prescriber. You should not depend on the "guess" of another colleague, even if it is a supervisor. If the medication is administered according to the charge nurse's belief, and the order is not correct, then you are accountable for the result.

Case Study III

In an emergency situation, treatment may be provided to an individual without obtaining consent. If there is sufficient opportunity to obtain consent, then the divorced parent who has legal custody of the child should be contacted.

Case Study IV

You should investigate the statutes to determine what information is required to be reported for a colleague in a suspected substance abuse situation. In many places, the nurse is held accountable if he or she is knowledgeable about an impaired practitioner but does not report the situation to the Board of Nursing. In most instances, the situation is not acted upon immediately but is investigated further by the appropriate authorities.

Self-Test

1. i

2. f

3. e

4. j

5. a

6. b

7. h

8. d

9. c

10. g

11. The nurse may avoid being liable by following the standards of care, providing competent care, communicating with other health care providers, documenting fully, and developing an empathetic rapport with clients.

12. Standards of care are defined in Nurse Practice Acts by Boards of Nursing, state and federal hospital licensing laws, professional and specialty organizations, and agency policies and procedures.

13. Informed consent requires the following:
    a. The person is a competent adult.
    b. Consent is given voluntarily.
    c. Options for care are understood.
    d. Opportunity was provided for questions.
    e. A physician-client relationship exists in which risks and alternatives are explained.
    f. A nurse witnesses the client's signature.

14. The nurse is obligated to report in the following circumstances: abuse, rape, gunshot wounds, attempted suicide, certain communicable diseases, and unsafe or impaired professionals.

15. a

16. c

17. d

18. c

19. a

20. b

CHAPTER 13

Case Study

a. The following techniques can be effective for an older individual with a moderate hearing impairment:
   - Reducing background noise
   - Checking and cleaning a hearing aid
   - Speaking slowly and clearly
   - Using a low rather than high-pitched voice
   - Avoiding shouting at the client
   - Using short, simple sentences
   - Facing the client and enunciating clearly to allow for lip reading
   - Not covering the mouth while talking
   - Talking toward the unaffected ear
   - Using facial expressions and gestures

b. The following techniques can be effective for individuals who do not speak English:
   - Speaking in a normal tone of voice
   - Establishing signals or methods of non-verbal communication
   - Obtaining an interpreter familiar with the language and culture
   - Allowing time for communication to take place
   - Developing a communication board, pictures, or cards for common requests
   - Having a dictionary available for reference

c. The following techniques can be effective for an individual who is blind:
- Announcing yourself when entering the room
- Communicating verbally before touching the client
- Orienting the client to the environment
- Explaining the procedure in advance
- Having the client handle the equipment, as appropriate
- Informing the client when you are done and leaving the room

d. The following techniques can be effective for an individual of another culture who is experiencing an invasive procedure for the first time:
- Explaining the procedure in advance, using an interpreter if necessary
- Recognizing possible discomfort with exposure and maintaining privacy
- Staying with the client to provide emotional support

Self-Test

1. c

2. h

3. g

4. i

5. e

6. j

7. f

8. d

9. b

10. a

11. The levels of communication that are demonstrated are as follows:
   a. Intrapersonal level
   b. Interpersonal level
   c. Public level

12. Examples of zones include the following:
   a. Intimate zone (0 to 18 inches): holding a baby, performing a physical examination, providing hygienic care for a client, changing a dressing
   b. Personal zone (18 inches to 4 feet): sitting at the bedside, taking a client's history, teaching an individual client, exchanging information with colleagues at change-of-shift
   c. Social zone (4 to 12 feet): making rounds with a physician, sitting at the head of a conference table, teaching a small class, or conducting a support session for a small group
   d. Public zone (12 feet or more): speaking at a community forum, testifying at a hearing, lecturing to a large class

13. Examples of how communication may be adapted include the following:
   a. Communication may be adapted for a toddler as follows:
      - Allowing the child to touch and examine objects
      - Focusing communication on the child
      - Avoiding analogies, using direct language the child can understand
      - Keeping unfamiliar equipment out of sight until necessary
      - Keeping facial expressions congruent with activities
      - Using dolls, puppets, or stuffed animals to communicate
   b. Communication may be adapted for an adolescent as follows:
      - Providing undivided attention and listening closely
      - Being courteous, calm, and open-minded
      - Avoiding judgment or criticism
      - Avoiding continuous questioning
      - Making expectations clear
      - Respecting privacy and views
      - Praising positive behaviors
      - Encouraging expression of ideas and feelings
   c. Communication may be adapted for an older adult as follows:
      - Maintaining a quiet environment, free of background noise
      - Allowing time for conversation
      - Listening attentively
      - Using short, simple sentences
      - Avoiding changing the subject frequently
      - Obtaining assistance, if necessary, to promote understanding (e.g., hearing aid)
      - Facing the individual directly
      - Speaking slowly and clearly, not shouting

14. Effective strategies not being used include the following:
    a. Courtesy is not being used. The client should be called by his or her name, such as Mrs. Jones or Mr. Brown.
    b. Courtesy is not being used. The client should be identified by name, not by room number and diagnosis.
    c. Confidentiality is not being applied. The client should not be discussed outside the immediate client area where anyone not involved in the client's care can overhear the conversation.
    d. Availability is not being applied. The nurse should spend time with the client or state when he or she will return to be with the client.
    e. Avoidance of medical jargon is not being considered. The nurse should explain to the client, in understandable terms, what to expect from the procedure.

15. c

16. b

17. d

18. a

19. d

20. a

CHAPTER 14

Case Study I

    a. A transfer report should include the following information:
        • Client's name, age, primary physician, and medical diagnosis
        • Summary of medical progress up to the time of transfer
        • Current physiological and psychological status
        • Current nursing diagnoses and plan of care
        • Critical assessments to be completed shortly after transfer
        • Any special equipment required
    b. More specifically, the primary nurse might want to know about the surgical procedure: how it was tolerated by the client, how the client responded to the anesthesia, what observations were made, and what treatments were completed in the PACU.

Case Study II

Sample SOAP documentation for Mrs. Q.:

S—States she is having intense pain in her right hip area and doesn't want to move because it really hurts
O—Grimacing and moaning in pain
A—Pain related to new surgical incision in right hip and postoperative positioning
P—Reduce or eliminate discomfort by administering analgesic medication as ordered and helping client to more comfortable position

Sample DAR documentation for Mrs. Q.:

D—Client is grimacing and moaning in pain. She states that she is having intense pain in right hip and does not want to move because it "really hurts." Dressing is dry and intact.
A—Client is assisted to more comfortable position, with leg supported. Analgesic is administered per order.
R—Client expressed reduction in discomfort to tolerable level.

Self-Test

1. d

2. e

3. a

4. b

5. c

6. Oral or written exchanges of information between care givers include change-of-shift and transfer reports, nursing conferences and client rounds, documentation, and consultation.

7. The following are purposes of the client record: communication, legal documentation, financial billing, education, assessment, research, auditing and monitoring.

8. The following are guidelines for completion of an incident report:
    a. The report is completed by the nurse who witnessed the incident or found the client.
    b. Concise, objective terms are used to complete the report.
    c. No interpretations or explanations are included.

d. The client's condition is objectively described.

e. Measures taken by the nurse, other nurses, or physician at the time of the incident are reported.

f. No blame is placed on anyone in the report.

g. The report is submitted to the appropriate person in a timely manner.

h. Photocopies for personal reference are not made.

9. Correct actions to be taken by the nurse include the following:

a. Draw a single line through the error, write the word *error* above the line, initial or sign the error, and complete the correct notation.

b. Use only objective descriptions of the client and use accurate quotes for client comments.

c. Use complete, concise descriptions of client interactions.

d. Draw a single line through the error, write the word *error* above the line, initial or sign the error, and complete the correct notation.

e. Use consecutive lines for charting and do not leave margins. Draw lines through unused space and sign your name at the end of the notation.

f. Only include factual information in the notation.

g. Identify that the physician was called to clarify an order for the client.

h. Have the other care giver document the information unless the individual calls with additional information. In that case, document that the information was provided by another individual.

i. Record pertinent information throughout the shift, signing each entry.

10. d

CHAPTER 15

Case Study

a. Mr. B. has no prior knowledge about his diagnosis or prescribed medication. He also has a prior family history of coronary disease—(his father died of a heart attack at 54 years of age.

b. Sample Teaching Plan for Mr. B.:

Learning Need	Resources	Objectives	Teaching Strategies
Knowledge deficit related to newly diagnosed hypertension and antihypertensive medication therapy	Educational media: videotape, audiotape information on hypertension Written materials on the diagnosis and the medication Information from the physician and other health care colleagues Nurse's knowledge of the diagnosis and treatment regimen	Mr. B. will be able to do the following: Describe the diagnosis, etiology, treatment, and complications Describe the actions, side effects, and time of administration for the antihypertensive Identify when to contact the physician for possible complications of the diagnosis or toxic effects of the medication Independently monitor and record his blood pressure daily and as necessary Develop a meal plan for a week that incorporates his therapeutic diet	Provide Mr. B. with available educational media and written information on hypertension and antihypertensive medication. Use illustrations to explain the function of the heart and circulatory system and the effects of hypertension. Demonstrate the technique for monitoring blood pressure, and have the client or significant other return and demonstrate the procedure. Involve significant others in the educational program.

Self-Test

1. d

2. c

3. e

4. a

5. b

6. a. Specific teaching methods that can be implemented for an infant include the following: maintaining consistency in routines (bathing, feeding), holding the child firmly while smiling and speaking softly, and having the infant touch different textures.

   b. Specific teaching methods that can be implemented for a school-age child include the following: teaching psychomotor skills needed to maintain health (using a syringe, changing a dressing) and offering opportunities to discuss health problems and answer questions.

   c. Specific teaching methods that can be implemented for an older adult include the following: teaching when the client is alert and rested, involving the individual in discussion or activity, focusing on wellness and strengths, using approaches to enhance sensory input, and keeping sessions short.

Family or significant others should be involved in the teaching process whenever possible, especially when working with children.

7. The nurse should consider the following factors when selecting an environment for teaching: privacy, room temperature, lighting, noise, ventilation, furniture, and space.

8. d

9. c

10. a

CHAPTER 16
Case Study

a. This adolescent client will most likely experience alterations in his self-concept, especially the perception of his body image and identity. Adolescents can be very sensitive about their physical appearance and social status, and now the client will have to cope with an alteration in his social and athletic activity in school. In addition, the paraplegia will significantly influence his sexual functioning, an area where he may have been exploring and now will have to adapt.

b. Sample Care Plan:

Nursing Diagnosis	Expected Outcomes	Nursing Interventions
Potential body image disturbance related to accidental injury and resultant lack of mobility and sensation to lower extremities (as manifested by his frequent verbalization of prior involvement in athletics and other school activities)	Client will adapt to change in body image by the following: • Discussing feelings about his injury and change in activity status • Participating in care as much as possible • Reflecting on personal strengths	Provide time for talking with the client and discussing feelings. Explore coping skills that the client has used before, and encourage and support those skills. Involve the client in health care activities.
Altered sexual patterns related to accidental injury and resultant lack of mobility and sensation to lower extremities	Client will learn and use measures to attain sexual satisfaction within limitations by doing the following: • Discussing feelings about sexual function and adaptation • Participating in an educational program on alternate measures to promote sexual response • Sharing his response to the measures and suggesting possible alternatives	Provide time to talk with the client and discuss feelings and concerns. Provide information on sexual response and stimulation for clients with paraplegia. Obtain a referral or consultation, if indicated, for additional support and information. Have another young paraplegic man speak with the client. Provide for client privacy.

Self-Test

1. b

2. e

3. d

4. a

5. c

6. Behaviors that can indicate an altered self-concept include the following: avoidance of eye contact, excessive apologizing, hesitant speech, excessive criticizing, excessive anger, frequent or inappropriate crying, putting self down, excessive dependence, hesitance to express views or opinions, lack of interest in what is happening, passive attitude, difficulty making choices, slumped posture, and unkept appearance.

7. Ways in which the nurse may promote self-concept include the following:
   a. Health promotion setting:
      • Supporting the development of health lifestyle measures with sound nutrition, regular exercise, adequate rest and sleep, stress reduction practices
      • Providing client education
      • Assessing alterations and making appropriate referrals
   b. Acute care setting:
      • Arranging visits with someone who has experienced similar problems or changes
      • Being sensitive to and supporting the client's needs.
   c. Restorative care setting:
      • Expanding the client's self-awareness
      • Encouraging self-exploration
      • Assisting the client in self-evaluation
      • Assisting the client in forming realistic goals, becoming committed to his or her achievement, evaluating the achievement, and reforming the plan as necessary

8. Alterations in sexual health include the following: infertility, sexual abuse, sexual dysfunction, and personal and emotional conflicts.

9. Client teaching for the promotion of sexual health may include instruction about the following:
   a. Refraining from drinking alcohol 1 to 2 hours before to sexual activity
   b. Discussing behavior that provides the most sexual stimulation and satisfaction
   c. Options available for contraception
   d. Side effects of medications that alter sexual function and response
   e. Use of usual positions and selection of times when client feels rested (for individuals with cardiac dysfunction)
   f. Safe sex practices

10. False

11. False

12. c

13. b

14. d

15. b

CHAPTER 17

Case Study

a. The nurse should obtain information about the extent to which the client practices Buddhism, including whether he or she is a vegetarian, fasts and refuses treatment on holy days, avoids alcohol, and hesitates to use medications. In addition, the client's advance directives should be obtained, since life support may be removed if indicated.

b. Depending on the degree to which the client practices his or her faith, adaptations may need to be made as follows:
   • Special dietary request for vegetarian meals
   • Scheduling of treatments and tests on days that are not considered holy
   • Determination of medications that are acceptable
   • Use of medications and mouthwash that do not contain alcohol
   • Providing contact with a Buddhist monk

Self-Test

1. Religion is seen as an organized way, through rules and rituals, that the individual demonstrates his or her spirituality and belief in or worship of God(s) or Supreme Being(s). Spirituality is the totality of the individual's beliefs, including faith, hope, spiritual health, and religion. The individual does not have to be religious to have spiritual well-being.

2. Intrapersonal connectedness: being connected or in touch with oneself
Interpersonal connectedness: being connected or in touch with others and the environment
Transpersonal connectedness: being connected or in touch with the unseen, God, or a higher power

3. Possible nursing diagnoses include the following:
   a. Potential for enhanced spiritual well-being
   b. Spiritual distress
   c. Ineffective individual coping
   d. Family coping: potential for growth
   e. Altered family processes
   f. Dysfunctional grieving
   g. Anxiety
   h. Hopelessness
   i. Self-esteem disturbance

4. Christian Scientists and Jehovah's Witnesses might refuse health care interventions.

5. c

CHAPTER 18

Case Studies

a. For a client from a culture that has a matriarchy social structure, the nurse should plan to have the wife, mother, or sister involved in the plan of care and the decision-making process.

b. Involvement of the family is important in helping the client to achieve an optimal level of well-being, but there might have to be limits placed upon the number of family members who may stay in the room, a reasonable time frame for visiting to allow the client to rest and receive treatment, and a determination of where the family may gather to conduct discussions.

c. The therapeutic diet might have to be adapted to avoid meat and meat products but still provide necessary nutrients (protein) or avoid unwanted ingredients (sodium). In an acute or restorative care setting, the dietitian should be involved in providing a menu that meets the client's cultural preferences but is also tasteful, satisfying, and within therapeutic guidelines.

d. A healer can provide emotional as well as health care support for the client. The nurse should work with the health care team to integrate, as much as possible, the actions of the healer. Traditional remedies or treatments should be investigated, however, to determine if there might be any interaction with the prescribed medications or therapies.

e. To promote communication with individuals and families who speak another language, the nurse should obtain an interpreter who is proficient in that language, use word signs or charts, use appropriate titles and greetings, be attentive to nonverbal communication, and clarify uncertain areas. Do not speak louder—this will not help!

Self-Test

1. a

2. c

3. b

4. e

5. d

6. Communication with individuals from other cultures may be promoted by the following:
   a. Respecting people as individuals
   b. Not treating people differently or in a patronizing manner
   c. Not assuming their emotional or intellectual status
   d. Addressing people appropriately
   e. Not trying to impress people by using phrases or saying that you have friends from their culture
   f. Explaining medical and nursing terms in understandable terms
   g. Including family members and recognizing cultural preferences in health care
   h. Clarifying areas that are uncertain
   i. Knowing when to initiate or avoid physical contact

7. Information that may be obtained from a client include the following:
   a. Heritage assessment—the degree to which a client identifies with and follows cultural beliefs and practices.
   b. Cultural phenomena—relocation, habits, customs, valued behaviors, cultural sanctions and restrictions, language and communication process, economic and educational status, social networks, family and community support.
   c. Health traditions—healing beliefs and practices, nutritional variables, and food practices.

8. Nursing diagnoses related to cultural needs may include the following:
   a. Impaired verbal communication
   b. Ineffective family coping
   c. Altered health maintenance
   d. Impaired social interaction
   e. Noncompliance

9. False

10. False

11. d

12. b

13. d

14. c

15. a

CHAPTER 19

Case Study

a. The client, who provides the major financial support to the family, has been hospitalized with a serious health problem. His wife has maintained a traditional role as homemaker while her husband has held a job. The younger daughter has assumed a family life that appears to be more acceptable to her parents, whereas her older sister is involved in an alternative family form. The younger daughter might be more involved in her parents' life because of her family pattern.

b. The family is apparently progressing from "launching children and moving on" to the "family in later life" stage. There are elements of both stages in this situation.

c. The nurse may hold discussions with the father and mother initially, moving toward a total family meeting at a later date. Providing opportunities for family members to express their feelings about both the health care and the family situations can facilitate open communication about family structure and relationships. The family may need to be referred for ongoing counseling if there is a negative impact on the health and recovery of the client.

d. The client might have feelings about his business and family roles and his ability to resume them when he is discharged. His wife will have to be involved in the educational process in order to follow through with the plan of care. She may also have to assume a greater decision-making role with the client to maintain the economic and emotional status of the family.

e. Possible family-oriented nursing diagnoses include the following:
   • Altered family processes
   • Altered role performance
   • Ineffective family coping

Self-Test

1. b

2. d

3. a

4. e

5. c

6. The family of today is facing the following issues: decrease in family size, marriage in later life, delay of childbirth, increase in divorce, increased need for child and older adult care, alternate lifestyles and family forms, increase in working women, increase in teenage pregnancy, and increase in the older population. In addition, major concerns of the family include a change in economic status, family violence, and AIDS.

7. The differentiation between the family as context and the family as client in relation to the nurse's primary focus includes the following:
   a. Family as context: The primary focus is the health and well-being of the individual family members.
   b. Family as client: The focus is on the health and well-being of the family as a whole unit.

8. "Family hardiness" is demonstrated by the internal strength and durability of the family unit, having a sense of control over the outcomes of life events, viewing change as beneficial and growth producing, and responding actively to stressors.

9. c

10. d

CHAPTER 20

Case Study I

a. Promotion of growth and development for the hospitalized infant should include the following:
  • Having the parents or guardians provide most of the care in order to avoid interfering with the attachment process
  • Limiting the number of caregivers and following the parents' directions for care to promote trust
  • Limiting negative experiences and providing pleasurable sensations

b. Promotion of growth and development for the hospitalized 5-year-old should include the following:
  • Creating a comfortable environment for the child and parents
  • Providing consistent and appropriate care if the parents are not available
  • Limiting the number of caregivers
  • Providing an environment of acceptance for regressive behavior and reassuring parents that the behavior is normal for children in this situation
  • Allowing children to examine equipment that might be used and to participate in procedures as appropriate
  • Providing comfort items, such as a tape with the parents' voices, pictures of family members, and favorite toys
  • Providing opportunities for play and social interaction with other children
  • Explaining routines in understandable language
  • Incorporating activities of daily living into the hospital routine

Case Study II

This client may benefit from reality orientation, which includes the following:
  a. Using time, date, place, and name in conversation
  b. Reinforcing reality and providing meaningful things to do
  c. Encouraging participation in activities
  d. Making sure that devices such as hearing aids and glasses are working properly
  e. Providing bowel and bladder training
  f. Reinforcing positive behaviors
  g. Being patient and allowing sufficient time for completion of activities
  h. Speaking slowly and clearly, repeating as necessary
  i. Providing clear, simple directions
  j. Maintaining a caring and stimulating environment

Case Study III

Children in this age group are usually interested in games and sports. For indoor recreation, board games, electronic games, or word games can be suggested. Hobbies and crafts are also appropriate if they stimulate and maintain the children's interest. If the children will be outdoors, supervised games such as volleyball, softball or baseball, kickball, tennis, or relay races can be organized. Some sports might need to be modified to meet the physical abilities of the age group. Swimming, bicycling, rowing or canoeing, walking, and hiking are activities that do not have to involve competition but promote exercise.

Case Study IV

Suicide is one of the main causes of death in adolescents and young adults. Parents should be aware of the following warning signs:
  a. Diminished performance in school
  b. Withdrawal from social activities with family and friends
  c. Substance abuse
  d. Changes in personality
  e. Disturbances in sleep, appetite, and usual activity levels
  f. Talking about death or suicide
  g. Giving away personal items

Case Study V

Individuals over the age of 40 should be instructed about the following recommendations for health screenings:
  a. Mammograms for women every 1 to 2 years, annually after age 50 (A baseline mammogram is usually done before age 40.)
  b. Proctosigmoidoscopic exams every 3 to 5 years and more frequently if necessary
  c. Rectal exam annually after age 40

Self-Test

1. d

2. a

3. c

4. e

5. b

6. Meanings of the terms are as follows:
  a. Growth—the measurable (quantitative) aspect of an individual's increase in physical dimensions as a result of an increase in the number of body cells.
  b. Development—the behavioral (qualitative) aspect of an individual's adaptation to the environment.
  c. Maturation—the genetically determined biological plan or sequence for an individual's growth and development.

7. The five external forces that influence growth and development are the family, peer group, life experiences, health environment, and living environment.

8. Play allows the child to develop motor, cognitive, and social skills. It also provides stimulation and an avenue for dealing with fears and frustrations. In the strange environment of the acute care center, play is an enjoyable and anxiety-reducing activity.

9. Toddlers like to explore their surroundings. This can lead to them putting unsafe foods, fluids, or items into their mouths and either choking or being poisoned. They also might try to stick objects into electrical outlets, which could result in electrocution. Their increased mobility allows them greater access to danger and makes them more prone to falls, burns, and drowning. Toddlers need to be carefully supervised in their activities. "Childproofing" the home environment is also very important. This includes covering electrical outlets, putting locks on cabinets with household chemicals or medications, and putting potentially dangerous items out of their reach.

10. Adolescents go through puberty, which is characterized by physical and sexual development. They usually experience an increase in height and weight during these years. Because of bodily changes, adolescents can have problems with skin blemishes or acne. Their psychosocial activities include greater interest in the opposite sex, development of personal and group or peer identity, sensitivity about their appearance, and investigation of careers.

11. The middle-age individual is concerned with career changes, the onset of menopause, marital changes, departure of children, and issues relating to aging parents.

12. Developmental tasks of older adults include physical changes, the loss of spouse and/or friends, a change in living arrangements, a change in relationships with their children, and the acquisition of new interests.

13. d

14. c

15. b

16. b

17. d

18. c

19. c

20. a

CHAPTER 21

Case Study

a. Mrs. R. may demonstrate the following behaviors indicative of complicated bereavement:
   - Overactivity without a sense of loss
   - Alteration in relationships with friends and family
   - Anger against particular individuals
   - Agitated depression—tension, guilt, feelings of worthlessness
   - Decreased participation in religious or cultural activities
   - Inability to discuss the loss without crying (even after a year or more)
   - False euphoria
   - Eliminating all signs of the deceased (e.g., pictures) or, conversely, creating a "shrine"
   - Alterations in eating and sleeping patterns
   - Regressive behavior

b. Possible nursing diagnoses for Mrs. R. include the following:
   - Dysfunctional grieving related to sudden loss of husband
   - Ineffective individual coping related to inability to deal with husband's suicide

   Possible goals include the following:
   - Mrs. R. will accept the reality of her husband's death.
   - Mrs. R. will renew her activities of daily living and complete a normal grieving process.

   Nursing interventions might include the following:
   - Using therapeutic communication to promote Mrs. R.'s verbalization of feelings about her husband's suicide
   - Demonstrating support of Mrs. R. by staying with her and using comfort measures such as touch
   - Referring Mrs. R. to support groups, clergy, or counseling as appropriate for her needs

Self-Test

1. The five types of loss are the loss of external objects, known environment, significant other, aspect of self, and one's own life.

2. Special circumstances that can influence grief resolution include suicide, sudden death, miscarriage or a child's death, and AIDS.

3. Examples associated with normal grieving include the following:
   a. Feelings: sadness, anger, guilt, anxiety, loneliness, fatigue, helplessness, shock, relief
   b. Cognitions: disbelief, confusion, preoccupation with or sense of presence of the deceased, hallucinations
   c. Physical sensations: hollowness in stomach, tightness in chest or throat, oversensitivity to noise, shortness of breath, muscle weakness, lack of energy, dry mouth
   d. Behaviors: sleep and appetite disturbances, absentmindedness, dreams of the deceased, sighing, crying

4. Factors that can influence a grief reaction include age, cultural or spiritual beliefs, sex roles, socioeconomic status, social support, the nature of the loss, the dying person's grief, the nature of relationships, and the goals of the individual.

5. A client who is to have surgery to remove a breast or other body part will experience anticipatory grief over the impending loss. A nurse who is working with clients who have terminal cancer or AIDS might also experience anticipatory grieving over their impending deaths.

6. Nursing interventions for the dimensions of hope include the following:
   a. Affective—showing an empathetic understanding of the client's and family members' strengths.
   b. Cognitive—offering information about an illness or treatment and correcting misinformation.
   c. Behavioral—helping the client to use personal resources.
   d. Affiliative—strengthening or fostering relationships with others.
   e. Temporal—promoting the client's experience of time and development of short-term goals.
   f. Contextual—encouraging development of achievable goals, reminiscing.

7. The nurse can involve the family or significant others of a dying client in the following ways:
   a. Helping them to schedule visits to avoid client fatigue
   b. Allowing young children to visit dying parents or grandparents
   c. Being willing to listen to complaints or other feelings about care
   d. Helping them to interact with the client

e. Helping them to get rest and "time off"
f. Supporting grieving and providing privacy as needed
g. Providing information about the client's condition
h. Communicating with them about the impending death
i. Providing a caring environment for them
j. Assisting them in decision making after death

8. b

9. c

10. c

CHAPTER 22

Case Study

a. This client might demonstrate the following:
   - Physical signs: increased heart rate, respirations, and blood pressure; headaches, fatigue, sleep disturbances, restlessness, gastrointestinal distress, weight gain or loss, backaches, amenorrhea, frequent or prolonged colds or flu
   - Psychological signs: forgetfulness, preoccupation, increased fantasizing, decreased creativity, slower reactions and thinking, confusion, decreased attention span
   - Emotional signs: crying tendencies, lack of interest, irritability, negative thinking, worrying
   - Behavioral signs: diminished activity or hyperactivity, withdrawal, suspiciousness, substance abuse, change in communication or interaction with others

b. A number of alternatives should be presented to this client so that she can select those that are most beneficial to her. The nurse can use guided imagery, biofeedback, progressive muscle relaxation, hypnosis, music or art therapy, humor, assertiveness training, and keeping a journal or diary.

Self-Test

1. c

2. e

3. a

4. b

5. d

6. The local adaptation syndrome involves a response of body tissue, an organ, or part of the body to a stressor such as trauma, illness, or other physical changes. The response is short-term and localized to one area. The general adaptation syndrome is a response by the entire body involving several organ systems. The response may continue until the individual is unable to defend against the effect of the stressor.

7. An individual's response to stress is influenced by the intensity, scope, duration, and number, and nature of the stressors that are present. In addition, the individual's level of personal control, feelings of competence, cognitive appraisal of the event, and availability of support systems will influence the response.

8. Indicators of stress include the following:
   a. Cognitive: forgetfulness, denial, increased fantasy life, poor concentration, inattention to detail, orientation to the past, decreased creativity, slower thinking and reactions, learning difficulties, apathy, confusion, lower attention span, calculation difficulties
   b. Gastrointestinal: nausea, diarrhea, vomiting, weight gain or loss, change in appetite, bleeding
   c. Behavior: change in activity level, withdrawal, suspiciousness, change in communication and interaction with others, substance abuse, excessive humor or silence, no exercise, hyperactivity
   d. Neuroendocrine: headaches, fatigue, insomnia or other sleep disturbances, feeling of uncoordination, restlessness, tremors, profuse sweating, dry mouth

9. c

10. b

CHAPTER 23

Case Study I

a. Generally, an individual who has a blood pressure reading of above 140/90 should be referred for medical follow-up. An average of two or more systolic readings above 140 mmHg, and diastolic readings above 90 mmHg are usually indicative of hypertension.

b. Additional information should be noted as to the arm used and the position (e.g., sitting, standing, lying down) of the client during the measurement, previous blood pressure readings, known medical problems, and any medical care being received or medications being taken by the client.

Case Study II

The client's pulse and blood pressure can be obtained in the lower extremities. The pulses available include the femoral, popliteal, posterior tibial, and dorsalis pedis. The blood pressure is assessed by placing the thigh-sized cuff over the posterior aspect of the middle thigh region while the client is in the prone position. The popliteal artery is used for palpation and auscultation of the blood pressure. Measurement in the lower extremities may be 10 to 40 mmHg higher in the systolic reading than that of the upper extremities.

Case Study III

A febrile client can exhibit the following signs and symptoms: increased body temperature; flushed, dry, warm skin; chills; feeling of malaise; or tachycardia. Nursing interventions for febrile clients should include the following:

a. Assessment of vital signs, especially temperature
b. Observation of client response, including skin color, temperature, and chills
c. Promotion of client comfort, responding to chills, and thirst
d. Collection of appropriate specimens, such as blood cultures
e. Promotion of rest and reduction of activities that increase heat production
f. Promotion of heat loss by removing coverings and keeping the client dry
g. Provision of care to meet increased metabolic demands, including oxygen, nutrition, and fluid requirements
h. Monitoring ongoing status

Case Study IV

If the pulse oximeter does not appear to be working, there can be a problem with light transmission or a reduction of the client's arterial pulsations. The site for measurement should be checked to determine that it is clean, warm, and dry, not directly near another light source, and receiving adequate circulation. The client should also be reminded to limit excessive motion of the extremity that is being used for measurement.

Self-Test

1. g
2. d
3. h
4. f
5. j
6. a
7. i
8. e
9. c
10. b
11. Vital signs should be taken at the following times:
    a. When the client is admitted to the health care agency
    b. On a routine schedule according to agency policy
    c. Before and after procedures, such as surgery and invasive diagnostic tests
    d. Before and after blood transfusions
    e. Before and after the administration of medications that can alter temperature regulation and cardiovascular or respiratory functioning
    f. When there are alterations in the client's status, such as change in the level of consciousness or indications of distress
    g. Before and after activities, including ambulation and exercises

12. False low readings can be obtained if the bladder or cuff is too wide, the arm is positioned above the heart level, the cuff is deflated too quickly (low systolic), the stethoscope is not working or is placed incorrectly, the assessment is repeated too quickly (low systolic), or different Korotkoff sounds are being used (low diastolic). False high readings can be obtained if the bladder or cuff is too narrow, the cuff is wrapped too loosely or unevenly around the arm, the cuff is deflated too slowly (high diastolic), the arm is not supported, or different Korotkoff sounds are being used (high systolic).

13. Conversions are as follows:
    a. $(97° F − 32) × 5/9 = 36°C$
    b. $9/5 × 38.4° C + 32 = 101.1° F$
    c. The nurse is alerted to temperature alterations of above 100.4° F or below 96.8° F on an oral Fahrenheit thermometer and measurements above 38° C or below 36° C on an oral Centigrade scale. Rectal temperature readings may be 0.9° F or 0.5° C higher than oral measurements, and axillary readings range within this same number of degrees lower than oral temperatures.

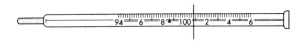

14. The pulses should be palpated as follows:

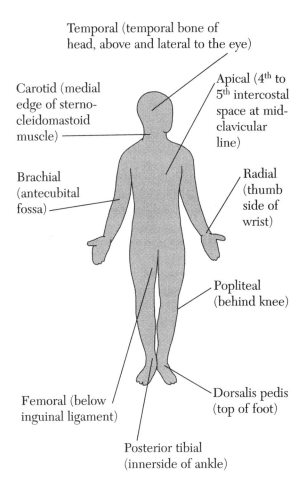

Temporal (temporal bone of head, above and lateral to the eye)

Apical (4th to 5th intercostal space at mid-clavicular line)

Carotid (medial edge of sterno-cleidomastoid muscle)

Brachial (antecubital fossa)

Radial (thumb side of wrist)

Popliteal (behind knee)

Femoral (below inguinal ligament)

Dorsalis pedis (top of foot)

Posterior tibial (innerside of ankle)

15. Aneroid scale:

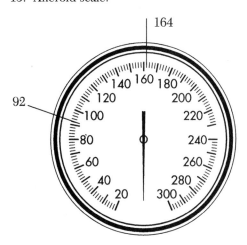

Mercury scale:

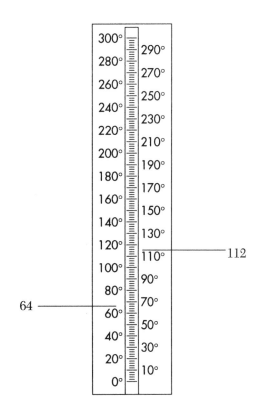

16. For older adults, the following should be considered:
    a. Temperature: usually lower, more sensitive to slight changes in self and environment, possible difficulty holding oral thermometer (with loss of teeth, muscle tone), decreased sweat gland function (prone to hyperthermia), diminished sensation to cold, and decreased insulation of subcutaneous fat (prone to hypothermia)

b. Pulse: may be difficult to palpate, arteries may feel stiff, heart rate decreased at rest, rate takes longer to return to normal after elevations, point of maximum impulse (PMI) may be difficult to palpate, sounds may be muffled. Pedal pulses may be difficult to palpate.

c. Respirations: more rigidity of the rib cage, possible spinal alterations (kyphosis or lordosis), decreased depth of respirations, increased use of accessory muscles, decreased efficiency of respiratory muscles, reduced response to increases in carbon dioxide and decreases in oxygen levels

d. Blood pressure: loss of upper arm mass, increase in BP range (particularly systolic), decreased BP after eating, sensitive to position changes (orthostatic hypotension)

17. a

18. c

19. c

20. b

CHAPTER 24

Case Study

For the 4-year-old boy, you are aware that the experience might be new and frightening. The child should be shown the assessment procedures on a doll or model while being given simple, understandable information, and he can handle the equipment that will be used (as appropriate). The exam should be conducted in a comfortable environment, with time allowed for the child to play. The child may be called by his first name, and he should be asked assessment questions that he will understand.

The older Hispanic woman may have responses to the examination that are influenced by her culture. She will need to be informed and prepared for the breast and pelvic assessments, with consideration given to her privacy. This client might desire another woman to be present during the examination or to actually conduct the examination. Care should be taken to determine that this client understands the information and instruction that is provided by an examiner who might speak only English. An interpreter may be obtained if the client is conversant in Spanish. The environment should be warm and comfortable. Ample time should be allowed for the client to answer questions and assume necessary positions for the examination.

For both clients, opportunities should be provided to use the bathroom before, during, and after the examination.

Self-Test

1. f

2. c

3. b

4. a

5. h

6. g

7. d

8. j

9. e

10. i

11. The examination should be systematic and well-organized, using a head-to-toe approach of all body systems. Both sides of the body are inspected for symmetry of appearance and function. If the client is experiencing difficulty, the area of abnormality is examined first. Adequate rest periods should be provided throughout the examination, and uncomfortable procedures should be performed near the end. Consideration should be given to the client's age and developmental status.

12. The purposes of performing a physical examination are the following:
    a. To gather baseline information about the client's health status
    b. To verify information obtained in the nursing history
    c. To verify nursing diagnoses
    d. To make clinical judgments about the client's health status and management
    e. To evaluate the physiological outcomes of care

13. Skills used in physical assessment include the following:
    a. Inspection—use of vision and hearing to detect characteristics of body parts and functions.
    b. Palpation—use of the hands to touch body parts in order to determine temperature, texture, position, and movement.
    c. Percussion—striking the body surface with the finger in order to produce a vibration and elicit sounds.
    d. Auscultation—listening to sounds created in the body organs (use of stethoscope).
    e. Olfaction—use of smell to determine the presence of characteristic odors.

14. Uses of positions for physical examination include the following:
    a. Lithotomy—examination of the external and internal female genitalia.
    b. Dorsal recumbent—examination of the head and neck, anterior thorax and lungs, breasts, axillae, heart, and abdomen.
    c. Knee-chest—examination of the rectum.
    d. Sims'—examination of the rectum and vagina.
    e. Lateral recumbent—examination of the heart.
    f. Prone—examination of the musculoskeletal system.

15. Preparation of the environment for a physical examination includes providing for privacy, adequate lighting, comfortable surroundings, and warmth. Explanations should be provided in advance, with time allowed for questions; the client should be approached in a calm and professional manner; and another individual may remain with the client during the examination if requested.

16. In a general survey, information is obtained on the client's general appearance and behavior (e.g., body type, posture, gait, hygiene, grooming, mood, speech), vital signs, height, and weight.

17. Client teaching includes the following:
    a. Skin: instruction on monthly self-examination, cancer warning signals (ABCD), reporting changes, prevention of overexposure to the sun, and treatment of dry skin
    b. Heart: instruction on risk factors for heart disease, nutritional information (fat and cholesterol reduction), and importance of medical follow-up

18. The pulses being palpated are as follows:
    a. Ulnar
    b. Posterior tibial
    c. Femoral
    d. Brachial
    e. Dorsalis pedis

19. The primary skin lesions are as follows:
    a. Papule
    b. Ulcer
    c. Macule
    d. Atrophy
    e. Wheal

20. The PMI is located in the left anterior chest wall at approximately the fourth to fifth intercostal space at the midclavicular line.

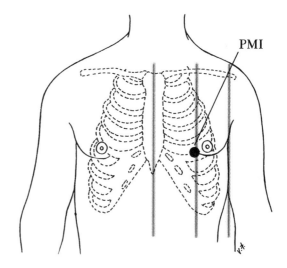

21. Common eye and visual problems include hyperopia, myopia, presbyopia, astigmatism, retinopathy, strabismus, cataracts, glaucoma, and macular degeneration. Descriptions may be found in Chapter 24 in the textbook.

22. With the use of olfaction (smell), the nurse can determine the presence of an infection, poor hygiene, gastrointestinal difficulties, acidosis, and the ingestion of alcohol.

23. The following are findings that may indicate abuse:
    a. Child Sexual Abuse
       Physical findings:
          Genital discharge, bleeding, pain, itching
          Difficulty sitting or walking
          Foreign bodies in genital tract or rectum

Behavioral findings:
Problems eating or sleeping
Fear of certain people or places
Regressive or acting out behavior
Preoccupation with own genitals
b. Domestic Abuse
Physical findings:
Injuries and trauma inconsistent with
reported cause
Multiple injuries, burns, bites
Old and new fractures
Behavioral findings:
Eating or sleeping disorders
Anxiety or panic attacks
Low self-esteem
Depression, sense of helplessness
Attempted suicide
c. Older Adult Abuse
Physical findings:
Injuries and trauma inconsistent with
reported cause
Bruises, hematomas, burns, fractures
Prolonged interval between injury
and treatment
Behavioral findings:
Dependent on caregiver
Physically and/or cognitively impaired
Combative, belligerent

24. Muscle strength can be assessed as follows:
    a. Biceps muscle strength is determined by
    pulling down on the forearm as the client
    attempts to flex the arm.
    b. Quadriceps muscle strength is determined
    while the client is sitting down, by applying
    downward pressure to the thigh while the
    client attempts to raise the leg.

25. The Glasgow Coma score for this client is 7.

    Eyes open to pain = 2

    Makes incomprehensible sounds = 2

    Demonstrates abnormal flexion of muscles = 3

    Total = 7

26. The patellar reflex is assessed with the client
    sitting and the legs hanging down freely or with
    the client lying down and supporting the knee
    in a flexed 90-degree position. The patellar ten-
    don is tapped briskly just below the patella.
    The normal response is an extension of the
    lower leg.

27. Inspection, auscultation, palpation, percussion

28. d

29. b

30. d

31. a

32. b

33. d

34. b

35. Expected or unexpected assessment findings
    are as follows:
    a. expected
    b. unexpected
    c. expected
    d. expected
    e. unexpected
    f. expected
    g. unexpected
    h. expected
    i. expected
    j. unexpected
    k. unexpected
    l. unexpected
    m. expected
    n. expected
    o. unexpected
    p. expected
    q. expected
    r. unexpected
    s. expected
    t. unexpected
    u. unexpected
    v. expected
    w. unexpected
    x. expected
    y. unexpected
    z. expected
    aa. unexpected
    bb. expected
    cc. expected
    dd. expected
    ee. expected
    ff. unexpected
    gg. expected
    hh. unexpected
    ii. expected

CHAPTER 25

Case Study I

The nurse should implement the following measures to prevent a urinary tract infection:
   a. Provide personal hygiene and perineal care.
   b. Use aseptic technique when manipulating the catheter and drainage equipment.
   c. Keep the drainage bag unobstructed and below the level of the bladder.
   d. Provide ample fluids, within client's limitations.

Case Study II

In order to prevent a wound infection, the nurse should do the following:
   a. Maintain a sterile technique during dressing changes.
   b. Use medical asepsis in all interactions with the client.
   c. Instruct the client in handwashing and asepsis.
   d. Dispose of contaminated materials appropriately and promptly.
   e. Assist in keeping the client and environment clean and dry.
   f. Limit the number of caregivers working with the client.
   g. Provide optimum nutrition and fluids, within client's limitations.
   h. Administer antibiotics, if prescribed.

Self-Test

1. j

2. e

3. f

4. i

5. c

6. b

7. h

8. d

9. g

10. a

11. The stages in the course of infection are as follow:
   a. Incubation period—interval between entrance of pathogen into the body and the appearance of symptoms.
   b. Prodromal stage of illness—interval from the onset of nonspecific signs and symptoms to more specific signs and symptoms; time when the client is more capable of spreading the disease to others.
   c. Full stage of illness—client manifests specific signs and symptoms of the infection.
   d. Convalescence—acute symptoms disappear; client begins recovery.

12. Normal flora, body system defenses, inflammation, and the immune response

13. The following are risks for nosocomial infection: multiple illnesses, compromised immune system, numerous invasive procedures or devices, use of broad-spectrum antibiotics, use of poor aseptic technique, multiple caregivers, and extended hospitalization.

14. Factors affecting susceptibility to infection include the following:
   a. Age: immaturity of the immune system in infants, greater susceptibility in children, refined defenses in adults, decline of immune system and change in organ function in older adults
   b. Nutritional status: increased susceptibility with inadequate dietary intake or reduction of protein, carbohydrates, and fats because of illness
   c. Personal habits: decreased resistance to respiratory infections from smoking, impairment of antibiotic effectiveness with alcohol ingestion, increased chance of sexually transmitted disease with risky sexual behavior (e.g., multiple partners)
   d. Environmental factors: increased exposure to pathogens through crowded and unsanitary living conditions
   e. Disease history: increased susceptibility for clients with other medical conditions or recent exposure to a communicable disease

15. Alterations in normal body system defenses include the following:
   a. Skin: cuts, abrasions, puncture wounds, insufficient or excessive bathing
   b. Respiratory tract: smoking, high concentrations of oxygen or carbon dioxide, decreased humidity, cold air

c. Urinary tract: catheterization, obstruction
d. Gastrointestinal tract: use of antacids, antibiotics, or birth control pills; impaction, obstruction

16. The proper procedure for collection of a urine sample is as follows:
    a. Apply gloves.
    b. Gather equipment—syringe (for catheter specimen) and sterile container.
    c. Instruct the client on how to obtain a clean voided specimen or aspirate urine from the indwelling catheter and transfer the urine from the syringe to the sterile container.
    d. Secure the top of the container and label and package the container per agency policy.
    e. Remove gloves and wash hands.

17. a. White blood cells (WBC): elevated in an acute infection and decreased in viral or overwhelming infections.
    b. Erythrocyte sedimentation rate: elevated with infectious processes
    c. Iron level: decreased in chronic infections
    d. Neutrophils: elevated with acute, suppurative infections and decreased with overwhelming bacterial infections
    e. Basophils: remain normal during infections

18. Infections in the home can be prevented by doing the following:
    a. Cleaning fequently in the kitchen with disinfectants (especially after using surfaces where raw meats have been cut)
    b. Discarding mops and sponges frequently
    c. Air drying, rather than towel drying, dishes
    d. Using disposable cups, utensils, and towels
    e. Keeping food properly refrigerated
    f. Washing all meats and vegetables before eating them; washing the hands and sink after handling them
    g. Thawing meats in the refrigerator
    h. Using pasteurized and processed milks and juices
    i. Cooking foods thoroughly

19. The nurse should bring an alcohol-based hand rub and/or detergent-containing towels or wipes
20. c—first; b—second and third; a —last
21. c
22. a
23. c
24. d
25. a

CHAPTER 26

Case Study I

To help this client maintain the medication regimen at home, you could create a large, colorful, easy-to-read schedule, chart, or calendar that the client can use to check off when medications have been taken. The client's medications can also be arranged, by time of administration, in a commercially available or homemade container so that the client can determine if the medications were taken as prescribed. (Some commercial devices will beep when it is time for medications to be taken.)

Case Study II

If the prescriber's handwriting is illegible, it is unsafe to make assumptions about the medication order. To avoid errors, you should contact the prescriber as soon as possible and clarify the order.

Case Study III

A client without an identification band should not receive medications. In order to verify the identity of the client, find another nurse or health care worker who is familiar with the client. Upon verifying the name of the client, obtain and provide the identification band for the client. Asking the client his or her name assists in verification but may be inaccurate if the client is not aware or oriented to the surroundings.

Self-Test

1. i
2. j
3. g
4. c
5. e
6. f
7. b
8. h
9. d
10. a
11. Federal and state legislation, State Nurse practice Acts, and agency policies and procedures

12. The following factors influence the actions of medications:
    a. Physiological variables: age, sex, weight, nutritional status, disease states
    b. Environmental conditions: stress, exposure to heat or cold, comfort of the setting
    c. Psychological factors: client's attitude, nurse's behavior

13. Definitions of terms are as follows:
    a. Side effects—secondary effects of medication, such as nausea.
    b. Toxic effects—accumulation of the drug because of impaired metabolism or excretion, usually severe in nature (e.g., myocardial depression).
    c. Anaphylactic reaction—severe allergic response, characterized by bronchiospasm, laryngeal edema, and dyspnea.

14. The routes for parenteral administration include intramuscular, intradermal, subcutaneous, and intravenous.

15. A drug order must include the following:
    a. Client's full name
    b. Date the order is written
    c. Drug name
    d. Dosage
    e. Route of administration
    f. Time and frequency of administration
    g. Signature of prescriber

16. The four common types of medication orders are the following:
    a. Standing order: carried out until prescriber cancels it
    b. Prn order: when the client requires it
    c. Single or one-time order: drug given only once at a specific time
    d. Stat order: dose of medication to be given immediately and only once

17. The nurse is knowledgeable about the medications, administers them correctly, monitors their effects, determines whether the client should receive them at a particular time, and assesses the client's ability to take the medications.

18. Right drug, right dose, right client, right route, and right time

19. The needle length is selected according to the client's height and weight and the type of injection to be given (e.g., subcutaneous or IM). A larger needle gauge may be needed for more viscous solutions. The size of the syringe is determined by the amount of medication that is to be given at one time. The usual size syringe for IM injections is 2 or 3 cc.

20. The three principles are the following:
    a. Do not contaminate one medication with the other.
    b. Ensure that the final dosage is accurate.
    c. Maintain aseptic technique.

21. Before injecting a medication, the nurse should consider the amount to be given, the characteristics and viscosity of the solution, and the location of anatomical structures.

22. The discomfort of an injection may be minimized by doing the following:
    a. Using a sharp-beveled needle of the smallest possible size
    b. Positioning the client comfortably
    c. Selecting the proper site
    d. Diverting the client's attention away from the procedure
    e. Inserting the needle quickly and smoothly
    f. Holding the syringe steady while injecting the solution
    g. Injecting the medication slowly and steadily
    h. Using the Z-Track technique
    I. Massaging the site unless contraindicated

23. The Z-Track technique should be used for medications that are irritating to the tissues.

24. The angles and types of injections are as follows:
    a. Intramuscular—90° angle
    b. Subcutaneous—45° angle
    c. Intradermal—5° to 15° angle

25. Medication may be administered intravenously through mixtures with large volumes of IV fluids, by injection (bolus) or intermittent access devices, or piggyback through an existing IV line.

26. a. $\dfrac{\text{Dose ordered}}{\text{Dose on hand}} \times \text{Amount on hand} =$
       Dose to be administered
    b. $\dfrac{\text{Child's surface area}}{1.7 \text{ m}^2} \times \text{Adult dose} =$
       Dose to be administered

27. A client having a mild allergic reaction could have urticaria (hives), a rash (eczema), itching (pruritus), or rhinitis (nasal discharge).

28. The meanings of the abbreviations are as follows:
    a. ac = before meals
    b. b.i.d. = twice a day
    c. prn = as necessary
    d. q4h = every 4 hours
    e. q.i.d. = 4 times a day
    f. stat = immediately
    g. hs = hour of sleep, bedtime

29. Volume-controlled administration set, miniinfusor pump, tandem set, and piggyback set

30. Calculations for medication orders are as follows:
    a. $\dfrac{150 \text{ mcg}}{75 \text{ mcg}} \times 1 \text{ tablet} = 2 \text{ tablets}$

To convert 0.150 mg to mcg, multiply by 1000.

    b. $\dfrac{150 \text{ mg}}{50 \text{ mg}} \times 1 \text{ ml} = 3 \text{ ml}$
    c. $\dfrac{20 \text{ mg}}{10 \text{ mg}} \times 1 \text{ ml} = 2 \text{ ml}$
    d. $\dfrac{250 \text{ mg}}{125 \text{ mg}} \times 1 \text{ tablet} = 2 \text{ tablets}$
    e. $\dfrac{75 \text{ mg}}{25 \text{ mg}} \times 0.5 \text{ ml} = 1.5 \text{ ml}$

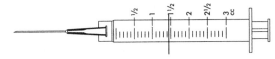

    f. $100 \text{ U} = 1 \text{ cc}$

    $\dfrac{24 \text{ U}}{100 \text{ U}} = 0.24 \text{ cc}$

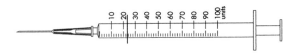

    g. $\dfrac{1.25 \text{ m}^2}{1.7 \text{ m}^2} \times 25 \text{ mg} = 18.4 \text{ mg}$

31. b

32. c

33. b

34. b

35. d

CHAPTER 27

Case Study

a. Mrs. T. should be assessed for her ability to move independently, including her posture, muscle strength, range of motion, gait (if able), balance, activity tolerance, and cognitive status. If Mrs. T. is able to bear weight on both legs and maintain an erect position, the nurse must determine if she is capable of ambulating safely. Initial assessment of Mrs. T.'s transfer out of bed should be accomplished with assistance in case that the client is unable to maintain a standing position.

b. If Mrs. T. is not able to ambulate independently, she may be able to use an assistive device, such as a cane or walker. If possible, one or more nurses can use a gait belt to assist Mrs. T. in ambulating. Should Mrs. T. not be able to ambulate safely, even with assistance, a wheelchair may be necessary. To assist Mrs. T. in gaining muscle strength, a program of exercise can be implemented.

Self-Test

1. j

2. h

3. i

4. g

5. f

6. b

7. e

8. d

9. a

10. c

11. Childhood and older adulthood

12. Physiological (e.g., musculoskeletal abnormalities, diminished cardiovascular function), emotional (e.g., anxiety, depression), pregnancy, and developmental (age and sex) factors influence activity tolerance.

13. Before and after client transfers, the nurse should do the following:
    a. Review the steps of transfer.
    b. Assess the client's mobility, strength, and cognitive status.
    c. Determine the necessary amount and type of assistance for transferral.
    d. Explain the procedure to the client.
    e. Raise the side rail on the other side of the bed.
    f. Position the bed at a safe and comfortable level.
    g. Assess the client for proper alignment and positioning.

14. Pathological conditions or events that can influence body mechanics include congenital disorders, neuromuscular diseases, musculoskeletal or neurological trauma, and prolonged immobility.

15. The devices are used as follows:
    a. Hand rolls maintain the hand, thumb, and fingers in a functional position.
    b. Hand-wrist splints are molded for the client to maintain alignment of the thumb and wrist.
    c. Trapeze bar allows the client to use the upper extremities to assist in moving around in bed, transfers, and exercises.
    d. Trochanter roll prevents external rotation of the hips.
    e. Foot board prevents foot drop by maintaining dorsiflexion of the foot.

16. The length of the crutch should be 3 to 4 finger widths from the axilla to a point 6 inches lateral to the client's heel.

17. The range of motion exercises being performed and the primary muscle groups that are involved are as follows:

a. Rotation of the neck	Sternocleidomastoid, trapezius
b. Abduction of the arm	Deltoid, supraspinatus
Adduction of the arm	Pectoralis major
c. Supination of the forearm	Supinator, biceps brachii
Pronation of the forearm	Pronator teres, pronator quadratus
d. Circumduction of the arm	Deltoid, coracobrachialis, latissimus dorsi, major
e. Hyperextension of the hip	Gluteus maximus, semitendinosus, semimembranosus
f. Flexion of the knee	Biceps femoris, semitendinosus, semimembranosus, sartorius
Extension of the knee	Rectus femoris, vastus lateralis, vastus medialis, vastus intermedius

18. c

19. b

20. a

CHAPTER 28

Case Study

a. You should assess some of the following areas regarding home safety:
   - Location of the home in the community
   - Security measures within the home
   - Environmental conditions— lighting, temperature, sanitation, stairways, floors and carpeting
   - Fire and electrical safety measures and hazards
   - Exposure to pollutants and pathogens

b. With a toddler and preschool child in the home, safety measures are extremely important. Accidents are one of the major problems for children, including falls and poisoning. If there are stairs in the home, gates should be in use or doors to the outside should be locked. For upper-level apartments or rooms, child safety devices should be in place on the windows. Any household chemicals or medications should be out of reach and locked up. There should also be locks on kitchen cabinets, drawers, and the refrigerator to prevent access. Electrical outlets should have covers, and plugs should be out of sight of the children. The family should have a fire safety plan, fire extinguishers, and smoke and fire alarms. Items that can be swallowed or broken should be out of reach. Additional safety measures should be in place in the kitchen and bathroom, such as faucet covers.

Self-Test

1. Oxygen, degree of humidity, nutrition, and optimal temperature

2. Inadequate lighting, clutter, lack of security, fire and electrical hazards

3. Air, water, noise, and land pollution

4. Diminished vision, hearing, mobility, reflexes, and circulation

5. The nurse can eliminate environmental threats by helping the client to meet basic needs, identifying and reducing physical hazards, reducing or eliminating pathogen and parasite transmission, and controlling the effects of pollution.

6. Risks for poisoning for various age groups are as follows:
   a. Toddler and preschool: hazardous substances, such as household chemicals or medicines, within reach of the curious youngster
   b. Adolescents and young adults: experimental ingestion of drugs or alcohol, suicide attempts, insect or snakebites
   c. Older adults: accidental ingestion of toxic substances because of poor vision, or overmedication due to forgetfulness

7. The objectives in the use of restraints are to reduce the risk of falls, prevent interruption of the treatment regime, prevent the removal of life support equipment (by a confused or combative client), and reduce the risk of injury to others by the client.

8. The following alternative measures may be implemented:
   a. Orienting clients and families to the surroundings
   b. Explaining routines and procedures
   c. Encouraging family and friends to stay with the client
   d. Providing adequate stimulation and diversional activity
   e. Using relaxation techniques
   f. Instituting exercise and activity plans
   g. Eliminating bothersome therapies as soon as possible
   h. Maintaining toileting routines
   i. Evaluating the effect of medications
   j. Performing regular assessments of the client's status

9. d

10. b

CHAPTER 29

Case Study I

Supplies needed for the newborn bath include the following: shirt or gown, diaper, safety pins (for cloth diaper), basin, soft washcloth, cotton balls, towel, and facial tissue. Additional supplies include: alcohol for cleaning the umbilical cord, petrolatum jelly or commercial preparation for prevention of diaper rash, and baby lotion. Plain water is best for the bath to avoid skin irritation and dryness. The newborn should be given a sponge bath until the umbilical cord falls off. The newborn should also be kept warm and covered throughout the bath, exposing only those areas that are being washed. Special care should be taken to prevent injury, including supporting the newborn's head and back, making sure the water is comfortably warm, and never leaving the child unsupervised. The sponge bath is provided in the same way as for an adult, with special attention to skin folds and creases. Eyes are wiped from the inner to outer canthus using plain water on a cotton ball. Cotton swabs are not used for cleaning the ears or nose. Fecal material can be removed with a facial tissue before washing the area. The circumcised area of the infant boy should be cleansed gently with water-moistened cotton balls. The newborn is always dried thoroughly to avoid heat loss. The diaper is placed so that it fits below the level of the umbilicus until the area is healed.

A tub bath may be given after the umbilicus is fully healed. The supplies required are the same as for the sponge bath. Special care is also given to safety, such as support of the newborn's head and back and testing of the water. The infant is lowered slowly into the tub to avoid startling.

Case Study II

The older adult client can experience changes in skin integrity. The skin is more fragile, so hot water and strong cleansing agents should be avoided. Older adults usually perspire less, so bathing does not have to be as frequent (unless personally desired). There can be an increased sensitivity or itching that might be relieved with the use of hydrocortisone cream, moisturizing soaps, or petrolatum jelly. Humidity should be higher in the environment to alleviate skin dryness. Care should be taken to avoid injury to the skin because wound healing is slower in this population.

Self-Test

1. The factors that influence hygienic care practices include body image, economic status, knowledge, sociocultural variables, personal preferences, and physical condition.

2. A back rub promotes relaxation, relieves muscular tension, stimulates circulation, and can promote a feeling of well-being.

3. Bathing allows for cleansing of the skin, stimulation of circulation, improved self-image, reduction of body odors, promotion of range of motion, and assessment of the client's integument, mobility, and state of mind.

4. The five guidelines are:
   a. Maintain privacy and dignity.
   b. Promote safety.
   c. Maintain warmth and comfort.
   d. Promote independence.
   e. Anticipate client needs.

5. Common skin problems include the following:
   a. Acne—inflammatory, papulopustular skin eruption, usually involving bacterial breakdown of sebum; appears on face, neck, shoulders, and back.
   b. Hirsutism—excessive growth of body and facial hair, especially in women.
   c. Contact dermatitis—inflammation of skin characterized by abrupt onset with erythema, pruritus, pain, and scaly oozing lesions; seen on face, neck, hands, forearms, and genitalia.
   d. Abrasion—scraping or rubbing away of epidermis; can result in localized bleeding and weeping of serous fluid.

6. Common hair or scalp problems include the following:
   a. Pediculosis capitis—tiny, grayish white parasitic insects that attach to hair strands; eggs look like oval particles, resembling dandruff; bites or putules may be observed behind ears and at hairline.
   b. Alopecia—balding patches in periphery of hair line; hair becomes brittle and broken; caused by improper use of hair care products or techniques.

7. Common foot or nail problems include the following:
   a. Tinea pedis—(athlete's foot) fungal infection of foot; scaliness and cracking of skin between toes and on soles of feet; small blisters containing fluid may appear.
   b. Paronychia—inflammation of tissue surrounding nail after hangnail or other injury; occurs in people who frequently have their hands in water; common in diabetic clients.

8. The client can be at risk for impaired skin integrity if he or she is immobile or has reduced sensation, vascular insufficiency, altered skin integrity, alterations in nutrition or hydration, reduction in skin moisture, or application of external devices.

9. a

10. b

CHAPTER 30

Case Study

a. To gather further information from the client about her current respiratory status, the nurse should ask the following questions:
   - "When do you experience shortness of breath or difficulty breathing?"
   - "What activities bring on the shortness of breath?"
   - "Does the shortness of breath interfere with your activities of daily living?"
   - "Do you find that it is hard to inhale or exhale?"
   - "Do you sleep with extra pillows at night?"
   - "Are you more tired than usual?"
   - "Do you smoke?" "Are you exposed to smokers or other environmental hazards at home or at work?"
   - "When does the cough start?"
   - "Are there times when your breathing/coughing is better or worse?"
   - "What are you bringing up when you cough?"
   - "Have you been exposed to anyone with a respiratory infection?"
   - "Have you recently had an upper respiratory infection?"
   - "Have you had pain in your chest when you breathe?"
   - "Are you currently taking any medications?"

b. Based on additional information from the client, nursing diagnoses for this client could be activity intolerance, ineffective airway clearance, impaired gas exchange, or risk of infection.

c. Nurse-initiated actions could include measurement of vital signs, auscultation of lung sounds, inspection of sputum, positioning for optimum respiratory function and comfort, and preparation of oxygen and suctioning equipment in case severe respiratory distress develops.

d. General teaching for health promotion should include the importance of the following:
   • Having the pneumococcal and influenza vaccines (if she has not had them)
   • Limiting exposure to crowds and environmental pollutants
   • Avoiding smoking or secondhand smoke
   • Covering the mouth and nose if out in cold air
   • Determining and improving activity and exercise tolerance
   • Taking medications regularly
   • Performing breathing and coughing exercises

Self-Test

1. c

2. f

3. g

4. d

5. b

6. j

7. a

8. i

9. h

10. e

11. The five behavioral factors that affect oxygenation are nutrition, exercise, cigarette smoking, substance abuse, and anxiety.

12. Conditions that can affect chest wall movement include pregnancy, obesity, musculoskeletal abnormalities, abnormal structural configuration, trauma, muscle diseases, and nervous system diseases.

13. Left-side heart failure is related to inadequate functioning of the left ventricle as a result of increased pressures and pulmonary congestion. Assessment findings can include decreased activity tolerance, breathlessness or dyspnea, dizziness, and confusion. Physical findings can include crackles on auscultation, hypoxia, shortness of breath on exertion, cough, and paroxysmal nocturnal dyspnea. Right-side heart failure is related to inadequate functioning of the right ventricle, usually as a result of pulmonary disease or left-side failure. Findings include weight gain, distended neck veins, hepatomegaly and splenomegaly, and dependent peripheral edema; all are signs of systemic venous congestion.

14. Assessment findings associated with a decrease in oxygenation include changes in breathing patterns, arrhythmias, altered heart and/or lung sounds, fatigue, weakness, dizziness, apprehension, restlessness, disorientation, headache, cyanosis, pallor, nonproductive or productive coughing, clubbing, alterations in chest movement, petechiae, and edema.

15. Lifestyle factors that contribute to cardiopulmonary health promotion include the following:
    a. Maintaining ideal body weight
    b. Eating a low-fat, low-salt diet
    c. Exercising regularly
    d. Avoiding smoking, secondhand smoke, and environmental pollutants
    e. Having regular check-ups
    f. Having pneumococcal and influenza vaccines
    g. Avoiding large crowds
    h. Covering the mouth and nose when sneezing and when out in cold weather

16. Abnormal chest wall movements are defined as follows:
    a. Retraction is the visible sinking in of the soft tissues of the chest between and around firmer tissue and ribs; seen often in the intercostal spaces.
    b. Paradoxical breathing is asymmetrical or asynchronous breathing where the chest contracts during inspiration and expands during expiration.

17. Physiological processes affecting oxygenation are as follows:
    a. Anemia affects oxygenation by decreasing the oxygen-carrying capacity of the blood.
    b. An airway obstruction limits the amount of inspired air that reaches the alveoli in the lungs.
    c. A fever increases the body's metabolic rate, which increases the oxygen demand of the tissues.

18. Surgical asepsis or sterile technique is used to suction the trachea.

19. Cardiopulmonary function test measurements include the following:
    a. Tidal volume measures the volume of air that is inhaled or exhaled per breath.
    b. Residual volume measures the volume of air that is left in the lungs after maximal exhalation.
    c. Vital capacity measures the volume of air that is exhaled after a maximal inhalation.
    d. An electrocardiogram measures the electrical activity of the heart.
    e. Scintigraphy is an imaging technique that uses radioisotopes to evaluate cardiac structures, myocardial perfusion, and contractility.
    f. An exercise stress test is used to evaluate the cardiac response to physical stress, providing information on myocardial response to increased oxygen needs.
    g. Echocardiography uses ultrasonic waves to evaluate the internal structures of the heart and motion of the heart wall.
    h. Cardiac catheterization is an invasive procedure that allows visualization of the heart and measures pressures and volumes within the heart itself.

20. Continuous bubbling in the chest tube water-seal chamber indicates an air leak.

21. Nursing interventions include the following:
    a. Dyspnea management—administration of medications (e.g., bronchodilators), supervision of oxygen therapy, and instruction in breathing and coughing techniques and relaxation measures.
    b. Patent airway—instruction in coughing techniques, suctioning, and airway placement.

    c. Lung expansion—positioning, administering chest physiotherapy, instruction in the use of incentive spirometry, and management of chest tubes.
    d. Mobilization of secretions—hydration of the client, humidification and nebulization of oxygen therapy, and administration of chest physiotherapy.

22. The nurse instructs the client and family and/or implements the following safety measures for home oxygen therapy:
    a. Place "no smoking" signs around the client area and inform visitors that smoking is prohibited where the oxygen is in use.
    b. Check the electrical equipment to determine that it is functioning properly and will not create sparks.
    c. Review fire procedures and location of extinguishers.
    d. Check the oxygen level to ensure a sufficient amount is present (an additional source may be obtained as a back up).
    e. Have an alternate source of oxygen in case of a power failure (if electrically operated unit).

23. d

24. d

25. b

26. b

27. a

28. c

29. a

30. d

CHAPTER 31

Case Study I

A client taking both digoxin and Lasix is more susceptible to fluid volume deficit (FVD) and hypokalemia. Digoxin strengthens the contraction of the heart muscle, improving the cardiac output and circulatory volume. Lasix is a potent diuretic that does not have a potassium-sparing effect. The client should be instructed to be alert to the signs of both decreased fluid and potassium as follows:

a. Hypokalemia—weakness, fatigue, decreased muscle tone, intestinal distention, change in pulse rate or rhythm.

b. FVD—poor skin turgor, thirst, sunken eyeballs, dryness, weakness, change in pulse rate or rhythm.

The client should also be instructed in the technique for taking her own pulse and on the importance of dietary replacement of potassium (e.g., bananas, oranges, potatoes) or administration of prescribed supplements.

Case Study II

The client on prolonged immobility is prone to hypercalcemia as a result of calcium being released from the bones into the bloodstream. The nurse should be alert to changes in the cardiac rate and rhythm (e.g., tachycardia), and increases in the blood urea nitrogen (BUN) and serum calcium levels. If the client is conscious, there can be anorexia, nausea, vomiting, low back pain, and a reduction in the level of consciousness.

Alcoholic clients are more susceptible to malnutrition and hypomagnesemia. The nurse should be alert to muscle tremors, hyperactive reflexes, confusion, disorientation, dysrhythmias, positive Trousseau's or Chvostek's signs, and a serum magnesium level below 1.5 mEq/L.

Case Study III

The nurse should anticipate that this client will have signs and symptoms of diminished oxygenation, including dyspnea, wheezing, coughing, activity intolerance, restlessness, pallor or cyanosis, and possible lack of concentration.

This client will most likely experience respiratory acidosis.

Self-Test

1. e

2. f

3. i

4. g

5. b

6. a

7. c

8. j

9. h

10. d

11. The terms identified are as follows:
    a. Extracellular fluid
    b. Interstitial fluid
    c. Intracellular fluid

12. Cations:
    Sodium (extracellular)
    Potassium (intracellular)
    Calcium (intracellular)
    Magnesium (intracellular)
    Anions:
    Chloride (extracellular)
    Bicarbonate (both)
    Phosphate (intracellular)

13. The three types of acid-base regulators within the body are chemical, biological, and physiological.

14. Infants, young children, and older adults are most susceptible to fluid and acid-base disturbances.

15. The solutions are identified as follows:
    a. Isotonic
    b. Hypotonic
    c. Isotonic
    d. Isotonic
    e. Hypertonic

16. Major risk factors for fluid, electrolyte, or acid-base imbalances include age, chronic disease, trauma, certain therapies and medications, and gastrointestinal losses.

17. The types of medications that can cause fluid, electrolyte, or acid-base disturbances include diuretics, steroids, potassium supplements, depressants, antibiotics, and antacids.

18. Nursing diagnoses for imbalances include the following:
    a. Ineffective breathing pattern
    b. Decreased cardiac output
    c. Fluid volume deficit
    c. Fluid volume excess

d. Impaired gas exchange
e. Impaired skin integrity
f. Impaired tissue integrity
g. Altered tissue perfusion

19. The nurse should implement the following for a client with a fluid restriction:
    a. Explain the rationale for the restriction.
    b. Identify the amount of fluid allowed and what is considered "fluid."
    c. Work with the client to determine the amount of fluid at meals, in between meals, at bedtime, and with medications.
    d. Use a standard as a starting point:
       • $\frac{1}{2}$ the total fluids during the active part of the day
       • $\frac{2}{5}$ of the fluid during the evening hours
       • Remainder for the night and prn
    e. Determine the type of fluids that are preferred by the client, unless contraindicated.
    f. Provide or assist with frequent mouth care.
    g. Avoid leaving extra fluids in the room, such as a full water pitcher.

20. The IV is discontinued, and warm, moist heat is applied to an area of phlebitis, with a warm towel applied to an infiltration for 20 minutes.

21. Teaching for clients and families with IV therapy in the home includes the following:
    a. The purpose of the therapy
    b. Aseptic technique
    c. Manipulation of the equipment
    d. Maintenance of the IV solution, tubing, and dressing
    e. Signs and symptoms of complications, and troubleshooting
    f. Indications for notification of the home health nurse
    g. Managing activities of daily living with the IV

22. Before a blood transfusion, the nurse checks the blood or blood product with another nurse to determine that the identification and blood type is correct. The nurse also assesses the following:
    a. IV site, needle size, patency of infusion, and presence of 0.9% NS solution
    b. Client's understanding of the procedure
    c. Client's vital signs to establish a baseline before the infusion begins

The nurse should stay with the client for at least the first 15 minutes of the transfusion in case of a possible reaction.

23. Autologous transfusions reduce the risk of mismatched blood and exposure to blood-borne infectious organisms. Perioperative blood salvage also contains more red blood cells than stored blood.

24. The associated electrolyte imbalances are as follows:
    a. Hyponatremia
    b. Hyperkalemia
    c. Hypocalcemia
    d. Hypomagnesemia

25. Calculations of IV infusion rates are as follows:
    a. $\dfrac{500 \text{ ml}}{5 \text{ hrs}} = \dfrac{500 \text{ ml} \times 15 \text{ gtt/ml}}{5 \text{ hrs} \times 60 \text{ min/hr}} = 25$ gtt/min
    b. $\dfrac{1000 \text{ ml}}{8 \text{ hrs}} = \dfrac{1000 \text{ ml} \times 10 \text{ gtt/ml}}{8 \text{ hrs} \times 60 \text{ min/hr}} = 21$ gtt/min
    c. $\dfrac{200 \text{ ml}}{4 \text{ hrs}} = \dfrac{200 \text{ ml} \times 60 \text{ gtt/ml}}{4 \text{ hrs} \times 60 \text{ min/hr}} = 50$ gtt/ml
    d. $\dfrac{2000 \text{ ml}}{18 \text{ hrs}} = 111$ ml/hr

26. TPN (total parenteral nutrition) is a nutritionally adequate hypertonic solution that contains glucose, other nutrients, and electrolytes.

27. b

28. c

29. d

30. c

31. b

32. b

33. d

34. c

35. b

36. d

37. c

38. c

39. d

40. a

CHAPTER 32

Case Study

a. A possible nursing diagnosis for this client is sleep pattern disturbance related to current life situation—stress at home and work.
Goals: Client will achieve an adequate amount of nightly sleep within 1 month.
Client will identify and verbalize current life stressors.
Client will practice stress reduction and relaxation techniques as needed.

b. The nurse may implement the following:
- Sit with the client and offer an opportunity for her to ventilate about her feelings and concerns.
- Instruct the client on stress reduction and relaxation techniques.
- Advise about the value of exercise and activity before sleep.
- Discuss manipulation of the environment to provide maximum comfort and minimum distraction.
- Instruct the client on the avoidance of heavy meals before bedtime and excessive caffeine or alcohol intake.
- Have the client maintain a log of sleep and rest patterns.

Self-Test

1. f

2. g

3. b

4. i

5. a

6. j

7. c

8. d

9. h

10. e

11. Stages 1 and 2 (NREM or nonrapid eye movement) are periods of lighter sleep, where the client is more easily aroused. Stages 3 and 4 (NREM) are periods of deeper, slow wave sleep, where the individual is more difficult to awaken. The individual also has phases of REM (rapid eye movement) sleep where vivid dreaming occurs, the eyes move rapidly, and the vital signs fluctuate up and down.

12. Sleep allows for the restoration and repair of physiological and cognitive processes. It preserves cardiovascular function, conserves energy, and prepares the individual for the next period of wakefulness.

13. Sleep can be affected by physical illness, medications or other substances, lifestyle changes, sleep pattern alterations, emotional stress, environmental variations, exercise, fatigue, and food and caloric intake.

14. Older adults have less stage 3 and stage 4 NREM sleep. REM sleep periods are shorter. Older adults tend to awaken more frequently during the night, and it might take longer to fall asleep. Naps during the day may increase. Sleep can also be influenced by the presence of chronic illnesses and discomfort.

15. The nurse can promote a restful environment by checking the following:
a. Is the client's bed clean and dry?
b. Are lights lowered and out of the client's eyes?
c. Are temperature and ventilation in the room at comfortable levels?
d. Is the amount of noise decreased?
e. Are the number of distractions decreased?

16. Safety measures for a client with nocturia include keeping a night-light on, removing clutter from the path to the bathroom, keeping a hospital bed at a level close to the floor, and placing a call bell within reach.

17. Bedtime rituals for adults include avoiding physical and mental stimulation right before bedtime, exercising 2 hours before, engaging in relaxing activities, using the bedroom only as a bedroom, and maintaining a consistent bedtime.

18. The components of a sleep history are the following:
a. Description of a client's sleep problem
b. Prior usual sleep pattern
c. Recent changes in sleep pattern
d. Bedtime routines and sleeping environment
e. Use of sleep and other medications
f. Dietary and substance (e.g., alcohol) intake

g. Symptoms during waking hours
h. Concurrent physical illness
i. Recent life events
j. Current emotional and mental status

19. A client's sleep may be altered by the following:
    a. Respiratory disease might necessitate additional pillows; breathing rhythm can be altered; nasal congestion and sore throat impair breathing and the ability to relax.
    b. Hyperthyroidism increases the time needed to fall asleep.
    c. Coronary heart disease frequently causes awakening during the night and changes in the stages of sleep.
    d. Gastric reflux or hiatal hernia can cause discomfort in the lower esophagus that is increased when lying flat; there will be a need for additional pillows to sit up or blocks to elevate the head of the bed.

20. c

21. d

22. b

23. c

24. a

25. c

CHAPTER 33

Case Study

a. In order to successfully use a patient-controlled analgesia (PCA) pump, the client must understand the purpose and use of the medication and pump and be able to locate and push the button on the pump that controls the administration of the medication.

b. Teaching for this client should include the following:
  • Use of the equipment
  • Purpose of PCA, action(s) of the medication, expected pain relief, precautions, and potential side effects of the medication (central nervous system depression)
  • General precautions for an IV infusion
  • Caution against family members or visitors operating the device for the client

Self-Test

1.
  a. Pain—a complex series of sensations; an unpleasant, subjective sensory and emotional experience associated with actual or potential tissue damage.
  b. Analgesic—classification of a medication used for pain relief.
  c. Local anesthesia—injection or application of a solution or substance that creates a loss of sensation to a particular body part or area.
  d. Exacerbation—increase in the severity of symptoms.
  e. Remission—partial or complete disappearance of symptoms.

2. a. Acute pain follows an injury, disease, or types of surgery. It has a rapid onset, varies in intensity (mild to severe), and lasts briefly. Chronic pain is prolonged, also varies in intensity, and usually lasts more than 6 months.
   b. Superficial pain results from stimulation of the skin. It is localized, of short duration, and usually a sharp sensation. Visceral pain results from stimulation of internal organs. It is diffuse, may radiate, usually lasts longer than superficial pain, and varies in sensation from dull to sharp.
   c. Referred pain is felt in a part of the body that is separate from the source of the pain. Radiating pain extends from the point of injury to another body part.

3. Behavioral responses to pain include the following:
   a. Vocalizations: moaning, crying screaming, gasping
   b. Facial expressions: grimace, clenched teeth, wrinkled forehead, lip biting, tightly closed or open eyes or mouth
   c. Body movement: restlessness, immobilization, muscle tension, increased hand and finger movements, pacing, rhythmic or rubbing motions
   d. Social interaction: avoidance of conversation or social contacts, focus on activities for pain relief, reduced attention span

   Physiological responses to pain include the following:
   a. Dilation of bronchial tubes, increased respiratory rate
   b. Increased heart rate

c. Peripheral vasoconstriction
d. Increased blood glucose level
e. Diaphoresis
f. Increased muscle tension
g. Dilation of pupils
h. Decreased gastrointestinal (GI) motility
i. Pallor
j. Nausea and vomiting
k. Weakness and exhaustion
l. Decreased heart rate and blood pressure (parasympathetic stimulation)

4. Influence of pain on activities of daily living include change of sleep patterns, inability to perform hygienic care, sexual dysfunction, alteration in home or work management, and interruption of social activities.

5. The level of pain may be assessed as follows:
   a. Toddler: use of words that the child can understand ("boo-boo"), pictures, dolls to act out with, pointing at areas of discomfort
   b. Speaker of a different language: use of an interpreter, pictures, gestures and pointing to areas of discomfort

6. Information to be obtained on the characteristics of pain includes onset and duration of the pain, location, severity, quality, pattern, relief measures, associated signs and symptoms, physical signs and symptoms, behaviors, effect on activities of daily living, and expectations of treatment.

7. The most appropriate nursing interventions are as follows:
   a. Attention level: distraction techniques
   b. Anxiety: relaxation techniques, imagery
   c. Fatigue: promotion of sleep and rest
   d. Internal control coping style: PCA

8. Nonpharmacologic interventions for pain relief include reduction or removal of painful stimuli, cutaneous stimulation, distraction, relaxation, guided imagery, anticipatory guidance, biofeedback, and hypnosis.

9. An ideal analgesic has a rapid onset and prolonged effectiveness, is effective with all age-groups, can be used orally or parenterally, lacks severe side effects, is nonaddicting, and is inexpensive.

10. Epidural anesthesia produces effective, longer-lasting pain relief with minimal sedation, eliminates the need for repeated injections, allows for earlier ambulation, has little effect on sensation or cardiovascular function, and produces fewer respiratory complications.

11. Individualizing a client's pain management can include the following:
    a. Using different types of pain relief measures
    b. Providing pain relief measures before the pain becomes severe
    c. Using measures that the client believes are effective
    d. Using the client's ideas for pain relief and scheduling
    e. Suggesting measures that are within the client's capability
    f. Choosing pain relief measures on the basis of the client's responses
    g. Encouraging the client to try measures more than once to see if they work
    h. Keeping an open mind about nontraditional measures
    i. Protecting the client from more pain
    j. Educating the client about the pain

12. The nurse can adapt or alter the client's environment to increase comfort by doing the following:
    a. Straightening wrinkled bed linen
    b. Positioning the client
    c. Loosening tight clothing or bandages (unless contraindicated)
    d. Changing wet dressings or bed linens
    e. Checking the temperature of hot or cold applications and bath water
    f. Lifting, not pulling, the client up in bed
    g. Positioning the client correctly on the bedpan
    h. Avoiding exposure of the skin or mucous membranes to irritants (e.g., urine)
    i. Preventing urinary retention by keeping the catheter patent
    j. Preventing constipation with fluids, diet, and exercise
    k. Reducing lighting that glares or shines directly on the client
    l. Checking the temperature of the room and the sensation of the client
    m. Reducing the level of noise and traffic

13. Three types of analgesics for mild to moderate pain are nonnarcotic and nonsteroidal: antiinflammatory drugs, opioids, and adjuvants or coanalgesics.

14. PCA allows for less total medication to be used by the client, with smaller amounts given at shorter intervals, and a more stable serum concentration of the medication being achieved. The overall effect is greater pain relief for the client.

15. A continuous IV narcotic analgesic drip is used for clients with severe pain (unrelieved with PO or intramuscular routes), severe nausea and vomiting, clotting disorders, inability to swallow, delirium, confusion, or change in mental status.

16. True or false
    a. True
    b. True
    c. True
    d. False
    e. False
    f. False

17. d

18. c

19. d

20. a

CHAPTER 34

Case Study

   a. To assist this client and the family with dietary planning, it is important to find out the following information:
      • Who prepares the food in the home?
      • Who buys the food, and where is the food purchased?
      • What foods are regularly eaten? Are there special foods for holidays or family occasions?
      • What are the client's food preferences?

In addition, the client should keep a record of dietary intake (usually recorded over 3 to 7 days).

   b. Teaching about foods that are high in sodium and saturated fat is an important part of the plan for this client. Reading labels and menus (if the client is eating out) will help in the selection of appropriate foods. The client and family should also be informed about possible substitutions for foods, spices, and oils that are high in sodium and

fat. Alternatives such as polyunsaturated oils, lean meats, and egg substitutes can be incorporated into meal preparation. A separate meal plan for the client is not usually necessary because flavorings like lemon can make foods attractive (as well as healthy) for the entire family. The most difficult times are often at holidays and other special occasions, when food plays a central role in the family's activities. Low-salt and low-fat substitutions, wherever appropriate, should be used. Fresh or frozen fruits and vegetables, without sodium or fat-based sauces or additives, are more flavorful than low-sodium canned foods. The client might also be able to eat traditional foods in moderation on these occasions. Realistic expectations work better for the client than harsh, uncompromising restrictions.

Self-Test

1. i

2. c

3. a

4. h

5. j

6. g

7. f

8. e

9. b

10. d

11. The factors that influence dietary patterns include developmental stage, culture and religion, socioeconomic status, personal preference, psychological factors, alcohol and drugs, and misinformation about food fads.

12. The goals are for individuals to increase their daily intake of fruits, vegetables, and grain products and decrease their intake of sodium.

13. The four basic food groups included milk, meat, bread and cereal, and fruits and vegetables. Individuals were to have selected servings from each of the four groups every day. The food pyramid guide identifies six different groups:

Fats, Oils, and Sugars (used sparingly)

Milk, Yogurt, and Cheese and Meat, Poultry, Fish, Beans, Eggs (2 to 3 servings/day)

Vegetables (3 to 5 servings/day) and Fruits (2 to 4 servings/day)

Bread, Cereal, Rice, and Pasta (6 to 11 servings/day)

14. General nutritional guidelines:
    a. Eat a variety of foods from the food pyramid; have plenty of grains, fruits, and vegetables.
    b. Balance the intake of food with the amount of physical activity.
    c. Reduce the intake of sugar, sodium, fat (especially saturated fat), and cholesterol.
    d. Moderate the intake of alcoholic beverages.

15. Specific nutritional needs include the following:
    a. Infant: fluid, vitamins C and D, iron, and fluoride
    b. School-age child: vitamins A and C and protein
    c. Adolescent: iron
    d. Older adult: vitamin D, reduced fat, and increased fiber, iron, and calcium

16. Laboratory studies include complete blood count (CBC), albumin, transferrin, prealbumin, electrolytes, blood urea nitrogen (BUN), creatinine, glucose, and triglycerides.

17. A client's nutritional intake can be influenced in the acute care setting by diagnostic testing (NPO, fatigue), stress, medications (taste, actions), food presentation ("hospital food"), and health status (not feeling well or not able to eat).

18. Nasogastric, jejunal, and gastrostomy routes are used for enteral feeding.

19. Concepts pertaining to TPN include the following:
    a. TPN (total parenteral nutrition) is used because the client is unable to ingest or digest enteral feedings.
    b. The nursing goals for TPN are to prevent infection, maintain the TPN system, prevent complications, and promote the client's well-being.
    c. Nursing interventions to prevent complications of TPN therapy include weighing the client daily, monitoring I & O (intake and output) and caloric intake, testing urine or blood for glucose, obtaining blood samples for nutritional assessment, observing for fluid and electrolyte balance, and maintaining the correct infusion rate.
    d. Acute care TPN is infused over 24 hours. Home care TPN is infused over 12 to 16 hours.
    e. The recommended infusion rate for lipids is 1 ml/min. Solutions should not be used if there is a separation of contents (oil or creamy layer on top) or it is more than 12 hours old.

20. Diet therapies for health deviations include the following:
    a. Congestive heart failure: sodium restriction
    b. Postoperative care: clear or full liquid diet
    c. Lack of teeth: mechanical or dental soft diet
    d. Diverticulosis or irritable bowel: high fiber diet

21. The nursing history focuses on the client's usual intake of food and fluid, food preferences, allergies, and any particular problems that the client might have with ingestion, digestion, or elimination.

22. b

23. b

24. d

25. a

26. b

27. d

28. b

29. d

30. a

CHAPTER 35

Case Study I

a. Before the IVP (intravenous pyelography), the client should be assessed for the following:
   - Allergies to shellfish, iodine, or contrast dyes
   - Fluid status (avoid dehydration from bowel preparation that can increase the potential toxicity of the contrast dye)
   - Medical conditions that increase risk (e.g., renal insufficiency)
   - Recent barium studies (tests within 2 to 3 days of the IVP will obscure findings)

The client should be instructed to do the following:
   - Take the cathartic the evening before
   - Remain NPO after midnight
   - Expect an IV infusion to be started for the injection of the dye
   - Expect a flushing sensation and a feeling of warmth, dizziness, or nausea when the dye is injected
   - Expect that a number of x-rays will be taken during the test and that voiding will be done near the end of the test

b. Following the IVP, the nurse will monitor I & O and report decreased or absent urination. The client will be informed that a normal diet may be resumed, fluid intake is encouraged, and any signs of an allergic reaction (itching, hives) should be reported.

Case Study II

The nurse may safely delegate the following urinary care measures: assisting the client with the use of the bedpan or urinal, monitoring I & O, maintaining aseptic technique, and promoting client privacy and dignity. In some institutions, the established policy might allow for additional measures to be delegated, such as routine catheter care and specimen collection. Delegation to unlicensed assistive personnel requires that the nurse evaluate their ability to safely and accurately perform the specified measures.

Case Study III

The action proposed by the primary nurse is unsafe to use because it could result in serious damage to the client's urethra. The correct procedure requires that you prepare a clean disposable towel, gloves, and a sterile syringe (same volume as the fluid in the catheter balloon). The client is positioned in the same way as for catheter insertion, the syringe is attached to the balloon port, and the entire amount of fluid is aspirated. The catheter is then slowly and smoothly pulled out. If resistance is encountered, an additional attempt is made to remove fluid from the balloon. The catheter is then wrapped in a waterproof pad and disposed of in an appropriate container along with the drainage tubing and bag (after emptying and measuring the remaining amount of urine). Perineal care is then provided to the client, and the nurse should carefully monitor the urinary output.

Case Study IV

The client is provided with a sterile specimen cup, sterile disinfectant wipes, and clean gloves. He is instructed to apply the gloves and wipe the urinary meatus in a circular motion, moving up from the meatus to the glans penis. He is also cautioned against using the contaminated wipe repeatedly. After cleansing, the client should discard the initial urination and begin collection in the sterile cup at the midstream portion of voiding. The cover of the specimen cup is then replaced, and the specimen is sent to the lab within 1 hour of the collection. To promote client understanding, the use of more understandable terms than meatus and voiding might be necessary.

Self-Test

1. d

2. g

3. i

4. h

5. a

6. j

7. e

8. b

9. f

10. c

11. Noninvasive procedures for examination of urinary function include abdominal roentgenogram (KUB), intravenous pyelogram (IVP), renal scan, and computerized axial tomography (CAT).

12. Nursing implications include the following:
    a. Monitoring vital signs frequently
    b. Promoting bed rest for 8 to12 hours
    c. Assessing peripheral pulses
    d. Observing for bleeding
    e. Maintaining a pressure dressing over the site for 24 hours
    f. Observing the client for a reaction to the dye
    g. Monitoring the client's I & O

13. Intermittent catheterization is used for immediate relief of bladder distention, long-term management of clients with incompetent bladders, sterile urine specimen collection, assessment of residual urine, and instillation of medication. Indwelling catheters are used for urinary outflow obstructions, clients having surgery of the urinary tract or surrounding structures, prevention of obstruction from blood clots, accurate monitoring of I & O and prevention of skin breakdown in critically ill or comatose clients, and provision of bladder irrigations.

14. A female client may be placed in the lithotomy or Sim's position for catheterization.

15. 2000 to 2500 ml/day is the recommended fluid intake.

16. Urination may be influenced as follows:
    a. Sociocultural: Privacy needs for urination and expectations (e.g., intermissions or recesses)
    b. Fluid intake: Increased intake will increase output (if fluid or electrolyte balance exists). Alcohol, caffeine, and foods with high fluid content promote urination.
    c. Pathological conditions: Diabetes mellitus and multiple sclerosis cause neuropathies that alter bladder function. Arthritis and joint diseases interfere with activity. Renal disease influences amount and characteristics of urine. Fevers reduce urinary output. Spinal cord injuries disrupt voluntary bladder emptying.
    d. Medications: Diuretics promote excretion of fluid and selected electrolytes. Some drugs change the color of the urine or influence the ability of the bladder to relax and empty.

17. Stress incontinence

18. Expected or unexpected characteristics of urine are as follows:
    a. ph 10 = unexpected
    b. Protein 4 mg = expected
    c. Glucose = unexpected
    d. Specific gravity 1.2 = unexpected

19. The condom catheter should be changed every day and the skin should be checked for signs of irritation and breakdown. Perineal care is provided with each catheter change. The tubing must be checked frequently to ensure that there are no kinks or other obstructions.

20. b

21. c

22. d

23. d

24. c

25. a

CHAPTER 36

Case Study

a. Nursing diagnosis: Constipation related to overuse of laxatives or enemas and inadequate dietary fiber (as manifested by client's statement that she is having difficulty with bowel elimination)
b. Goal: Client will establish a regular defecation pattern within 1 to 2 months.
c. Outcomes: Client will have a regular bowel movement within 3 days, her abdomen will be nondistended and nontender, and she will pass soft, formed stools at least every 2 to 3 days.
d. Goal: Client will maintain a diet that incorporates an adequate amount of fiber and fluids.
e. Outcomes: Client will identify and eat foods that are high in fiber and drink an adequate amount of fluid on a daily basis.
f. Nursing interventions:
   • Instruct on foods high in fiber.
   • Instruct on the importance of an adequate fluid intake.
   • Encourage to allow ample or regular time for defecation.
   • Instruct on the adverse effects of reliance on laxatives or enemas.

- Investigate family and social contacts for stimulation of appetite.
- Identify that daily bowel movements are not absolutely necessary.

Self-Test:

1. d

2. e

3. a

4. b

5. c

6. Dietary recommendations for constipation include the following:
   a. Increased intake of fiber (vegetables, fruits, whole grains) and fluids
   b. Chopped foods rather than pureed (for poor dentition)
   c. Mashed foods with fruit juices and hot tea (for difficulty swallowing)

7. Dietary recommendations for diarrhea include the following:
   a. Avoidance of spicy or high-fiber foods
   b. Avoidance of milk and milk products (for lactose-intolerant)
   c. Increased intake of low-fiber foods (chicken, beef, pasta)
   d. Fluid and electrolyte replacement

8. Bowel elimination is influenced by the following:
   a. Diet: Regular food intake, high-fiber and gas-producing foods promote peristalsis, low-fiber foods slow peristalsis, and lactose or selected food intolerance can lead to diarrhea and cramping.
   b. Positioning: Squatting or sitting allows for intraabdominal pressure to be exerted and thigh muscles to be contracted to aid in defecation.
   c. Pregnancy: Constipation commonly occurs because of pressure of the fetus on the rectum.
   d. Diagnostic tests: Some tests require NPO or enemas in advance, and barium can harden and cause constipation if not eliminated after the test.
   e. Activity: Immobilization decreases peristalsis, and regular exercise increases it.

f. Psychological status: Stress, anxiety, or fear can increase nervous stimulation and lead to diarrhea; depression can decrease peristalsis. Excessive pressure placed on children to become toilet trained can lead to chronic constipation.

9. The nurse can provide local application of heat, sitz baths, or topical medications (as prescribed) to promote comfort for the client with hemorrhoids.

10. Causes for the laboratory results include the following:
    a. Increased stomach gastrin—pernicious anemia.
    b. Increased total bilirubin—biliary tract obstruction.

11. Clients should be cautioned against straining (Valsalva's maneuver) on defecation if they have cardiovascular disease, glaucoma, or increased intracranial pressure.

12. Risk factors for colon cancer include the following:
    a. Age over 50 years
    b. Family history of colorectal cancer
    c. Ethnocultural background
    d. Personal history of inflammatory bowel disease
    e. Urban residence
    f. High dietary intake of fats and low fiber intake

13. Adults are assisted to a left-lying Sim's position.

14. Kayexalate enema

15. Hypertonic enema
    a. A hypertonic enema works by exerting osmotic pressure, pulling fluid from the interstitial spaces and filling the colon with fluid. The distention in the colon promotes defecation.
    b. Hypertonic enemas are indicated for clients who are not able to tolerate a large-volume fluid enema. They are contraindicated for infants and for individuals who are dehydrated.
    c. Fleets enema.

16. Factors that lead to diarrhea include the following:
    a. Emotional stress increases intestinal motility.
    b. Medications irritate the intestinal mucosa (iron), increase intestinal motility (laxatives), or allow an overgrowth of normal intestinal flora that inflames and irritates the mucosa (antibiotics).
    c. Tube feedings: Hyperosmolarity of enteral solutions draws fluid into the intestine and promotes defecation.
17. c
18. c
19. b
20. b

CHAPTER 37

Case Study

Mrs. B. might benefit the most from discussing her feelings, needs, and concerns with the nurse and being involved as much as possible in the decision-making process for her plan of care. In addition, Mrs. B. might benefit from the following interventions:

    a. Orienting her to the environment, routine and schedule, and staff members
    b. Placing her with mobile clients who can interact with her
    c. Encouraging frequent visits from family members and friends
    d. Providing her with materials she enjoys, such as books and magazines
    e. Providing stimulating diversional activity for her, such as music and games
    f. Engaging in conversation with her during meals and implementation of nursing actions
    g. Encouraging her to use any necessary assistive aids, such as glasses
    h. Encouraging and helping her (as necessary) to attend to daily grooming
    i. Providing a stimulating physical environment by changing her view, setting up personal objects, and so on

Self-Test

1. Nervous, muscular, and skeletal systems

2. The objectives of bed rest are to decrease physical activity and oxygen needs, allow the ill or debilitated client to rest, and prevent further injury.

3. Bed rest might be required for clients with cardiovascular conditions (e.g., myocardial infarction, congestive heart failure), neurological conditions (e.g., head injuries, spinal cord trauma), musculoskeletal conditions (e.g., fractures), pulmonary conditions (e.g., chronic lung disease), and other conditions where the client is severely weakened (e.g., terminal phase of cancer).

4. Fluid and electrolyte imbalances that occur with immobility include hypercalcemia and hypovolemia (initial phases).

5. An immobilized client might react to the experience by exhibiting hostility, belligerence, inappropriate moods, withdrawal, confusion, anxiety, and depression.

6. Anthropometric measurement allows for the evaluation of muscle atrophy and determination of decreased protein (negative nitrogen balance).

7. Cardiovascular system changes:
    a. Orthostatic hypotension: Move the client slowly from one position to another.
    b. Increased cardiac workload: Place the client in an upright position (if possible) and provide regular exercise and adequate fluid intake.
    c. Thrombus formation: Provide regular exercise, adequate fluid intake, and antiembolitic stockings.

8. Respiratory system changes:
    a. Pneumonia and atelectasis: coughing and deep breathing, turning, upright positioning, chest physiotherapy, adequate fluid intake, and exercise

9. Exercise for hospitalized clients may include, dependent on their abilities, light walking, stretching, and range of motion.

10. The nurse assesses for deep venous thrombosis (DVT) by removing TED or elastic stockings, socks, or other clothing and checking for redness, warmth, tenderness, or pain in the calf area. Homan's sign may be noted if the client experiences calf pain on dorsiflexion of the foot. In addition, calf and thigh circumferences may be measured to check for edema.

11. General teaching for a client with limited mobility should include the following:
    a. Explanation of the need for position changes
    b. Explanation of the importance of, and demonstration and performance of, range of motion exercises
    c. Description of the effects of immobility and risk for pressure ulcers
    d. Discussion of stimulating diversional activities
    e. Explanation of fluid and nutritional intake needs
    d. Encouragement of participation in the plan of care

12. Dietary needs of the immobilized client are influenced by the presence of infection, need for wound healing, food intolerance, gastrointestinal functioning, and daily caloric requirements.

13. a

14. d

15. b

CHAPTER 38

Case Study

a. Nursing diagnosis: Risk for impaired skin integrity related to prolonged pressure on bony prominences, as manifested by reddened areas (reactive hyperemia) to sacrum, elbows, and heels

b. Goal: Integrity of skin and underlying tissues will be maintained.

c. Outcomes: Reactive hyperemia will subside and client's normal skin coloration will return within 2 days. Client will assist, as possible, with q1-2h turning and positioning.

d. Nursing interventions:
   - Reposition or assist with repositioning q1-2h.
   - Encourage the client to shift weight when out of bed in a chair.
   - Assess skin and underlying tissues with each position change.
   - Use supportive devices—padding for mattress and bony prominences.
   - Keep sacral area clean and dry.
   - Measure, document and report reddened areas.

1. g

2. h

3. b

4. c

5. j

6. a

7. i

8. d

9. e

10. f

11. Sites marked should include the occipital bone, scapula, spine, elbow, iliac crest, sacrum, ischium, Achilles tendon, and heel.

12. Stages of pressure ulcer development:
    a. Stage I
    b. Stage II
    c. Stage III
    d. Stage IV

13. The following increase a client's risk for pressure ulcer development: shearing force, friction, moisture on the skin, poor nutrition, cachexia, infection, impaired peripheral circulation, obesity, and advanced age.

14. The older adult's skin is usually less tolerant to pressure, friction, and shearing forces. It is also drier and thinner, with a reduced rate of epidermal cell renewal. Circulation to the extremities may also be reduced.

15. The three major areas of nursing intervention include: hygienic and topical care, positioning (30-degree angle), and application and maintenance of supportive surfaces and mattresses.

16. Documentation should include notation of the following:
    a. Hyperemia: location, size, color, and hourly reassessment
    b. Any blisters, pimples, or scabs
    c. Client mobility
    d. Nutritional status

17. Wound healing is influenced by the following:
    a. Age: Infants and older adults might have decreased circulation, oxygen delivery, clotting, and inflammatory responses, with an increased risk of infection. Older adults have slower cell growth and differentiation, and scar tissue is less pliable.
    b. Obesity: Individuals have a decreased supply of blood vessels in fatty tissue (impaired delivery of nutrients to the site), and suturing of adipose tissue is more difficult.
    c. Diabetes: Individuals have small blood vessel disease (reduced oxygen delivery), and elevated glucose levels impair macrophage function.
    d. Immunosuppression: A reduced immune response leads to poor healing. Steroids also mask signs of inflammation or infection, and chemotherapeutic agents interfere with leukocyte production.

18. Possible complications are hemorrhage, infection, dehiscence, evisceration, and fistulas.

19. Types of wound drainage include the following:
    a. Serous—clear, watery plasma.
    b. Sanguineous—fresh bleeding.
    c. Serosanguineous—pale, more watery, with plasma and red cells.
    d. Purulent—thick, yellow, green, or brown, with dead/live organisms and white blood cells.

20. To obtain an aerobic wound culture, the nurse should do the following:
    a. Cleanse the wound.
    b. Place the tip of a sterile swab into fresh wound drainage.
    c. Return the swab to the culturette tube.
    d. Cap the tube.
    e. Crush the inner ampule so that the medium coats the tip of the swab.
    f. Send the culturette tube to the lab as soon as possible.

21. The steps for caring for a traumatic wound are the following:
    a. Stabilize the client's cardiopulmonary function.
    b. Promote hemostasis (stop any bleeding).
    c. Cleanse the wound.
    d. Protect the site from further injury.

22. The use of dressings allows for decreased exposure to microorganisms, hemostasis (pressure dressing), better healing, support or immobilization of a body part, coverage of an unattractive wound, and thermal insulation.

23. The nurse can increase the client's comfort level by carefully removing any tape, gently cleansing the wound and manipulating the dressings and drains, positioning the client, and providing the prescribed analgesic medication before the procedure.

24. The principles for wound cleansing are the following:
    a. Cleanse in a direction from least to most contaminated.
    b. Use friction when applying local antiseptics.
    c. Allow irrigating solution to flow from the least to most contaminated area.

25. The technique taught to the client and family at home is clean rather than sterile. A "no touch" method should be used where only the edges of the dressings are contacted.

26. a. The use of heat is contraindicated in an area of active bleeding, in an acute localized inflammation, or for an individual with cardiovascular problems.
    b. Cold therapy is contraindicated for edematous injuries, in areas of diminished circulation, and for a client who is shivering.

27. Paraffin bath or warm soak

28. Bandages applied to the extremities:
    a. Bandages are applied starting from the distal site and moving toward the torso.
    b. Bandages to the extremities promote venous return and decrease edema.

29. Small body part: circular bandage turn
    Joints: figure eight turn
    Head: recurrent turn
    Wrist or upper arm: spiral turn

30. Total score = 13 points
    Client risk = "at risk" status

31. d

32. a

33. c

34. d

35. a

CHAPTER 39

Case Study I

For this client, you could implement the following interventions:

a. Assist in arranging the environment so that the client knows where everything is and so that clutter is out of the way.

b. Recommend or assist in obtaining books with larger print, audiotaped books, and music.

c. Allow time for discussion of feelings, needs, and concerns.

d. Refer the client to community agencies (e.g., Foundation for the Blind).

e. Instruct or assist in improving the lighting in halls and stairways and the use of color-coding (edges of stairs, medication bottles, appliance dials).

f. Instruct in the importance of follow-up visits to the ophthalmologist.

g. Investigate family and social contacts.

Case Study II

A client in an intensive care unit (ICU) can experience sensory overload from the intensity of sounds and activity or sensory deprivation from restricted visits of family and friends. The nurse should try to organize care so that the client is allowed the opportunity for uninterrupted rest whenever possible. Monitors at the client's bedside should have volume controls so that they can be turned down to a lower level. Time should also be taken by the nurse to sit with the client, either quietly or for verbal stimulation. Visits from family members and friends should be encouraged, but not to the point of client fatigue. The environment should be arranged so that the client has a different or more pleasant view, and personal items (e.g., photos) should be placed within the client's field of vision. It might be a challenge for the nurse in this setting to adapt the client's sensory input; therefore creativity, within realistic limits, is recommended.

Self-Test

1. Other terms are as follows:
   a. Visual
   b. Auditory
   c. Gustatory
   d. Olfactory
   e. Tactile
   f. Kinesthetic

2. Sensory deprivation is an inadequate quantity or quality of stimulation that impairs perception. Sensory overload occurs when the individual receives multiple stimuli and the brain is not able to disregard or selectively ignore some of the stimuli.

3. Clients at risk for sensory alterations include older adults, immobilized clients, and clients with known sensory deficits.

4. The correct terms for the descriptions are as follows:
   a. Cerumen accumulation
   b. Presbyopia
   c. Presbycusis
   d. Cataract

5. Sensory function is influenced by the following:
   a. Age (older adulthood) can cause the following:
      • Decreased hearing acuity, speech intelligibility, and pitch discrimination
      • Increased dryness of cerumen and obstruction of the auditory canal
      • Reduced visual fields; increased glare sensitivity; impaired night vision; reduced accommodation, depth perception, and color discrimination
      • Reduced sensitivity to odors and diminished taste discrimination
      • Difficulty with balance, spatial orientation, and coordination
      • Diminished sensitivity to pain, pressure, and temperature
   b. Medications can cause ototoxicity, optic nerve irritation (Chloramphenicol), or reduce sensory perception (analgesics, sedatives, antidepressants).
   c. Smoking can cause atrophy of the taste buds and interference with olfactory function.

6. Assessment of vision:
   a. Ask the client to read.
   b. Use the Snellen chart to check visual acuity.
   c. Assess visual fields and depth perception.
   d. Assess pupils.
   e. Ask the client to identify colors.

   Assessment of hearing:
   a. Use ticking watch, whispering, tuning fork.
   b. Observe client's conversation and interaction with others.
   c. Compare ability to distinguish consonants and vowels.
   d. Inspect external ear canal.

   Assessment of touch:
   a. Check for sensitivity to light touch and temperature.
   b. Assess client's ability to distinguish sharp and dull stimuli.
   c. Assess client's ability to distinguish objects in the palm of the hand.
   d. Ask if client feels unusual sensations.
   e. Ask the client to tie shoelaces or a bow

7. Sensory deprivation can lead to the following:
   a. Cognitive function: decreased learning capacity, poor problem solving and task performance, disorientation, strange thinking, and regression
   b. Affective function: boredom, restlessness, increased anxiety, emotional lability, and increased need for socialization
   c. Perceptual function: decreased attention span, disorganized visual and motor coordination, temporary loss of color discrimination, disorientation, and confusion

8. Child eyesight safety includes the following: avoiding toys with long, pointed handles or sharp edges; keeping the child from running with a pointed object; and keeping pointed objects and tools out of reach.

9. Sensory stimulation can be increased in the acute care environment by the following:
   a. Increasing the client's view outside and within the room
   b. Arranging decorations, plants, photos, greeting cards, and the client's personal items
   c. Providing audiobooks and large-print reading material
   d. Spending time with, listening to, and conversing with the client
   e. Playing pleasant music or putting on television shows that the client enjoys

   f. Providing correct temperature and attractive meals
   g. Providing a variety of textures and aromas to enhance the client's appetite

10. The nurse may communicate with a hearing-impaired client by the following:
   a. Making sure that a hearing aid, if needed, is in place and in working order
   b. Approaching the client from the front to get his or her attention
   c. Facing the client on the same level, with adequate lighting
   d. Making sure that glasses, if needed, are worn and are clean
   e. Speaking slowly and articulating clearly, using a normal tone of voice
   f. Rephrasing, rather than repeating, information that is not heard
   g. Using visible expressions and gestures
   g. Talking toward the client's better ear
   h. Using written information to reinforce spoken words
   I. Not restricting a deaf client's hands
   j. Avoiding eating, chewing, or smoking while speaking with the client
   k. Avoiding speaking while walking away, in another room, or from behind the client

11. Ototoxicity may be caused by the following:
   a. Antibiotics: aminoglycosides, vancomycin, minocycline
   b. Diuretics: ethacrynic acid, furosemide, torsemide
   c. Analgesics: indomethacin, aspirin, ibuprofen, naproxen

12. Adaptations to sensory alterations include the following:
   a. Hearing deficit: Amplify low-pitch sounds, use lamps with sound activation, use assistive devices for telephones, and obtain closed-captioning for the television.
   b. Diminished sense of smell: Use smoke and carbon monoxide detectors, take special care with disposal of matches and cigarettes, and check the expiration dates on foods.
   c. Diminished sense of touch: Lower the temperature of the water heater, and use caution when checking the bath or shower water.

13. c

14. c

15. c

CHAPTER 40

Case Study I

Explain and demonstrate coughing and deep breathing exercises with splinting of the abdominal incision. Assist in and encourage turning and positioning every 2 hours. Reinforce the use of the incentive spirometer. Explain and demonstrate range of motion exercises. Provide prescribed analgesia prior to activities, keeping in mind the action and dosage of the medication and its possible effect on the client.

Case Study II

Preoperative teaching for the client who is having ambulatory surgery can be done when the client comes for preoperative tests and physical assessment. There can also be telephone contact with the client on the evening before the surgery, as well as a 24-hour resource line for the client to use for questions. Additional teaching may be conducted immediately before the procedure and before the client's discharge. Information provided to the client usually includes instructions specific to the surgery and anesthesia (e.g., dressings, activity and dietary restrictions), signs and symptoms of complications, and time frame for follow-up visits.

Case Study III

Any significant change in the client's status should be reported to the surgeon and/or anesthesiologist immediately. Because of the effects of general anesthesia, temperature alterations are especially critical before surgical procedures. Surgery should be postponed until the client's temperature has returned to normal.

Case Study IV

The client should be informed that, under usual circumstances, all loose items are removed before surgery. If the client will be adversely affected by the removal of his "lucky" medallion, it may be pinned inside of the client's gown or surgical cap, depending on the type of surgery. It is very important, however, that the operating room personnel be informed before to the surgery that the client has the medallion in place. It might be the policy of the agency that the client will have to sign a form stating that he has kept the medallion, or other jewelry, on his person in case of a loss.

Self-Test

1. Classifications for surgical procedures are as follows:
   a. Elective surgery
   b. Major surgery
   c. Diagnostic surgery
   d. Emergency surgery
   e. Palliative surgery
   f. Transplant surgery

2. The following medical conditions can increase a client's surgical risk: bleeding disorders, diabetes mellitus, heart disease, upper respiratory infection, cancer, liver disease, fever, chronic respiratory disease, immunological disorders, and abuse of street drugs.

3. The factors that place the older client at risk for surgery are as follows:
   a. Cardiovascular: Changes in structure and function reduce cardiac reserve and predispose the client to postoperative hemorrhage, increased blood pressure, and clot formation.
   b. Pulmonary: Changes in structure and function reduce vital capacity, increase the volume of residual air left in the lungs, and reduce blood oxygenation.
   c. Renal: Changes in structure and function increase the possibility of shock with blood loss, limit the ability to metabolize drugs or toxic substances, increase the frequency of urination and the amount of residual urine, and reduce the sensation of the need to void.

4. Implications for surgical clients taking medications are as follows:
   a. Heparin alters normal clotting factors, increasing the risk of hemorrhage. It should be discontinued at least 48 hours preoperatively. It further alters clotting factors if it is used with other medications, such as aspirin and ibuprofen.
   b. Insulin: The diabetic client's need for insulin is reduced preoperatively because of NPO. Dose requirements might increase postoperatively because of stress response and IV administration of glucose solutions.

5. General information in preoperative teaching includes the following:
   a. Pre- and postoperative routines
   b. Expected sensations
   c. Pain relief measures available (e.g., PCA)
   d. Postoperative exercises
   e. Activity and dietary restrictions

6. An ambulatory surgery PACU (postanesthesia care unit) usually has two phases. The first phase is similar to the inpatient PACU, where the client is monitored closely and stabilized. The second phase of the ambulatory surgery PACU differs in that it prepares the client for discharge and self-care. Clients receiving local anesthesia may move directly to the second phase of recovery. Clients in the ambulatory surgery setting will be gradually progressed to sitting up, taking fluids, eating light snacks, and ambulating to the bathroom. When the client's condition becomes stable, he or she will be discharged home.

7. On the day of surgery in an acute care setting, the nurse should do the following:
    a. Complete the preoperative checklist documentation.
    b. Monitor vital signs.
    c. Provide or assist with hygienic care.
    d. Remove prostheses and cosmetics and provide client with gown and surgical cap.
    e. Complete preparation of the bladder and bowel (e.g., enemas, catheterization).
    f. Apply antiembolic stockings.
    g. Complete any special procedures.
    h. Safeguard the client's valuables.
    i. Provide emotional support and promote dignity.
    j. Administer preoperative medications.

8. Routine screening tests include complete blood count, serum electrolyte analysis, coagulation studies, serum creatinine test, urinalysis, 12-lead electrocardiogram, and chest x-ray.

9. Commonly used types and purposes of preoperative medications include the following:
    a. Sedatives: used for relaxation and decrease in nausea
    b. Tranquilizers: used to decrease anxiety and relax skeletal muscles
    c. Narcotic analgesics: used to sedate, decrease pain and anxiety, and reduce the amount of anesthesia required
    d. Anticholinergics: used to decrease mucous secretions in the oral and respiratory passages and prevent laryngospasm

10. The circulating nurse cares for the client in the operating room by completing other preoperative assessments, establishing and implementing the intraoperative plan of care, evaluating the care, and providing for the continuity of care postoperatively. The circulating nurse assists with the operation of nonsterile equipment, provision of additional instruments and supplies, calculation of blood loss and urinary output, and documentation of the procedure. The scrub nurse is primarily responsible for maintaining the sterile field during the procedure and adhering to strict medical asepsis. This nurse applies sterile drapes, provides sterile equipment to the surgeon, and keeps count of supplies used during the operation.

11. The uses and side effects for medications are as follows:
    a. General anesthesia: used for major procedures that require extensive tissue manipulation. Side effects include cardiovascular depression or irritability, respiratory depression, and liver and kidney damage.
    b. Regional anesthesia: used when operating on a specific body area. Side effects include a sudden fall in blood pressure and respiratory paralysis.
    c. Local anesthesia: used for minor procedures, especially in ambulatory surgery, and after general anesthesia for postoperative pain relief. Side effects include local irritation and inflammation.

12. Injury to the client can be prevented during the operation by ensuring that the equipment count is accurate, the client is monitored carefully, special equipment is properly managed (e.g., lasers, cautery), and emergency equipment is available.

13. Typical postoperative orders include the following:
    a. Frequency of specific assessments
    b. Types of intravenous fluids and infusion rates
    c. Postoperative medications
    d. Oxygen therapy or incentive spirometry
    e. Dietary and activity restrictions
    f. Positioning in bed
    g. Intake and output
    h. Laboratory tests and x-ray studies
    i. Additional special instructions

14. Postoperative complications for each system include the following:
    a. Respiratory: atelectasis, pneumonia, hypoxia, pulmonary embolism
    b. Circulatory: hemorrhage, hypovolemic shock, thrombophlebitis, thrombus or embolus formation

c. Gastrointestinal: abdominal distention, constipation, nausea or vomiting

d. Integumentary: wound infection, dehiscence, evisceration, skin breakdown

15. The five postoperative exercises are diaphragmatic breathing, incentive spirometry, controlled coughing, turning, and leg exercises (range of motion).

16. c

17. b

18. d

19. c

20. c

Test Bank

CHAPTER 1

Health and Wellness

1-1. What is one of the goals of The Healthy People 2000 initiative?
a. Provide insurance to all United States citizens
b. Identify gaps among ethnic minorities in regard to disease prevention behaviors
c. Increase the life expectancy of Americans
d. Reduce the percentage of communicable diseases in childhood

1-2. The health-illness continuum has what purpose?
a. It can be used to compare one client's health to another client's health
b. It helps the nurse define health and illness as absolute states
c. It defines health as a dynamic state that fluctuates as a person adapts to changes
d. It does not consider a client's risk factors in identifying level of health

1-3. What are risk factors in the health-illness continuum model?
a. More common in adolescents than adults
b. Modifiable traits that health care providers can assist a client to change
c. Variables that increase the vulnerability of a client to develop illness
d. Direct indicators of the presence of disease

1-4. Pender's health promotion model focuses on what?
a. Assessing a family's response to illness in its members
b. Detecting the presence of illness in an individual
c. Interventions that nurses can use to assist a client's journey toward self-actualization
d. The development of wellness in a client

1-6. In McCabe's model of healing, which of the following is true?
a. Nursing interventions are manipulations of energy fields
b. Disease is measured by direct observations and laboratory tests
c. Illness is defined as a normal process within an individual
d. Abnormal chest pain is a signal that summons the healing response

1-7. External variables that influence health beliefs and practices include all of the following except which one?
a. Developmental stage
b. Family practices
c. Socioeconomic factors
d. Cultural background

1-8. Which of the following is an example of primary prevention?
a. Taking medication daily to control high blood pressure
b. Physical therapy on the affected arm and leg of a client recovering from a cerebrovascular accident
c. Teaching abstinence in the public school system
d. Exploring the hiring of a client with a known disability

1-9. Risk factors are described in what way?
a. Variables that increase the vulnerability of an individual to an illness
b. Generally modifiable
c. Direct indicators that specific diseases will develop in an individual
d. Most commonly used in the assessment of tertiary prevention

1-10. Which of the following is *not* a step in the change process as described by Haber and Lacy?
a. List the benefits of the change
b. Detail the steps involved in implementing the change
c. Regularly evaluate the change process
d. Describe specific alternatives if the change does not occur

1-11. An adult client has recently been diagnosed with emphysema resulting from his long history of smoking. This diagnosis is an example of what?
a. Acute illness
b. Tertiary disease
c. Chronic illness
d. Internal variable

B   C   C   D   B   D   A   C   D   D   C
1   2   3   4   5   6   7   8   9   10 11

CHAPTER 2

The Health Care Delivery System

2-1.   The State Farm Insurance Company is an example of what?
a.   Seamless care delivery model
b.   Form of Medicare
c.   Health Maintenance Organization
d.   Third-party payer

2-2.   A client's mother is being discharged home with the services of a home health agency. The client is worried about the cost of home health care. The nurse explains to the family that under Medicare and Medicaid regulations, government funds can be used to pay for which of the following?
a.   Private duty nursing care
b.   Housekeeping services
c.   Medical supplies such as syringes and dressings
d.   Companion services

2-3.   A prenatal client is in her second trimester of pregnancy. She is unemployed and financially impoverished. To obtain prenatal care, what is one method of federal funding?
a.   Medicare
b.   An individual state plan of health care
c.   A nonprofit organization
d.   Medicaid

2-4.   An adult client is selecting a health care plan. The client wants one person to be in charge of all health care needs. What is the program that will best meet the client's needs?
a.   Managed care
b.   Captivation care
c.   Long-term insurance
d.   Catastrophic health insurance

2-5.   An adult client has developed chronic bronchitis and believes it is associated with working in a florist business. The client should be seen by whom?
a.   Acute care nurse
b.   Occupational nurse
c.   Nurse entrepreneur
d.   Infection control nurse

2-6.   All the following are primary characteristics of a nursing center *except* which one?
a.   Direct access by the client to the nurse
b.   Nursing model of care
c.   Board of directors to establish sound policies
d.   Holistic reimbursed care services

2-7.   An adult client receives assistance from a nurse living in the neighborhood. This type of nursing practice best describes which of the following?
a.   Nursing as a caring profession
b.   Parish nursing
c.   Block nursing
d.   Volunteer nursing

2-8.   An adult client has been seeing a family nurse practitioner for gastrointestinal discomfort. Suddenly the client develops intense pain and is hospitalized for a perforated ulcer. Hospitalization in this circumstance is an example of what?
a.   Primary prevention
b.   Ambulatory surgical services
c.   Managed care services
d.   Secondary health care services

2-9.   An adult client is recovering from a "brain attack." The client does not require intravenous feedings but still needs considerable nursing interventions during this rehabilitation time. Being single and unable to be cared for at home, this client could best be cared for at which of the following?
a.   Primary prevention center
b.   Subacute care facility
c.   Convalescent care center
d.   Crisis intervention center

2-10.   An adult client is cared for by a restorative health care team. The restorative health care team concept means what?
a.   The team will meet and tell the client what to do after discussing the case
b.   The client and the family will be included in the team meetings to discuss options of care
c.   The client will not have to go to a respite care center
d.   The client will be referred to a home health care team

2-11.   An adult client has pancreatic cancer and has a prognosis of survival of 3 to 6 months. The client's family should seek what services?
a.   Respite care
b.   Adult day care
c.   Hospice care
d.   Long-term care

2-12.   The nurse asks a patient care assistant to bathe a client. This action is an example of what?
a.   Managed care
b.   Delegation
c.   Work redesign
d.   Residential community care

2-13.   A care map is designed for a client who is recovering from cardiac surgery. One day the client develops an unexpected complication. This complication is an example of what?
a.   Variance
b.   Critical pathway
c.   Patient focused care model
d.   Discharge plan

2-14.   Discharge planning begins when a client is at what stage?
a.   Has a discharge order written by the physician
b.   Is admitted to the hospital
c.   Knows that discharge is likely to be within a day or two
d.   Is within 1 day of being discharged

CHAPTER 3

Nursing Management of Client Care

3-1.   An effective leader has which quality?
a.   Does not make any independent decisions
b.   Encourages others to perform to the best of their ability
c.   Has natural leadership qualities and "is born that way"
d.   Primarily functions from an autocratic leadership style

3-2.   According to Gustafson, all of the following are common management functions *except* which one?
a.   Controlling
b.   Decision-making
c.   Evaluating
d.   Staffing

3-3.   The nurse manager asks a staff nurse to provide comfort measures in whatever manner the nurse chooses. This is an example of what style of leadership?
a.   Primary care
b.   Autocratic
c.   Democratic
d.   Laissez-faire

3-4.   An ambulatory clinic is managed by the nurse and everyone says, "She runs a pretty tight ship." This best describes what style of leadership?
a.   Primary care
b.   Autocratic
c.   Democratic
d.   Laissez-faire

3-5.   The nurse manager frequently explains new inservice procedures to nursing staff in the home health agency. This is an example of what style of situational leadership?
a.   Directing
b.   Coaching
c.   Supporting
d.   Delegating

3-6.   A delivery of care model is which of the following?
a.   Staffing plan that specifies the number of registered versus licensed practical nurses
b.   Framework for providing nurses with goals for assessment, diagnosis, and intervention
c.   System for organizing the relationships and roles of all nursing care personnel
d.   System that dictates the total number of staff necessary for a particular nursing division

3-7.   What is one important advantage of primary nursing over team leading?
a.   Decreased length of hospitalization
b.   Increased time with the physician
c.   Personal care assistants doing more client care
d.   Improved continuity of client care

3-8.   In case management, a nurse functioning as a case manager has what role?
a.   Frequently gives direct client care
b.   Is responsible for selected tasks based on qualifications and skills
c.   Coordinates care of groups of clients, facilitating referrals and discharge planning
d.   Administers all medications and treatments for a group of clients

3-9. In one acute care facility, the various nursing units do not share their nursing staff with the other nursing units. This is an example of what type of staffing?
a. Centralized management
b. Accountability
c. Active responsibility
d. Decentralized management

3-10. The physician is normally accompanied by a staff nurse when assessing clients. This is an example of what type of practice?
a. Caring
b. Continuous quality improvement
c. Collaborative practice
d. Interdisciplinary collaboration

3-11. All the following are leadership skills required of the student nurse *except* which one?
a. Aggressiveness
b. Team communication
c. Knowledge building
d. Clinical care coordination

3-12. The nurse always makes a list of interventions that should be implemented during the upcoming shift of care. This is an example of what?
a. Setting priorities
b. Goal setting
c. Evaluating the situation
d. Utilizing interruption control

CHAPTER 4

15 Critical Thinking and Nursing Judgment

4-1. According to the American Philosophical Association, all the following are critical thinking skills *except* which one?
a. Inference
b. Self-regulation
c. Implementation
d. Interpretation

4-2. The nurse asks a client to recount the details of the spouse's death. This is an example of what type of exercise?
a. Grieving
b. Reflection
c. Long-term memory
d. Engagement

4-3. The nursing student is learning essential clinical skills. The student tells the nursing instructor, "I can't remember whether I should put on sterile gloves or exam gloves." This is probably an example of: what type of thinking?
a. Complex critical thinking
b. Commitment critical thinking
c. Basic critical thinking
d. Problem-solving

4-4. The nurse tells a colleague, "I'm going to ask my clients with jugular vein distention if they also have dependent edema." This is an example of what action?
a. Problem identification
b. Data collection
c. Formulation of a hypothesis
d. Testing the hypothesis

4-5. A clinical nurse specialist decides to advise the critical care staff to ambulate their postoperative cardiac clients sooner to see if the clients can decrease the incidence of pneumonia. This is an example of what type of action?
a. Formulating a hypothesis
b. Problem-solving
c. Decision-making
d. Diagnostic reasoning

4-6. All the following are components of the nursing process *except* which one?
a. Taking action
b. Evaluating the results of the action
c. Gathering client data
d. Documenting the results of the action

4-7. The nurse manager states, "I am confident that our new critical pathways will make a positive difference in the recovery of the cholecystectomy clients." According to Kataoka-Yahiro, this is an example of what component of critical thinking?
a. Specific knowledge base
b. Standards for critical thinking
c. Critical thinking competencies
d. Attitudes for critical thinking

4-8. A staff nurse decides to question the hygienic practices of the respiratory therapists in the intensive care unit. This is an example of what type of questioning?
a. Fairness
b. Risk taking
c. Creativity
d. Curiosity

4-9. The nurse manager is attempting to develop mutual trust between the day shift and the night shift. The nurse manager is trying to enhance which critical thinking attitude?
a. Integrity
b. Humility
c. Discipline
d. Perseverance

4-10. The nurse writes three goals for a client with an alteration in tissue perfusion of the lower extremities. This is an example of what nursing process?
a. Assessment
b. Nursing diagnosis
c. Planning
d. Implementation

CHAPTER 5

Nursing Assessment

5-1. What is the primary source of information for a data base concerning a client?
a. Physician
b. Chart
c. Client
d. Family

5-2. A client discusses a change in employment due to a recent back injury. According to Gordon's health patterns, this is an example of which pattern?
a. Nutritional-metabolic
b. Coping-stress tolerance
c. Cognitive-perceptual
d. Role-relationship

5-3. What is an example of objective data?
a. The client's statement of being in pain
b. Heart rate of 66 beats per minute
c. Itching from a histamine response
d. Headache from photosensitivity

5-4. A client tells you that there is continual abdominal cramping. This is an example of what type of data?
a. Subjective
b. Objective
c. Disputable
d. Personal

5-5. Which of the following statements would be appropriate in the working phase of the interview?
a. "Good morning, I will be your nurse today."
b. "Why didn't you come into the hospital earlier, Mrs. Vas?"
c. "I've just got one more question, Mr.Leif."
d. "Tell me about the diet you eat at home."

5-6. All the following are elements of a nursing health history except which one?
a. Past health history
b. Biographical information
c. Present insurance coverage
d. Environmental history

5-7. What is an environmental aspect of the health history?
a. Presence of a caring atmosphere set by the nurse
b. Drawing the curtains around the client's bed while interviewing
c. Direct questioning techniques that encourage open communication
d. Asking the client to clarify statements to enhance the interview process

5-8. A client states, "I'm burning up, and I think I have a temperature." The nurse takes the client's temperature, observes the skin for flushing, and feels the skin temperature. Why does the nurse perform these assessment activities?
a. Validation of subjective data
b. Clustering of subjective data
c. Review of subjective data
d. Documentation of subjective data

5-9. The nurse feels the chest for vocal fremitus in a client suspected of having lung consolidation. This action is an example of what?
a. Inspection
b. Auscultation
c. Percussion
d. Palpation

5-10. After assessing a client, the nurse determines a diagnosis of decreased cardiac output. This is an example of what type of data action?
a. Validation
b. Clustering
c. Documentation
d. Verification

5-11. What is a basic rule for nursing documentation?
  a. Use previous client experience to generalize specific nursing diagnoses for each client
  b. Make a nursing diagnosis as soon as possible after collecting the data
  c. Be factual in recording observations
  d. Do not be excessively descriptive of client symptomology

CHAPTER 6

Nursing Diagnosis

6-1. What is a nursing diagnosis?
  a. Statement of a client response to a health problem that requires nursing intervention
  b. Identification of nursing problems
  c. Derivation of the physician's history and physical
  d. Unchanged during the course of a client's hospitalization

6-2. A client has a decreased respiratory rate, moist breath sounds, and labored breathing. These are what type of data?
  a. Cluster of similar signs and symptoms
  b. Examples of nursing diagnoses
  c. Risk factors
  d. NANDA grouping

6-3. What is an exception to one of the types of nursing diagnoses?
  a. Risk nursing diagnosis
  b. Wellness nursing diagnosis
  c. Syndrome nursing diagnosis
  d. Potential nursing diagnosis

6-4. A nursing diagnosis is "decreased cardiac output related to interstitial excess in the extremities." What is the "decreased cardiac output" of this diagnosis?
  a. More debilitating symptomology of the diagnosis
  b. Medical diagnosis
  c. Diagnostic label of this nursing diagnosis
  d. Problem area that can be treated with nursing interventions

6-5. A client has been successfully treated for "hyperthermia related to noncompliance in taking adequate antipyretics." What can be said of the first nursing diagnosis?
  a. It should not be changed
  b. It should be crossed out on the progress record, and the word "error" should be written above it
  c. It was the more important diagnosis
  d. It can be modified as new data is provided to the nurse

6-6. What is a nonnursing diagnosis category?
  a. Anxiety
  b. Activity intolerance
  c. Respiratory failure
  d. Hopelessness

6-7. What nursing diagnosis has the highest priority?
  a. Anxiety related to outcome of diagnostic bronchoscopy
  b. Social isolation related to impaired mobility
  c. Impaired skin integrity related to leakage of ileostomy drainage
  d. Ineffective airway clearance related to incisional pain

6-8. Assessment reveals that a client has lost 10 lb in the last 2 months. Weight loss is one of the three defining characteristics of the diagnostic category "altered nutrition: less than body requirements." Knowing this, what should the nurse do?
  a. State the nursing diagnosis "altered nutrition: less than body requirements, related to poor dietary habits"
  b. Examine the assessment data to see if other signs and symptoms of altered nutrition exist
  c. Ignore the data on the weight loss because 10 lb is not that much
  d. State the diagnosis "weight loss related to decreased food intake"

6-9. A client's nurse is unable to insert a peripheral IV because of decreased circulation and poor respiratory status. How should the nurse document this situation?
  a. "Inability to initiate peripheral IV due to poor veins"
  b. "Decreased cardiac output that does not allow IV insertion"
  c. "Hopeful of starting IV when patient circulation improves"
  d. "Decreased cardiac output related to altered ventilation"

6-10. What is a valuable use of nursing diagnoses?
a. Allowing the nurse to compete with physicians
b. Developing individualized care plans
c. Treating nursing problems and medical problems
d. Managing client care for the entire health care team

CHAPTER 7

Planning for Nursing Care

7-1. A client smokes and has emphysema. From this data alone, what level of priority should the nurse establish?
a. High level
b. Moderate level
c. Intermediate level
d. Low level

7-2. Which client goal is written correctly?
a. Client will state the purpose of the medication before discharge
b. Client will feel better by morning
c. Client's pulse will be normal
d. Nurse will establish IV access by the beginning of day shift

7-3. Which expected outcome statement is correctly written?
a. Nursing assistant will set client up for a bath every morning
b. Client will eat at least 80% of meals and gain 1 lb by October 1
c. Client will have improved airway clearance by November 15
d. Client will identify need to increase dietary intake of fiber by July 4

7-4. Which nursing intervention is correctly stated?
a. Listen to breath sounds frequently
b. Nurse will offer 3 oz water to client every 2 hours while awake
c. Increase ambulation in the room
d. Nurse will encourage coughing and deep breathing

7-5. A client is suffering from gastric reflux and shortness of breath. Which of the following is the correct goal statement concerning this condition?
a. "Client will have no acid indigestion after meals and a respiratory rate of 14 to 18 breaths per minute."
b. "Client will breathe unlabored at 14 to18 breaths per minute by the end of this shift."
c. "Client will not complain of stomach pain or breathing problems within the next 8 hours."
d. "Client will be comfortable by morning."

7-6. Which of the following is true concerning nurse-initiated interventions?
a. Developed after evaluating the interventions for the recent medical diagnoses
b. Supervised by the entire health care team
c. Determined by the local state nursing practice acts
d. Made in concert with the plan of care authorized by the physician

7-7. The staff nurse asks the clinical nurse specialist (CNS) to consult in developing an individualized teaching plan for a client. Which action of the staff nurse is *not* appropriate in the consultation process?
a. Giving the CNS a brief history of the client's illness
b. Telling the CNS that the client is uncooperative and will be hard to teach
c. Describing to the CNS the teaching strategies tried thus far
d. Incorporating the CNS's recommendations into the care plan

7-8. What is the nursing care plan?
a. Written guideline for implementation and evaluation
b. Documentation of client care
c. Projection of potential alterations in client behaviors
d. Tool to set goals and project outcomes

7-9. Which factor should a nurse *not* consider when choosing interventions for a client?
a. Research base for the interventions
b. Competency of the nurse
c. Viability of the client
d. Feasibility of the intervention

7-10. The student nurse is writing a care plan for a weekly clinical experience. Which example best compares the care plan to the one written by the staff?
   a. The care plan is less specific than the nurse's care plan
   b. The assessment section of the student nurse's care plan is not as thorough
   c. The student nurse's care plan is probably more elaborate
   d. The nurse's care plan includes the medications and the lab results

CHAPTER 8

19 **Implementing Nursing Care**

8-1. What is the basis for nursing implementation?
   a. Medical diagnosis
   b. Nursing criteria
   c. Outcome criteria
   d. Nursing care plan

8-2. The physician leaves orders for the client to receive an analgesic via either IV, IM, or PO routes. The nurse can evaluate the client and decide which route. This practice is an example of what?
   a. Standing order
   b. Protocol
   c. Intervention
   d. Assessment regimen

8-3. The nurse listens to the change-of-shift report and then tells an LPN to provide total client care for five clients, with a nursing assistant to help. This type of nursing care is an example of what kind of system?
   a. Functional nursing
   b. Total client care
   c. Case management
   d. Team nursing

8-4. The nurse walks into a room and finds the client lying on the floor. What step of the nursing process is necessary at this time?
   a. Implementation
   b. Planning
   c. Assessment
   d. Nursing diagnosis

8-5. The nurse attends an inservice on using a new infusion pump, which requires an entirely new tubing system. This type of learning for the nurse is an example of what?
   a. Cognitive skill learning
   b. Psychomotor skills
   c. Interpersonal skill training
   d. Communication and education

8-6. A client requires assistance in ambulating to the bathroom each morning. This type of activity is an example of what?
   a. Activity of daily living
   b. Setting goals
   c. Critical decision-making
   d. Behavior modification

8-7. Checking the patency of an IV before administering the medications is an example of what?
   a. Preventing adverse reactions
   b. Assisting with activities of daily living
   c. Counseling
   d. Compensating for adverse reactions

8-8. The nurse administers a medication to the client that has a known side effect of causing dizziness. The nurse informs the client not to get up without help and raises the side rails. These activities are examples of what?
   a. Arranging the environment to reduce distractions
   b. Making the client physically comfortable
   c. Identifying situations in which the nurse needs assistance
   d. Anticipating complications and initiating preventive measures

8-9. As the nurse works with a client in the achievement of goals, what is an inappropriate action?
   a. Keeping the care plan flexible
   b. Maintaining the privacy of the client
   c. Adhering to the plan of care by both client and family
   d. Encouraging the client to achieve the goals quickly to enhance movement toward being discharged

8-10. The level of assistance that clients require in the implementation phase of the nursing process is exemplified by what?
   a. Two clients with the same medical diagnoses that require the same level of assistance in the provision of nursing care
   b. Unconscious clients who will require total care in their physical needs
   c. The nurse supplementing the client's capabilities when necessary
   d. Hospitalized clients receiving total care from the nursing staff

CHAPTER 9

Evaluation

9-1. The stated expected outcome is "heart rate will be below 90/minute by 4/21." On April 21, the nurse identifies tachycardia and a rate of 110/minute. On the basis of this the nurse should first do what?
   a. Discontinue the care plan
   b. Reassess the client
   c. Review the appropriateness of the nursing diagnosis
   d. Revise the expected outcome

9-2. All the following are examples of evaluative measures *except* which one?
   a. Observing the amount the client eats at each meal
   b. Taking the client's temperature
   c. Questioning a client about pain
   d. Administering medication as ordered

9-3. A client has met the goals set for improvement of ventilatory status. The nurse can now do what?
   a. Modify the care plan
   b. Reassess the client's response to care and evaluate the implementation step of the nursing process
   c. Discontinue the care plan
   d. Create a nursing diagnosis that states the goals have been met

9-4. What is the overall goal of quality assurance?
   a. Find nursing errors
   b. Document excellence of nursing care
   c. Discover ways to improve health care
   d. Ensure excellent health care

9-5. A client has received several nursing interventions. To evaluate the interventions, what should the nurse examine?
   a. Appropriateness of the interventions and the correct application of the implementation process
   b. Nursing diagnoses to ensure they are not medical diagnoses
   c. Care planning process for errors in other health care team members' judgment
   d. Interventions of each nurse to enable the nurse manager to correctly evaluate his or her performance

9-6. What does "doing the right thing" mean?
   a. Evaluating the caring process of the nurses responsible for client care
   b. Assessing the efficacy of a procedure in relation to a client's condition
   c. Critiquing the continuity of care in services provided
   d. Showing the relationship between outcomes and resources used to deliver client care

9-7. JCAHO's steps for quality improvement include all of the following *except* which one?
   a. Reevaluating to determine if a plan was successful
   b. Collecting and analyzing data from monitoring activities
   c. Defining the key aspects of service for the clinical area
   d. Assessing the financial appropriateness of the client interventions

9-8. "Clients extubated early will have fewer postoperative complications" is an example of what?
   a. Structure indicator
   b. Responsibility indicator
   c. Outcome indicator
   d. Process indicator

9-9. A correctly stated threshold for evaluation in the quality improvement process is:
   a. "Incidence of skin breakdown in clients with strokes"
   b. "Clients are able to discuss home medication regimes"
   c. "Ninety percent of clients will express satisfaction with the quality of their meals"
   d. "Most of the clients who are on bedrest will maintain skin integrity"

9-10. The nurse decides to use the Focus-PDCA model. What is the nurse most likely doing?
a. Implementing a new policy on the nursing unit
b. Organizing a team to evaluate a current clinical problem of the nursing staff
c. Examining the infrastructure of the acute care facility
d. Evaluating the nursing staff using a centralized program of study

CHAPTER 10

Professional Nursing Roles

10-1. Who was the first professor of nursing?
a. Florence Nightingale
b. Isabel Hampton Robb
c. Mary Adelaide Nutting
d. Mary Agnes Snively

10-2. How did the 1980 American Nurses Association Congress for Nursing Practice define nursing?
a. Performance for compensation of any act in the observation, care, and counsel of the ill
b. Administration of medications and treatments prescribed by licensed physicians or dentists
c. Promotion or restoration of client health and the prevention of illness
d. Diagnosis and treatment of human responses to actual or potential health problems

10-3. How is a conceptual model's nursing value viewed?
a. Assisting nurses in the application of their clinical skills
b. Providing knowledge to improve practice and to guide research
c. Directing the health care team in its collaborative approach to client care
d. Promoting solid values from which to build the precepts of professional nursing

10-4. Which theorist purports that the goal of nursing is to work independently with other health care workers?
a. Hall
b. Rogers
c. King
d. Henderson

10-5. A client asks the nurse, "What is the difference between the 2-year (A.D.N.) and the 4-year (B.S.N.) nurse?" What is the nurse's best response?
a. "The 2-year nurse can begin practicing earlier and pay off college debts more easily."
b. "The 4-year nurse implements research projects."
c. "The 2-year nurse does not participate in as many theoretical courses."
d. "The 4-year nurse is educated in a broader manner and has a better foundation for graduate education."

10-6 An adult client loses balance easily. The nurse explains to the x-ray technician that the client should have physical assistance when standing for the upcoming x-ray procedure. This action is an example of what?
a. Caring
b. Case management
c. Protector role
d. Client advocate role

10-7. A client requires a prescription for osteoarthritis. Who is the individual most likely to fulfill this need?
a. LPN
b. RN
c. APN
d. Nurse educator

10-8. A client requires a surgical intervention for a diseased gallbladder. Which nurse is most likely to provide care during the intraoperative setting?
a. Clinical nurse specialist
b. Certified Registered Nurse Anesthetist
c. Nurse practitioner
d. APN

10-9. The least likely setting in which the client of the 21st century will receive care is the:
a. Acute care setting
b. Home care setting
c. Ambulatory care setting
d. Short-term care setting

10-10. Which statement is true concerning UAPs?
a. They usually practice under the license of the RN.
b. They are allowed to perform those skills that the RN is able to teach them in the clinical setting.
c. They are in the second year of their nursing education.
d. They provide basic care skills.

CHAPTER 11

Ethics and Values

11-1.   What is bioethics?
a. Personal belief about the worth of a given idea, attitude, or object that sets standards and influences behavior
b. Judgment of behavior
c. Study of ethics within the field of health care
d. Study of right and wrong behavior, which often evolves from social life

11-2.   The nurse decides to withhold a client's medication because it will lower the respiratory rate of the client. This action is an example of what?
a. Responsibility
b. Accountability
c. Competence
d. Ethical behavior

11-3.   Nonmaleficence refers to:
a. Displaying respect for all persons
b. Supporting the client's right to informed consent
c. Preventing or removing harm to client when possible
d. Considering how the client can best be helped

11-4.   An older client believes that life should not be prolonged when hope is gone. The client has decided that "extra lifesaving measures" should not be taken when physical life is at the end. The client has discussed these desires with family members, completed a living will, and left directions with the physician. This scenario is an example of what?
a. Affirming a value
b. Choosing a value
c. Prizing a value
d. Reflecting on a value

11-5.   The nurse is working with a 12-year-old who has diabetes. The nurse often overhears the parents telling the child, "We were meant to take good care of our bodies" or "Going off your diet is irresponsible and childish; you should be ashamed of yourself." What is the mode by which the parents are attempting to transmit values?
a. Modeling
b. Moralizing
c. Laissez-faire
d. Responsible choice

11-6.   In what age-group is the characteristics of redefinition and testing of values most evident?
a. Preschool child
b. School-age child
c. Adolescent
d. Adult

11-7.   A client states, "I deserve to have the bed next to the window because I am one of the hospital board members." This statement is an example of what?
a. A cultural value
b. Ethnocentrism
c. Values clarification
d. Deontology

11-8.   The community health nurse states, "I wish we had just a portion of the dollars we spend repairing atherosclerotic hearts to teach this community about cardiovascular risk factors." This statement is an example of what?
a. Deontology
b. Feminist ethics
c. Utilitarianism
d. An ethical dilemma

11-9.   A nurse is working with the parents of a seriously ill newborn. Surgery has been proposed for the infant, but the chances of success are unclear. In helping the parents to resolve this ethical conflict, the nurse knows that the first step is what?
a. Exploring reasonable courses of action
b. Collecting all available information about the situation
c. Clarifying values related to the cause of the dilemma
d. Identifying people who can solve the difficulty

11-10. A nurse decides to tell the adult children that they need to decide what to advise their father about his taking analgesics during the terminal phase of his illness. This action is an example of what?
a. Evaluating the action
b. Articulating the problem
c. Determining one's own values on the ethical dilemma
d. Negotiating the outcome

C B C C B D B C B D
1 2 3 4 5 6 7 8 9 10

CHAPTER 12

23 Legal Concepts in Nursing Practice

12-1. A client receives $350,000 for wrongful care in a regional trauma center. This settlement is most likely the result of what?
a. Violation of criminal law
b. Tort
c. Breach of conduct in statutory law
d. Misbehavior contradicting common law

12-2. A confused client rolls out of bed because both side rails were not raised. This is an example of what?
a. Felony
b. Assault
c. Battery
d. Negligence

12-3. The nurse puts a restraint vest on a client without the client's permission and without a physician's order. The nurse may be guilty of what?
a. Assault
b. Battery
c. Invasion of privacy
d. Neglect

12-4. In a malpractice suit against a nurse, a client must prove any of the following except which one?
a. Client was injured
b. Client's injury was caused by the nurse's failure to carry out a duty
c. Nurse's intention was not favorable
d. Nurse did not carry out that duty or breached the duty

12-5. Good Samaritan laws encourage health care providers to render assistance in accidents because they do what?
a. Supply funds for first aid training
b. Limit legal liability in emergency situations
c. Establish standard treatments for emergency aid
d. Provide for reimbursement for first aid services rendered

12-6. A state with child abuse legislation requires that a nurse who suspects abuse or neglect must do what?
a. Report it to the proper legal authority
b. Inform the parents that their acts are illegal
c. Call the security department to handle the problem
d. Prevent the parents from seeing the child during hospitalization

12-7. A student nurse who is employed as a personal care assistant may perform which type of client care?
a. Learned in school
b. Expected of a nurse at that level
c. Identified in the position's job description
d. Requires technical rather than professional skill

12-8. The nurse is about to administer a medication and notices that the physician's order looks incorrect regarding the amount of medication. What should the nurse do?
a. Administer the medication with extreme caution and observe for adverse reactions in the client
b. Document the suspicion that the dosage amount is incorrect, and withhold the medication
c. Notify the physician and withhold the medication
d. Write a progress note to the physician explaining why the medication was withheld

12-9. A client with increased intracranial pressure is operated on without the client's consent. What can be said about this procedure?
a. It is an example of informal consent
b. It makes the care providers liable for malpractice
c. It should not have been done without the expressed and informed consent of a close family member
d. It is valid due to the emergent condition of the situation

12-10. A client states, "I don't want any more surgeries. I just want to die." The nurse provides the client with information about the levels of life-sustaining procedures that could be provided. This action is an example of what?
a. Advanced directives
b. Passive euthanasia
c. Living will
d. Assisted suicide

B D B C B A C C D A C D
1 2 3 4 5 6 7 8 9 10 11 12

12-11. A client falls while ambulating, and the staff nurse is asked to complete an incident report. What happens with this document?
a. It is part of the permanent medical record
b. It will be used as evidence if the client pursues criminal negligence
c. It serves as a means of quality improvement and risk management
d. It is only examined by the nurse managers on the staff nurse's unit

12-12. A prenatal client is considering an abortion. What are the nurse's options?
a. Present the potential problems associated with this procedure
b. Inform the client that she will have to wait a week before she will be allowed to have the procedure
c. Objectively care for the client and attempt to discourage her from having the procedure
d. Inform the physician to enable the appropriate communication to the parents, if the client is a minor

CHAPTER 13

Communication

13-1. A nurse makes the statement, 'I don't want to care for the client in room 224 after hearing what you have told me." This statement is an example of not being what?
a. Self-confident
b. Analytical
c. Open-minded
d. Inquisitive

13-2. A nurse decides to talk to another staff nurse at the nursing station about a client for which they are caring. This activity is an example of what?
a. Public communication
b. Gossip
c. Validation
d. Interpersonal communication

13-3. How is metacommunication best defined?
a. Saying something that you really don't believe
b. A complete form of the sender's message, which includes attitudes and content
c. Having one's physical appearance match one's verbalization
d. Communicating many ideas at once

13-4. The nurse is conducting an admission interview with a client. To maintain the client's territoriality and maximize communication, where should the nurse sit?
a. 0 to 18 inches from the client
b. 18 inches to 4 feet from the client
c. 4 to 12 feet from the client
d. 12 feet or more from the client

13-5. To facilitate communication with a preschooler, what should the nurse do?
a. Demonstrate how equipment works
b. Provide close physical contact
c. Allow time to talk
d. Tell the child exactly what he or she can do

13-6. A client recently had a bowel resection, resulting in a colostomy. When the nurse enters the room to begin teaching about care of the ostomy, the nurse finds the client crying and decides to delay the teaching session. Why?
a. Possible differences in connotative meaning
b. Pacing of the conversation
c. Timing and relevance of the information
d. Environmental setting of the conversation

13-7. In what phase are contracts for the therapeutic helping relationship formed?
a. Orientation
b. Preinteraction
c. Working
d. Termination

13-8. The nurse is caring for a client who is obese and has hypertension. Which statement by the nurse will promote effective communication?
a. "Why haven't you stayed on your diet in the past?"
b. "From what you've told me it seems that cutting out fried foods was the hardest part of your diet plan. Is that right?"
c. "The best thing for you to do would be to join Weight Watchers."
d. "It's really not good for your weight to keep going up and down like this."

13-9. The nurse informs a client, "I will be back in 15 minutes." This action is an example of what?
a. Availability
b. Empathy
c. Trust
d. Confidentiality

13-10. While a client is being questioned, his son states, "My father really means that he doesn't know what the respiratory therapist means." This communication statement is an example of what?
a. Focus
b. Summarizing
c. Paraphrasing
d. Clarifying

13-11. All the following are "blockers" to effective communication *except* which one?
a. Triangulation
b. False reassurance
c. Socializing
d. Approval

CHAPTER 14

Documentation and Reporting

14-1. The home health nurse forgets to chart some of the skills provided for a client. This action could result in what?
a. Questions from the client and family
b. Concern from the patient care assistant about the knowledge level of the nurse
c. Lack of reimbursement to the home health care agency
d. Malpractice on the part of the nurse

14-2. The purpose of the client record includes all the following except which one?
a. Financial billing
b. Research
c. Assessment
d. Ethical guidelines

14-3. Which statement is correctly documented according to the six guidelines for quality recording?
a. "Crying. States she doesn't want visitors to see her like this."
b. "Respirations rapid, lung sounds clear."
c. "Was depressed today."
d. "Had a good day. Up and about in room."

14-4. For a written report to be accurate, it must include which of the following?
a. Interpretations of client behavior
b. The nurse's objective observations
c. Abbreviations familiar to the nurse
d. Lengthy entries using lay terminology

14-5. The nurse records, "Client states he is experiencing more stress today than yesterday due to his new diagnosis." This statement is an example of what?
a. SOAP documentation
b. Narrative documentation
c. PIE documentation
d. Charting by exception

14-6. In a source record, the traditional form of the medical record, which of the following is true?
a. Each discipline has a separate section to record data
b. Information is well organized according to client's problems
c. Entries are made in random order throughout the client chart
d. There is a decrease in the fragmentation of data

14-7. The nurse reads in a chart that the client had a small bowel resection 10 years ago. The nurse probably found this data in which part of the chart?
a. Flow sheet
b. Kardex
c. Admission nursing history form
d. Focus chart entry

14-8. The nurse manager assesses the clients on the orthopedic unit and verifies that four clients require a higher nurse-to-client ratio. This type of assessment is most likely an example of what?
a. Standardized care plan
b. Acuity charting system
c. Critical pathway
d. Charting by exception

14-9. The nurse uses a new computer software package that enables visualization of wounds similar to a client's on the nursing unit. The use of computer software is an example of what?
a. Automated speech recognition
b. Computer-based patient records
c. Virtual reality
d. Graphic user interface

14-10. During a change-of-shift report, which of the following occurs?
a. Two or more nurses always visit all clients to review their plan of care
b. Nurses should exchange judgments they have made about client attitudes

c. The nurse should identify nursing diagnoses and clarify client priorities

d. Client information is communicated from the nurse on a sending unit to a nurse on a receiving unit

14-11. The physician telephones a new prescription to a nurse for one of the clients on the neurological unit. What should the nurse do?

a. Not give the medication until the physician is able to write the medication prescription in person

b. Verify the physician's new medication order with another registered nurse

c. Clarify the new medication order with the pharmacy

d. Document the new prescription in the client's chart

14-12. The nurse writes an incident report on a client who fell in the rest room. What is the purpose of this documentation?

a. Keep the nurse from being sued

b. Assist in the quality improvement program of the nursing unit

c. Assure proper care for the client

d. Add to the medical record of the client

CHAPTER 15

Client Education

15-1. What accrediting body establishes general guidelines for client and family education?

a. JCAHO

b. HEW

c. AACN

d. AMA

15-2. Health education should focus primarily on what?

a. Motivating the client to comply with a given health care regimen

b. Allowing the entire health care team to give a variety of strategies for the client to follow

c. Determining the client's level of knowledge and perception of what learning is needed

d. Preventing diseases and learning good health promotion activities

15-3. The nurse observes a client self-administer an insulin injection. Administration of insulin is an example of what?

a. Cognitive learning

b. Affective learning

c. Motivational learning

d. Psychomotor learning

15-4. A 3-year-old client is scheduled for an invasive test. During a short teaching session, what should the nurse use?

a. Short story

b. Play

c. Discussion

d. Self-expression

15-5. A client is unable to use certain orthotics due to slight paralysis of the upper extremities. What is the physical attribute necessary for learning psychomotor skills relating to this problem?

a. Size

b. Strength

c. Coordination

d. Sensory acuity

15-6. Which of the following clients is most ready to begin a patient teaching session?

a. A client with a recent back injury who is unwilling to accept that the injury may result in permanent paralysis

b. A newly diagnosed diabetic who is complaining of being awake all night because of a noisy roommate

c. A client with irritable bowel syndrome who has just returned from a morning of testing in the GI lab

d. A client who had myocardial infarction 4 days ago and now seems somewhat anxious about how this will affect the future

15-7. A client does not know how the renal system can be responsible for hypertension. Which diagnostic statement best describes this problem?

a. Altered self-concept

b. Decreased cardiac output

c. Knowledge deficit

d. Inaccurate knowledge base

15-8. The nurse tells a client that stopping smoking for the past 3 days is a tremendous accomplishment. This teaching approach is called what?

a. Selling

b. Participating

c. Reinforcing

d. Entrusting

15-9. The nurse tells a client with a recent back injury that damage to the nerves is like a watering hose that has been pinched off and needs time to allow normal nerve transmission. This statement is an example of what?
a. Analogy
b. Role-playing
c. Discovery
d. Demonstration

15-10. The nurse is teaching a 74-year-old client how to apply dressings to a recent abdominal incision. What should the nurse remember?
a. The client is unable to think abstractly compared to younger years.
b. Independence is a character quality to accentuate in the teaching process.
c. The teaching sessions should be longer than for younger adults.
d. This client will probably not learn as fast as the middle-age adult.

15-11. Who or what is the referent in communication strategies?
a. Learner
b. Person who conveys the message
c. Idea that initiates the reason for communication
d. Method used to transmit the message

CHAPTER 16

27 & 28 **Self-Concept and Sexuality**

16-1. A client has a colostomy in repairing a benign tumor of the bowel. This surgery is most appropriately called what?
a. Role stressor
b. Body-image stressor
c. Identity stressor
d. Gender stressor

16-2. An older adult client retired last year and is struggling emotionally. This situation is most likely a problem of which component of self-concept?
a. Role
b. Identity
c. Self-esteem
d. Body image

16-3. The nurse shares personal problems with gender development as a child. This is an example of critical thinking related to what?
a. Knowledge
b. Experience
c. Attitudes
d. Standards

16-4. After assessing a client, the nurse states, "You seem to not think you can do this procedure at home." This statement is an example of what?
a. Cultural variation
b. Lack of critical thinking
c. Client's expectations
d. Judgmental attitude

16-5. What is the first step in planning in the nursing process?
a. Assessing
b. Developing a nursing diagnosis
c. Gathering data
d. Developing goals and outcome criteria

16-6. Sex education should begin when?
a. Infancy
b. Adolescence
c. Midchildhood, before puberty
d. Puberty

16-7. Which contraception method is 100% effective?
a. Sterilization
b. Oral contraceptives
c. Abstinence
d. IUD

16-8. What is one of the least effective methods of contraception?
a. IUD
b. Oral contraceptive
c. Condom
d. Diaphragm

16-9. Which of the following is untrue about sexual abuse?
a. It can cause victim guilt.
b. It is sometimes provoked by the child.
c. It can cause sexual dysfunction.
d. It can be evidenced by excessive clinging to parents.

16-10. In taking a client's health history, it is important that the nurse do which of the following?
a. Discuss sexual concerns only if the client brings them up
b. Use emotionally laden terms when discussing sexual concepts
c. Focus on physical factors that affect sexual functioning
d. Routinely include a few questions related to sexual functioning

16-11. What is the most likely physical change that comes with age concerning sexual function?
a. Increased vaginal secretions in women
b. Prolonged erection time in men
c. Shorter vagina in women
d. Quicker arousal times in men

CHAPTER 17

Spiritual Health

17-1. How is the concept of faith best defined?
a. Emotional expression of a belief
b. Individual's belief that one's will efficaciously causes things to happen
c. Belief in the concept of God as defined in monotheistic religions
d. A belief that gives a person meaning and purpose in life

17-2. A client has been newly diagnosed with a terminal illness. What will this diagnosis create?
a. Time for the client to face fears about life
b. Change that will cause spiritual distress
c. Religious problems
d. Time to pray for spiritual healing

17-3. A client who is a Buddhist asks the nurse if Buddhism allows the circumcision of male infants. How should the nurse respond?
a. Attempt to learn the basic principles of Buddhism and tell the client she will try to find the information
b. Tell the client she does not practice the Buddhist faith and does not know
c. Ask a clergy member to come and visit the client
d. Tell the client that advice related to a belief system is outside the nurse's practice

17-4. Why does a nurse utilize the Jarel spiritual well-being scale?
a. Determine the type of religious affiliation of the client
b. Measure the satisfaction the client has with their religious activities
c. Evaluate a client's perceptions about a given personal condition
d. Assess the nurse's concerns about the spirituality of the client

17-5. A client of a Far Eastern religion says, "I want to die on the floor." This request is an example what?
a. Cultural norm
b. Ritual practice
c. Radical belief
d. Practice associated with fellowship and community

17-6. A client is newly diagnosed with multiple sclerosis. This diagnosis, according to NANDA, can be labeled as what?
a. Potential for negative spiritual well-being
b. Spiritual distress
c. Risk of fear and anxiety
d. Chronic illness with spiritual implications

17-7. The nurse is establishing presence with the client. As a foundation, the nurse must first do what?
a. Develop a complete nursing history of the client
b. Inform the client that they will be working together toward common goals
c. Create an environment of trust with the client
d. Assess whether the client is comfortable discussing health-related issues

17-8. A client and nurse are establishing a healing relationship with one another. What is the least likely central step in this process?
a. Mobilizing hope for the nurse and the client
b. Determining the physiological or psychological cause of the client's disorder
c. Finding an interpretation of the illness that is acceptable to the client
d. Assisting the client in using social, emotional, or spiritual resources

17-9. A client informs the nurse that he or she does not eat pork because of religious beliefs. Which religion does this person most likely practice (of the following)?
a. Jehovah's Witness
b. Buddhism
c. Islam
d. Baha'i

17-10. A client asks the nurse if they can "pray together right now." What is the nurse's best response?
a. "I think that is a wonderful idea."
b. "I don't know how, but I can try."
c. "I will go get our chaplain."
d. "I'm somewhat uncomfortable with praying with my clients."

17-11. If a client refuses to remove a specific religious garment for daily bathing, what should the nurse do?
a. Remove it anyway
b. Ask the client if it won't hurt to remove it, just during the hospitalization
c. Tell the client that other people of the same faith have allowed the clothing item to be taken off
d. Respect the client's wishes

CHAPTER 18

9 Cultural Care in Nursing

18-1. Which characteristic is not included in evaluating the heritage consistency in a client?
a. Ethnicity
b. Religion
c. Gender
d. Culture

18-2. Who is the traditional healer of the Puerto Rican culture?
a. Medicine man
b. Partera
c. Talisman
d. Señora

18-3. To respect a client's personal space and territoriality, the nurse must do what?
a. Avoid the use of touch
b. Keep the curtains closed around the client's bed

c. Stand at least 8 feet away from the client if possible
d. Carefully explain nursing care and procedures

18-4. A client needs respiratory treatment as an outpatient every other day but does not value adhering to a time schedule. What can the nurse do?
a. Schedule the appointments and tell the client to be there
b. Ask the client to call the clinic if an appointment must be canceled
c. Explain the importance of the treatments and the consequences of not having them regularly
d. Ask the respiratory therapy department to call the client each day as a reminder of the appointment

18-5. A client who speaks English as a second language informs a translator that healing remedies are used instead of the prescribed medications. What is the best nursing diagnosis?
a. Impaired socialization related to lack of assimilation
b. Altered health maintenance related to health care beliefs
c. Ineffective coping related to language differences
d. Noncompliance related to lack of knowledge regarding necessary medical care

18-6. South American cultures believe that health is what?
a. Reward for good behavior
b. Balance of yin and yang
c. State of emotional and physical well-being
d. Ability to live in harmony with nature

18-7. To avoid cultural conflicts with a client, what should the nurse do?
a. Assure the client that quality health care is being received
b. Provide the client with information about the dominant culture
c. Ask the client about expectations of nursing care and procedures
d. Avoid nursing interventions that might cause the client embarrassment

18-8. If a client does not speak English well, what should the nurse do?
a. Call the client by first name
b. Not attempt to interpret nonverbal movements because of their different meanings
c. Use slang terms in the client's language learned from hearing the client's verbalizations
d. Ask the client to clarify what has been said when it was misunderstood

18-9. The swamp root is a traditional remedy of which country?
a. France
b. Germany
c. Cuba
d. Haiti

18-10. Tactile relationships are important to which group of cultures?
a. Hispanic
b. Asian
c. European
d. North American

CHAPTER 19
Family Context in Nursing

19-1. Which is true about the majority of families today?
a. They consist of a mother, a father, and one or more children
b. They include a stepchild
c. They include a mother who works outside the home
d. They have health insurance coverage

19-2. If a client's family functions as context, on what does evaluation focus?
a. If the client is meeting psychophysiological and social needs
b. If individual family members are concerned and caring about one another
c. If the family is meeting its developmental tasks
d. If the family is satisfied with its new level of functioning

19-3. What is a family form called that includes relatives other than nuclear family members?
a. Blended
b. Communal
c. Extended
d. Homogenous

19-4. When planning family goals, what should the nurse do?
a. View the family as a system
b. Make the goals as broad as possible
c. Not incorporate the developmental stages of members not closely associated with the client
d. Assess the availability of the family members

19-5. In gerontological nursing practice, what must the nurse do?
a. Recognize that greater physical health impairments decrease the risk of the older adult's depression
b. Be aware of the fact that in the older stages of life, developmental tasks are not as important in setting goals
c. Consider the effects of caregiver strain on the family members
d. Realize that older adults have very similar social networks as younger family counterparts

19-6. Families with adolescents must do what?
a. Increase their boundaries to include the children's independence
b. Adjust to their new roles as parents
c. Deal with the realignment of relationships with extended families to include the spouse
d. Develop adult-to-adult relationships between the children and their parents

19-7. How can family structure best be described?
a. A basic pattern of predictable stages
b. Flexible patterns that contribute to adequate functioning
c. The pattern of relationships and ongoing membership
d. A complex set of relationships

19-8. Which is true about family health practices?
a. They are very similar within each culture.
b. They might not value good health, and consequently they can be detrimental to the family members.
c. They can be important to some but not all families.
d. They usually include adaptive behaviors in the event of a health crisis.

19-9. How is cultural sensitivity best defined?
a. Recognition that most family members are similar to each other because of their cultural backgrounds
b. Accurate knowledge about the norms of a given culture
c. Assessment of the effects of culture on each individual, making each client unique
d. Determination of the amount of bias that a health care provider has for the different ethnic backgrounds of clients

19-10. "Launching children" as a stage in the family life cycle involves what?
a. Joining new family members through marriage
b. Accepting the shifting of generational roles
c. Allowing children independence as they begin school
d. Dealing with the disabilities and death of parents

CHAPTER 20

11-14 **Growth and Development**

20-1. The Apgar scale is an assessment tool that is used to do which of the following?
a. Rate physiological characteristics of the newborn
b. Predict psychosocial development of the newborn
c. Measure effectiveness of respiratory drive in the infant
d. Determine potential for fetal survival after delivery

20-2. When a hospitalized child shows a greater than usual reliance on parents, what should the nurse tell them?
a. That this behavior is normal
b. That they should help the child to become independent
c. That they should let the child know this is unacceptable
d. That regressive behavior will prolong the recovery period

20-3. A parent asks the nurse about toilet training a toddler. What should the nurse tell the parent?
a. Boys are typically toilet trained earlier than girls
b. Nighttime control takes longer than daytime control

c. The toddler age is a little young for toilet training
d. The toddler seldom learns this skill to please the parents

20-4. What is the age of beginning to understand moral development?
a. Toddler
b. Preschool
c. Early school age
d. "Middle years" of childhood

20-5. What is the developmental behavior most characteristic of the school-age child?
a. Formal and informal peer group membership as the key in forming self-esteem
b. Fear centering around the loss of self-control
c. Need for positive feedback from parents and teachers
d. Rationalization and intellectualization used as defense mechanisms

20-6. When developing a teaching plan for a young adult, the nurse should be aware that an important aspect of learning in this stage is what?
a. The decision-making process
b. Communication based on subjective criteria
c. Concrete operations rather than abstractions
d. An attention span limited by awareness of need

20-7. The percentage of height attained by girls by the age of menarche is what?
a. 75% to 80%
b. 80% to 85%
c. 85% to 90%
d. 90% to 95%

20-8. What are the major causes of adolescent mortality?
a. Injuries, substance abuse, and suicide
b. Injuries, homicide, and suicide
c. Homicide, motor vehicle accidents, and suicide
d. Motor vehicle accidents, eating disorders, and suicide

20-9. What is the climacteric?
a. Decline of reproductive capacity and changes associated with the decrease in sexual hormones
b. Transition time from middle to late adulthood
c. Time when cognitive performance begins to peak in middle-age adults
d. Ability of the older adult to achieve sexual arousability

A A B B C A D B A B C B
1 2 3 4 5 6 7 8 9 10 11 12

20-10. What is reminiscence, to the nurse working with geriatric clients?
a. An alteration often seen in Alzheimer clients
b. The ability of older adults to recall their past
c. Adjustment of one's reality orientation to the present time period
d. An important cause of social isolation

20-11. What is the genital period, according to Freud?
a. An infant stage of development
b. A fixation of the child on one's genital regions
c. An adolescent and adult stage of development
d. A time when manipulation of the genitalia results in pleasurable sensations

20-12. When, according to Erikson, is intimacy vs. isolation a major issue?
a. Puberty
b. Young adulthood
c. Middle adulthood
d. Older adulthood

CHAPTER 21

Loss and Grief

21-1. A client describes being depressed because the children have all moved away from home. This type of depression is classified as what?
a. Perceived loss
b. Situational loss
c. Maturational loss
d. Actual loss

21-2. According to Kübler-Ross, at what stage of dying is it important for the nurse to offer regressive care such as food, drink, and safety?
a. Acceptance
b. Bargaining
c. Denial
d. Anger

21-3. A client's daughter dies in a traumatic accident. The client states, "I can't believe my daughter is dead." According to Worden, this is what?
a. Task I
b. Task II
c. Task III
d. Task IV

21-4. Which age-group has the most difficulty accepting death because of the developmental task of establishing identity?
a. Toddler
b. School-age
c. Adolescent
d. Young adult

21-5. A college-age person dies in the emergency room after a motor vehicle accident. What should the nurse do?
a. Isolate the parents from the other relatives in the initial grieving process
b. Include all the family members in working through the grieving process
c. Separate out those family members closest to the deceased victim and counsel them
d. Be prepared for a realistic acceptance by some of the family members of this crisis

21-6. To be effective in assisting clients with problems related to loss and grief, the nurse should do what?
a. Know when there is a need to take care of oneself
b. Believe in God and life after death
c. Complete a course in death and dying
d. Share personal feelings and be sympathetic

21-7. As nurses develop a comprehensive plan of care for a terminal client, they should do what?
a. Focus on the data collected from the family and the client
b. Use the expertise of the hospital chaplain
c. Implement counseling strategies from a wide variety of theoretical perspectives
d. Access other professionals within the health care team as resources for developing the plan

21-8. Which statement is *not* one of Worden's principles for effective mourning?
a. Encourage the establishment of new relationships
b. Provide continuing support
c. Encourage movement through the stages of grieving
d. Interpret "normal" behavior

21-9. After the death of a client, which of the following does a nurse's responsibility *not* include?
   a. Insisting that the family view the body to say "goodbye" even if they are reluctant
   b. Placing the body in a supine position to make it look natural and as comfortable as possible
   c. Inserting the client's dentures to maintain normal facial features
   d. Discussing organ donation with the family if the client is a medically suitable donor

21-10. A client states, "My uncle died because of me." The client is most likely what age?
   a. Toddler
   b. Preschooler
   c. School-age child
   d. Adolescent

CHAPTER 22

Stress and Adaptation

22-1. What is an example of the local adaptation syndrome?
   a. Inflammatory response
   b. Alarm reaction
   c. Reflex pain response
   d. Ego defense mechanisms

22-2. The general adaptation response to stress would include which of the following?
   a. Increased appetite
   b. Increased respiratory rate
   c. Decreased perspiration
   d. Decreased heart rate

22-3. A client is unable to compensate for a stressor. This response is part of what?
   a. Fight-or-flight response
   b. Resistance stage
   c. Exhaustion stage
   d. Alarm reaction

22-4. A client asks a nurse for help. This request is an example of what?
   a. Roy's adaptation model
   b. Paterson and Zderad's humanistic nursing model
   c. Orem's self-care theory
   d. Neumon's model of nursing

22-5. A client dies and the family is able to continue with its daily employment activities. This response is labeled as what?
   a. Denial
   b. Suppression
   c. Cognitive appraisal
   d. Task-oriented behaviors

22-6. A client suffers a job loss and then contracts an illness. This response is classified as what?
   a. Natural response
   b. Environmental factor
   c. Mind-body interaction
   d. Stressor

22-7. A client asks the nurse to describe health-enhancing habits that can reduce the impact of stress. What is the best response of the nurse?
   a. "Avoid vigorous exercise because it will decrease your energy reserve."
   b. "Eat a diet high in meat and sugar to provide for body fuel reserves."
   c. "Reduce your social and personal contacts to save time for more important things."
   d. "Try developing a list of tasks to be performed in order of priority."

22-8. What is a subjective finding of stress?
   a. Increased appetite
   b. Stomach pain
   c. Tachycardia
   d. Hypertension

22-9. A client becomes depressed after a job loss. This type of crisis is identified as what?
   a. Maturational
   b. Developmental
   c. Stress-crisis sequence
   d. Situational

22-10. The nurse asks a client to make appropriate changes as part of the crisis intervention treatment. This change is identified as what?
   a. First step
   b. Second step
   c. Third step
   d. Fourth step

22-11. A client thinks of a relaxing situation every time stress increases. This action is called what?
   a. Restorative care
   b. Guided imagery and visualization
   c. Progressive muscle relaxation
   d. Assertiveness training

CHAPTER 23

Vital Signs

23-1.   Temperature control is integrated by what?
  a. Medulla oblongata
  b. Pituitary gland
  c. Thyroid gland
  d. Hypothalamus

23-2.   A client is shivering. What is this physiological response?
  a. Involuntary body response that increases heat production
  b. Psychological body response of regulating body temperature
  c. Movement of skeletal muscle that decreases body temperature
  d. Response of the endocrine system to increase the basal metabolic rate

23-3.   The nurse bathes a client who is febrile. How does this intervention increase heat loss?
  a. Radiation
  b. Convection
  c. Condensation
  d. Conduction

23-4.   The nurse takes a rectal temperature. What is normal for rectal temperature?
  a. Between 37° and 38.5° C
  b. 1° lower than Fahrenheit temperatures
  c. 5° C higher than oral temperatures
  d. Usually performed with a glass thermometer

23-5.   The client is given corticosteroids for a febrile state. The corticosteroid's mechanism of action is to
  a. decrease the production of the pathogen response
  b. interfere with the hypothalamus response
  c. increase the metabolic response of the hepatic system
  d. decrease the lymphocytic response of the immune response

23-6.   What is the pulse site located below the inguinal ligament, midway between the symphysis pubis and the anterior superior iliac spine?
  a. Temporal
  b. Brachial
  c. Posterior tibial
  d. Femoral

23-7.   A client is obese and the nurse takes the blood pressure with a standard-size cuff. How will this affect the reading?
  a. Falsely low
  b. Accurate
  c. Falsely high
  d. Indistinct

23-8.   A postoperative client stands up and begins to feel faint. What should the nurse do?
  a. Take an orthostatic blood pressure reading
  b. Expect the sitting blood pressure to be higher than the standing blood pressure
  c. Attempt to listen to the Korotkoff sounds
  d. Listen to the client's apical pulse with the diaphragm of the stethoscope

23-9.   A client has a CVP inserted. How is the placement verified?
  a. By the wave form it creates
  b. By the measurement numbers it creates
  c. With peripheral blood pressure readings
  d. With a chest x-ray

23-10.   While assessing the vital signs of an infant, the nurse should be aware of what?
  a. They are essentially the same as an adult's
  b. The pulse and respirations will be higher than an adult's
  c. All the measurements are labile during the first months of life
  d. Babies are highly sensitive to changes in nursing personnel

23-11.   A client begins breathing very rapidly. The nurse documents this as what?
  a. Eupnea
  b. Increased tidal volume
  c. Tachypnea
  d. Hypoxemia

CHAPTER 24

33 Health Assessment and Physical Examination

24-1.   In physical assessment the term baseline data refers to what?
  a. Pattern of findings identified when client is first assessed
  b. Physiological outcomes of care
  c. Normal range of physical findings
  d. Clinical judgments made about a client's changing health status

24-2. The nurse assesses a client for lung consolidation. What is the technique that vibrates the chest wall?
a. Inspection
b. Palpation
c. Percussion
d. Auscultation

24-3. What position is most often used for assessment of the female genitalia?
a. Supine
b. Dorsal recumbent
c. Knee-chest
d. Lithotomy

24-4. While performing an assessment, what should the nurse do?
a. Stereotype the elderly concerning their common physical characteristics
b. Specifically interview clients for suspected abuse histories
c. Disregard racial differences in the physical qualities of the client
d. Continue to ask questions, even if they obviously make the individual uncomfortable

24-5. Upon examining a client, the nurse finds a circumscribed elevation of skin filled with serous fluid on the upper lip. The lesion is 0.4 cm in diameter. What is this type of lesion called?
a. Macule
b. Nodule
c. Vesicle
d. Pustule

24-6. A client's skin does not return to its normal shape after being assessed. What could this finding be?
a. Poor skin turgor
b. Edema
c. Pallor
d. Erythema

24-7. The nurse notes that PERRLA has been documented for a client. This observation is an assessment of what?
a. Condition of lacrimal apparatus
b. Condition of the conjunctiva and sclera
c. Pupillary reflexes to light and accommodation
d. Visualization of the internal eye structures

24-8. The nurse assesses the internal ear of an infant. How is the ear pulled?
a. Back and down
b. Up and forward

c. Very gently up
d. Down and forward

24-9. A client has a suspected condition of hyperthyroidism. To assess this condition the nurse does what?
a. Asks the client to recount normal gastrointestinal habits
b. Palpates the trachea for any abnormalities
c. Has the client swallow water while palpating for abnormalities
d. Compares the cervical lymph node chains with those of the supraclavicular area

24-10. While auscultating a client with pneumonia, the nurse hears low-pitched, continuous musical sounds over the bronchi on expiration. What are these sounds called?
a. Crackles
b. Rhonchi
c. Wheezes
d. Friction rubs

24-11. In assessing a client's abdomen, the nurse begins with what?
a. Inspection
b. Auscultation
c. Palpation
d. Percussion

24-12. An adolescent client does not want the genitalia to be examined. What is the best statement by the nurse?
a. "Don't worry, we can defer this part of the examination."
b. "We need to do this anyway, so please lie still."
c. "This is a necessary part of your assessment, but I will keep you covered up as much as possible."
d. "Just tell me if your private parts have had any unusual conditions or look different recently."

24-13. The nurse uses the Glasgow Coma Scale to do what?
a. Assess the client's mental status
b. Compare a client to norms for his or her age
c. Evaluate the memory capability of a client
d. Measure the level of consciousness of a client

CHAPTER 25

Infection Control

25-1.   A client obtains *E.coli* from lake water. The water acts as what?
a.   Reservoir
b.   Infectious agent
c.   Mode of transmission
d.   Portal of exit

25-2.   What is the action of normal flora?
a.   Participation in maintaining a person's health by inhibiting multiplication of disease-carrying microorganisms
b.   Assistance with the formation of antibodies
c.   Assistance with the digestion and absorption of nutrients
d.   Effect on the methods of transmission of disease

25-3.   The nurse throws away a glove and states that it is not sterile. This action is an example of what?
a.   Medical asepsis
b.   Prevention
c.   Surgical asepsis
d.   Safe practice

25-4.   The nurse advocates safe practice for isolation related to the TB agent by wearing what?
a.   Mask
b.   Gloves, and mask
c.   Gloves, mask, and gown
d.   Gloves, mask, gown, and eye covering

25-5.   The nurse sets up a nonbarrier sterile field on a client's overbed table. In which situation is the field contaminated?
a.   Nurse keeps the top of the table above the waist
b.   Sterile saline solution is spilled on the field
c.   Sterile objects are kept within a 1-inch border of the field
d.   Nurse, who has a cold, wears a double mask

25-6.   The nurse dons sterile gloves. In which situation are the gloves incorrectly removed?
a.   Outside of one cuff is grasped with the other gloved hand
b.   Fingers of the bare hand tuck inside the remaining glove's cuff
c.   Glove is peeled off, turned inside out, and discarded
d.   Inside of one cuff is grasped with the other gloved hand

25-7.   A client has a pressure ulcer. What is an intrinsic risk factor for this alteration?
a.   Improper positioning
b.   Incontinence
c.   Restraints
d.   Poor hygiene

25-8.   A home health client self-injects with insulin daily. What is the concentration of bleach to place in a disposal container?
a.   1:5
b.   1:10
c.   1:20
d.   1:50

25-9.   An infected client is in an interval period of time, experiencing nonspecific signs and symptoms. This period of time is known as what?
a.   Incubation period
b.   Prodromal period
c.   Full stage of illness
d.   Convalescence

25-10.   The nurse is taking care of contaminated client care items. Which semicritical item only requires a disinfectant?
a.   Surgical instruments
b.   Bedpans
c.   Gastrointestinal endoscopes
d.   Linens

25-11.   The nurse is obtaining a stool specimen. What is the correct safety equipment for the nurse to wear?
a.   Mask
b.   Gloves
c.   Gloves and mask
d.   Gloves, mask, and gown

CHAPTER 26

35 Administering Medications

26-1.   A clear fluid containing water and alcohol that is designed for oral use is what?
a.   Suspension
b.   Elixir
c.   Syrup
d.   Cocktail

26-2.   A client's medication is transformed into an inactive substance. What is this action termed?
a.   Absorption
b.   Distribution
c.   Metabolism
d.   Excretion

26-3. The nurse administers a medication for its local effects. Which route of administration is most likely?
a. Oral
b. Subcutaneous
c. Inhalation
d. Topical

26-4. A client receives 3500 mg of a medication. What is this dosage in grams?
a. 0.35 g
b. 3.5 g
c. 35 g
d. 350 g

26-5. A client is to receive chloramphenicol, 125 mg PO. Chloramphenicol 250 mg/ml is available. What should the client receive?
a. 0.05 ml
b. 0.4 ml
c. 0.5 ml
d. 1 ml

26-6. A child weighs 12 kg. Using the body surface formula, the dose of a drug that the child should receive, if the normal adult dose of the drug is 300 mg, is what?
a. 50 mg
b. 90 mg
c. 100 mg
d. 200 mg

26-7. The nurse documents a medication given to a client. What should the nurse record?
a. Rationale for giving a questionable wrong dosage of medication
b. Medication before giving it
c. Prescriber's intention for ordering a given medication
d. Medication after giving it

26-8. The nurse instills a medication into a specific anatomical location. What is the correct statement?
a. "Ear medications are best administered by pulling the adult's ear down and back."
b. "Nasal medications also have the advantage of a systemic effect from swallowing a portion of the medication."
c. "Opthalmic medications should not be applied to the cornea."
d. "Topical applications are seldom systemic."

26-9. A client is to receive two different kinds of insulin. What is the correct method of insulin administration?
a. Prepare the unmodified insulin first
b. Never mix lente and ultralente insulin in the same syringe
c. Administer the mixed insulins within 30 minutes of their placement into a syringe
d. Ultralente insulin is much more potent than regular insulin and therefore should be given alone

26-10. The nurse will be giving a drug by intravenous bolus through an existing IV line. The nurse has correctly drawn the medication into the appropriate syringe. What should the nurse do next?
a. Check the manufacturer's directions for specified time recommendation for administration of the medication
b. Wash hands and apply gloves
c. Aspirate for blood return and inject medication
d. Occlude intravenous line by pinching tubing just above the injection port

26-11. The nurse is administering a medication that is very irritating to the muscle. What should the nurse use?
a. Intradermal injection technique
b. Deltoid muscle for the site of injection
c. Dorsogluteal site on the buttocks
d. Z-track technique of injection

26-12. A medication is ordered to be intravenous and is mixed with 100 ml of compatible IV fluid. This type of medication administration is what?
a. Piggyback method of administration
b. Volume controlled infusion
c. Intermittent venous access
d. Intravenous bolus method of infusion

26-13. The nurse is administering medications. In which situation should the nurse wear gloves?
a. Administering eye drops
b. Giving an IM injection
c. Adding medication to an existing IV bag
d. Applying medication to a client's sublingual space

CHAPTER 27

Body Mechanics

27-1.   Which bones of the skull provide contour?
   a. Long
   b. Short
   c. Flat
   d. Irregular

27-2.   Chemicals such as acetylcholine, which transfer the electrical impulse from the nerve across the myoneural junction to the muscle, are known as what?
   a. Neurotransmitters
   b. Proprioceptors
   c. Isometrics
   d. Synergistics

27-3.   A client has a disorder that is characterized by inadequate and delayed mineralization in the bone. What is this disorder?
   a. Osteoporosis
   b. Inflammatory joint disease
   c. Osteomalacia
   d. Arthritis

27-4.   The nurse is lifting a client. To prevent back strain, what should the nurse do?
   a. Twist the upper torso to enhance the use and strength of the upper extremities
   b. Keep the weight of the client as close to the body (of the nurse) as possible
   c. Keep the knees stiff to encourage their lifting strength potential
   d. Loosen the stomach muscles to keep from injuring the pelvic region

27-5.   A client has pneumonia and must be placed in a position that will assist in the drainage of lung secretions. This position is known as what?
   a. Sim's
   b. Semi-Fowler's
   c. Lateral
   d. Prone

27-6.   When are transfer belts used?
   a. When moving a client up in bed
   b. With all clients
   c. By physical therapists only
   d. To allow the nurse to maintain stability of a client during a transfer

27-7.   A client has a casted right leg and requires crutch walking, which restricts any pressure from the affected leg. What is the method of preferred crutch walking?
   a. Four-point alternating
   b. Tripod position
   c. Three-point gait
   d. Two-point gait

27-8.   A client is diagnosed with a dislocated hip. In order to *not* externally rotate the legs, the nurse should use what device?
   a. Trapeze bar
   b. Foot boot
   c. Sandbags
   d. Trochanter roll

27-9.   A client in balanced suspension traction needs assistance by two people to move up in bed. What should the nurses do?
   a. Face the middle of the bed while pulling the client
   b. Face the top of the bed while moving the client
   c. Keep their feet close together for balance
   d. Place a pillow under the client's head while moving

27-10. A client with hemiplegia is transferred from the bed to a chair. What should the nurse do?
   a. Grasp the client underneath the arms while assisting with the transfer
   b. Support the affected side of the client
   c. Stand on the stronger side of the client to ensure less strain for the caregiver
   d. Encourage the client to not use the chair handrests because of their restrictions on movement

27-11. An extremely obese client requires the use of a mechanical lift to have a sitz bath. What should the nurse do?
   a. Leave the client's glasses in place to encourage visualization of the movements
   b. Position the lifting machine 1 m from the bed to allow easier body movements of the nurse
   c. Place the sling from the shoulders to the knees of the client to support the client's weight
   d. Ask the client to grasp the shoulders of the nurse during the transfer movements

27-12.   A client requires adduction movements of the shoulder during range-of-motion exercising. The degrees of the movement of this positioning are normally what?
a.   45 to 60
b.   60 to 90
c.   180
d.   320

CHAPTER 28

38   **Safety**

28-1.   What organization enforces regulations that protect consumers from harmful effects of products used in health care agencies?
a.   FCCA
b.   FDA
c.   FRD
d.   FIC

28-2.   Which developmental stage has the highest risk of injury from falls?
a.   Preschooler
b.   School-age child
c.   Adult
d.   Older adult

28-3.   What is an example of a procedure-related accident?
a.   Burn
b.   Poisoning
c.   Medication error
d.   Food allergy

28-4.   A confused client is pulling at an IV line during hospitalization. What is the nurse's best intervention for the client's safety?
a.   Encourage the family to visit and remain in the room with the client
b.   Use elbow restraints
c.   Apply bilateral wrist restraints
d.   Dress the client with a vest-type restraint

28-5.   Parents call the ER about their child, who has swallowed an acid substance. Most likely the parents will be instructed to have the child drink what?
a.   Lemon juice
b.   Water
c.   Vinegar
d.   Milk

28-6.   A client falls asleep while smoking in bed. What is the nurse's first responsibility?
a.   Report the fire
b.   Attempt to extinguish the fire
c.   Assist the client to a safe place
d.   Close all the windows and doors to contain the fire

28-7.   A child might choke on food unless it is cut up into small pieces. This risk of injury is most likely to occur beginning at what age?
a.   10 months
b.   11 months
c.   12 months
d.   13 months

28-8.   A client accidentally spills grease on an open burner. What is the most appropriate fire extinguisher to use?
a.   Dry chemical extinguisher
b.   Water extinguisher
c.   Carbon dioxide extinguisher
d.   Soda and acid extinguisher

28-9.   A parent instructs the child not to eat a certain part of the holly plant. What is the toxic part of this plant?
a.   Berry
b.   Seed
c.   Foliage
d.   Leaf

CHAPTER 29

39   **Hygiene**

29-1.   Sweat glands, sebaceous glands, and hair follicles are found where?
a.   Epidermis
b.   Dermis
c.   Subcutaneous layer
d.   Fat

29-2.   Increased androgen levels cause what?
a.   Hirsutism
b.   Acne
c.   Dwarfism
d.   Decreased secondary sex characteristics

29-3.   How is perineal care done?
a.   With a partial bed bath
b.   With an indwelling Foley catheter
c.   In combination with a sitz bath
d.   At the same time as a sponge bath

B   A   B   C   A   D   B
1   2   3   4   5   6   7

29-4. A client with diabetes requires meticulous foot care. What should the nurse do?
a. Use nailclippers to avoid tearing the nail
b. Apply hot water bottles to the feet to soften the nail beds
c. Wash and dry any cuts immediately
d. Apply commercial corn removers as needed

29-5. The nurse is performing mouth care for an unconscious client. What is the first intervention that the nurse should employ?
a. Assess for a gag reflex
b. Retract the upper and lower teeth with a padded tongue blade
c. Position the client in a Sim's position
d. Obtain a portable suction machine

29-6. What should be done with a client's facial hair?
a. Shaved prior to the bath
b. Shaved by the client
c. Trimmed and any mustaches removed if the client is unconscious
d. Shaved with an electric razor if clotting times are prolonged

29-7. What should be done with a client's contact lenses?
a. Removed while the client is in acute care
b. Left in place for a maximum of 1 week if they are extended-wear lenses
c. Cleaned with antimicrobials on a daily basis
d. Removed daily unless they are gas permeable

29-8. When making a bed, how should the nurse position the bed?
a. With the head of the bed slightly raised
b. At its lowest level to ensure the safety of the client
c. Close to the overbed table to enable easy retrieval of linen supplies
d. At its highest level to ensure proper body mechanics

29-9. A hair and scalp assessment reveals that a client has head lice. What would be an appropriate intervention?
a. Shave the hair off the affected area
b. Place oil on the hair and the scalp and repeat until all lice are dead
c. Shampoo with Kwell shampoo and repeat 12 to 24 hours later
d. Shampoo with regular shampoo and dry with hair dryer set at the hottest setting

29-10. An immobilized client is scheduled to go to the operating room (OR). What bed should the nurse make?
a. Occupied bed immediately before bathing the client
b. Unoccupied bed after the client is taken to the OR
c. Occupied bed immediately after bathing the client
d. Postoperative bed after the client is taken to the OR

29-11. A client is pregnant. What can the pregnancy cause?
a. Dental caries and increased tendencies to halitosis
b. Gums to lose vascularity and tissue elasticity
c. Increased tendency to develop gingivitis
d. Increased incidence of loss of teeth

CHAPTER 30

Oxygenation

30-1. A client's preload is decreased. A decrease in preload can be interpreted as what?
a. Output of the left ventricle is decreased.
b. Amount of ventricle filling at rest is decreased
c. Length of time for the cardiac cycle is decreased
d. Resistance to the cardiac ejection volume is decreased

30-2. The movement of gases into and out of the lungs depends on what?
a. 50% oxygen content in the atmospheric air
b. Pressure gradient between the atmosphere and the alveoli
c. Use of accessory muscles of respiration during expiration
d. Amount of carbon dioxide dissolved in the fluid of the alveoli

30-3. A client has hyaline membrane disease. What is the most likely age of this client?
a. Infant
b. Toddler
c. Preschooler
d. School-age child

30-4.　A client has left-side heart failure. What is a common sign of this alteration?
a. Jugular vein distention
b. Peripheral edema
c. Weight gain
d. Lung field congestion

30-5.　During hyperventilation, what happens to a client?
a. Decreased pH level
b. Should be told to decrease rate of inhalation
c. Serum carbon dioxide level lowered
d. Becomes acidotic

30-6.　A client is sitting up in bed with the upper torso resting on the overbed table. This type of positioning is an example of what?
a. Orthopneic positioning
b. Deoxygenation
c. Dyspnea
d. Pain relief

30-7.　A client with advanced alcoholism has hemorrhaging esophageal varicies. This condition will most likely lead to what?
a. Respiratory infection
b. Respiratory distress
c. Productive cough
d. Fatigue

30-8.　A client is asked to inhale and perform a series of coughs during exhalation. This is known as what type of coughing?
a. Quad
b. Huff
c. Cascade
d. Postsurgical

30-9.　The use of chest physiotherapy to mobilize pulmonary secretions involves the use of what?
a. Hydration
b. Percussion
c. Nebulization
d. Humidification

30-10.　The nurse is observing the chest tubes of a client who recently had thoracic surgery. What should the nurse expect to see?
a. Clamped tubes with two hemostats
b. 1500 cc of bright red drainage noted in the drainage bottle
c. Bubbling in the suction-control chamber
d. Chest drainage system sitting on top of the client's overbed table

30-11.　A client is "pursed-lip breathing." This type of breathing means that the client is what?
a. Breathing slowly
b. Very anxious
c. Using ISRBD
d. Controlling exhalation

CHAPTER 31

41 Fluid, Electrolyte, and Acid-Base Balances

31-1.　A client has intracellular dehydration. What concentration of solution is used to restore this deficit?
a. Hypotonic
b. Hypertonic
c. Isotonic
d. Oncotic

31-2.　A client is febrile and consequently very diaphoretic. This condition is an example of what?
a. Sensible water loss
b. Extracellular overload
c. Insensible water loss
c. ADH deficit

31-3.　A client has renal insufficiency and develops metabolic acidosis. The pH of the arterial blood does what?
a. Elevates
b. Decreases
c. Remains the same
d. Compensates independently

31-4.　A client has hypocalcemia. This condition results in what?
a. Decreased phosphorus
b. ECF dehydration
c. Magnesium imbalances
d. Neuromuscular excitability

31-5.　A client's arterial blood gases are as follows: $pH = 7.51$, $PaCO_2 = 42$, $PaO_2 = 84$, $HCO_3 = 30$. The client is in what condition?
a. Metabolic acidosis
b. Metabolic alkalosis
c. Respiratory acidosis
d. Respiratory alkalosis

Ch 30

B B A D C A B C B C D
1 2 3 4 5 6 7 8 9 10 11

31-6. A client with a head injury has had a urine output of 1000 cc for the past 24 hours, despite a 3000 cc IV fluid intake. In addition, the sodium level is 24. These symptoms are indicative of what?
a. Secretion of inappropriate ADH (SIADH)
b. Diabetic insipidous
c. Hypernatremia
d. Metabolic alkalosis

31-7. A client has a urine specific gravity of 1.007. What does this means about the urine?
a. It is very concentrated
b. Its output indicates renal failure
c. Its concentration level suggests a high hematocrit
d. It has few solutes in it

31-8. A client is on fluid intake restrictions. The larger portion of input should be between what hours?
a. 2300 and 0700
b. 0700 and 1500
c. 1500 and 2300
d. 0700 and 1900

31-9. When selecting a site for placement of an intravenous needle, what should the nurse do?
a. Try the dominant hand first
b. Elevate the extremity on a pillow
c. Use the most distal portion of a vein
d. Locate the vein that is over a bony prominence

31-10. A client is to receive Kefzol, 1 gm diluted in 100 cc NS, over 30 minutes. The macrodrip set delivers 15 gtts/ml. What will the drip rate be?
a. 25 drops/min
b. 50 drops/min
c. 75 drops/min
d. 100 drops/min

31-11. A client has an infiltrated peripheral IV. What is the primary difference in the symptoms of the infiltration versus the phlebitis regarding infiltrated areas?
a. Swollen
b. Uncomfortable
c. Cooler
d. Infected

CHAPTER 32

42 **Sleep**

32-1. A client is sleeping and the vital signs are significantly lower than normal. These findings are consistent with what?
a. Stage 1 of the sleep cycle
b. Stage 2 of the sleep cycle
c. Stage 3 of the sleep cycle
d. Stage 4 of the sleep cycle

32-2. A child has difficulty going to bed at night because of a fear of separation. The child is most likely what age?
a. Infant
b. Toddler
c. Preschooler
d. School-age child

32-3. A 73-year-old client is experiencing difficulty staying asleep. What is characteristic of the older adult?
a. Has a longer period of stage 3 than stage 4 NREM
b. Has an increased need for sleep
c. Awakens more during the night
d. Stays awake later at night because of frequent day napping

32-4. A client has sleeping problems and wishes to increase normal sleeping patterns. What is a suggested sleep aid?
a. l-tryptophan
b. Beta-blockers
c. Alcohol
d. Narcotics

32-5. The nurse is planning care for a client with sleep pattern disturbance. What is the most appropriate intervention?
a. Turning off all the lights in the client's room
b. Synchronizing schedules for the medications
c. Encouraging exercise immediately before bedtime
d. Discussing with the client the advantages of long-term benzodiazepine use

32-6. A client has a sleeping pattern disturbance. What might an MSLT reveal?
a. A change in the EEG
b. That stress is accentuating the sleep problem
c. That some of the problem is attributed to the medication regimen
d. That it takes an average of almost an hour for the individual to fall asleep

32-7. A client has a lack of airflow during sleep for 1 to 2 minutes. This condition is most likely what?
a. Insomnia
b. Narcolepsy
c. Sleep apnea
d. Cataplexy

32-8. A client expresses concern that a newborn child is sleeping too much. What should the nurse's initial response be?
a. "Don't worry, most newborns sleep a lot."
b. "You sound concerned; let's examine how many hours the child is actually sleeping."
c. "You need to discuss this with your pediatrician."
d. "Please have your spouse call me to discuss this problem."

32-9. A nurse asks the parent of a hospitalized child what the normal bedtime routine is. What is the best rationale for asking this question?
a. Determining why the child is not sleeping normally in the acute care setting
b. Evaluating whether the parent is using proper techniques for helping the child's sleep pattern
c. Designing appropriate measures to help the child sleep during hospitalization
d. Assessing whether the child requires medicinal assistance in falling asleep

32-10. A client has a hiatal hernia and has difficulty sleeping. What is a nursing intervention specific to this disorder?
a. Applying stress reduction techniques
b. Providing bedtime routines that are consistent
c. Administering analgesics just before the client's hour of sleep
d. Eating small meals before bedtime

32-11. A client in restorative care is having difficulty sleeping. What should the nurse do?
a. Restrict lengthy daytime napping
b. Encourage regularly scheduled nap times
c. Limit the client's activity in the evening
d. Discourage strenuous exercising during the day

CHAPTER 33

 Comfort

33-1. Pain is a protective mechanism warning of tissue injury and is largely what?
a. Symptom of a severe illness or disease
b. Subjective experience
c. Objective experience
d. Acute symptom of short duration

33-2. A client states that abdominal pain is lessened while watching television. This response is an example of what?
a. Nociceptor stimulation
b. Positive protective reflex response
c. Application of the gate control theory
d. Perception of pain

33-3. A client with multiple sclerosis is feeling euphoric because of being asymptomatic for more than 2 years. This example indicates the client is in what?
a. Remission
b. Intractable type of pain
c. Exacerbation
d. Chronic pain problem

33-4. A nurse asks a client to label the pain level from "0 to 10." What is this?
a. Reference to PCA
b. VAS
c. CRIES scale
d. NRS

33-5. A client states that a headache occurs every time arthritic pain exacerbates. The headache is an example of what?
a. Assessment sign
b. Behavioral effect
c. Concomitant symptom
d. Severe form of pain

33-6. A client complains of sharp pain along the chest and down the right arm. What is this type of pain?
a. Recurring
b. Referred
c. Radiating
d. Radiohumeral

33-7. A client has an epidural catheter in place and is receiving morphine sulfate for postoperative pain control. When the nurse enters the room, the client is complaining of pain. What should the nurse do first?
a. Call the physician immediately
b. Speak to the client in a quiet tone of voice and reassure the client that the anxiety will ease
c. Stop the morphine infusion
d. Ask the client to describe the pain

33-8. The nurse describes the specific details of upcoming surgery. The details are an example of what?
a. Guided imagery
b. Relaxation
c. Biofeedback
d. Anticipatory guidance

33-9. A client has a large laceration from an MVA and is in the ER. Why does the physician choose a local anesthetic to use during suturing?
a. The local anesthetic produces temporary loss of sensation by inhibiting nerve conduction
b. The client looks very anxious
c. The medication in the local has very few side effects
d. The potential for hemorrhage precludes the use of IV anesthesia

33-10. The nurse uses the "ABCDE" approach to pain assessment and tells the client to select a pain control method that seems best. This selection of pain control is an example of which approach?
a. "A"
b. "B"
c. "C"
d. "D"

33-11. An elderly client is experiencing chronic joint pain. The nurse should remember that the older adult has what?
a. Less risk of developing gastric toxicity
b. More problems with pain as part of the aging process
c. Shorter period of pain relief from opioid drugs
d. Greater risk for lowered pain tolerance

CHAPTER 34

 Nutrition

34-1. A client's liver stores glucose in the form of glycogen. What is this type of synthesis?
a. Lipogenesis
b. Glycogenesis
c. Gluconeogenesis
d. Catabolism

34-2. A client is told to eat foods that keep blood cholesterol down. What lipid group is the best from which to select foods?
a. Saturated fatty acids
b. Fat-soluble vitamins
c. Polyunsaturated fatty acids
d. Unsaturated fatty acids

34-3. Which food is high in biological protein value?
a. Cereal
b. Peanuts
c. Eggs
d. Spinach

34-4. The major portion of absorption of nutrients occurs where?
a. Mouth
b. Large intestine
c. Stomach
d. Small intestine

34-5. A client is to perform a diet history at home to provide baseline nutritional information. This history should include an intake of what?
a. Solid foods for 3 days
b. Food for 3 days, including a weekend day
c. Solid foods for 3 days, including a weekend
d. Food for 3 to 5 days

34-6. What enteral tube feeding involves surgical placement?
a. Gastrostomy tube
b. PEG tube
c. RAG tube
d. Nasogastric tube

34-7. What are parenteral nutrition feedings?
a. Hypotonic in nature
b. Hyperosmolar in nature
c. Usually infused through peripheral IV lines
d. Always made of lipid solutions

34-8. What is a good food source high in folic acid?
a. Milk
b. Potatoes
c. Fruit
d. Liver

34-9. An infant usually triples birth weight at what age?
a. 6 months
b. 9 months
c. 12 months
d. 18 months

34-10. The nurse is evaluating lab results on a newly admitted client. A protein deficit is indicated by what?
a. Elevated hemoglobin level
b. Decreased hematocrit level
c. Elevated transferrin level
d. Decreased albumin level

34-11. A postoperative cardiac surgery client is on a prudent diet. The foods that are consistent with this diet have what quality?
a. Reduce serum lipid levels
b. Are easily swallowed
c. Do not require chewing
d. Are clear and bland in nature

CHAPTER 35

45 **Urinary Elimination**

35-1. Urine is initially formed in which body part?
a. Nephron
b. Kidney
c. Glomerulus
d. Ureter

35-2. A client has a urinary diversion created with a reservoir formed from a bowel segment. What is this reservoir called?
a. Ureterostomy
b. Ileal loop
c. Ilium reservoir
d. Continent pouch

35-3. After birth, an infant should micturate within what period of time?
a. 12 hours
b. 18 hours
c. 24 hours
d. 48 hours

35-4. A client requires urinary output measurements. What should the nurse use to measure collected urine?
a. Graduated measurement container
b. Urine hat
c. Urinal
d. Bedpan

35-5. The nurse notes that the Foley bag has remained empty for 3 hours. What should the nurse's first action be?
a. Notify the physician
b. Check for kinks in the tubing
c. Insert a new Foley catheter
d. Increase the fluid intake

35-6. A nurse helps a client to void by compressing downward with both hands below the umbilicus and above the symphysis pubis. What is this procedure called?
a. Crede's maneuver
b. Kegel exercise
c. Micturition
d. Trigone stimulation

35-7. The nurse collects a midstream urine sample. What is the primary difference between the midstream collection method and a urinalysis sample?
a. Midstream sample has fewer contaminants
b. Urinalysis sample does not require gloves to be used by the care provider
c. Midstream sample is sterile
d. Urinalysis sample requires less urine

35-8. A client requires an indirect scan of the urinary tract. What is this test?
a. Renal ultrasound
b. Computerized axial tomography
c. Intravenous pyelogram
d. Renal scan

35-9. To perform an indwelling catheterization, when are sterile gloves applied?
a. Before washing the perineal area with soap and water
b. After positioning the client but before draping the client
c. Before testing the catheter balloon
d. Before opening the catheterization kit

35-10. A client has a condom catheter in place. What is the primary advantage of the condom catheter?
a. It is more easily applied
b. It does not cause urinary tract infections as easily as indwelling catheters
c. It does not require surgical intervention
d. It does not require a drainage bag

35-11. A client has stress incontinency. What is this condition?
a. Involuntary passage of urine after a strong sense of urgency to void
b. Total uncontrollable and continual loss of urine
c. Involuntary loss of urine occurring at somewhat predictable intervals
d. Increased intraabdominal pressure that causes leakage of a small amount of urine

CHAPTER 36

Bowel Elimination

36-1. Most nutrients and enzymes are absorbed in which organ?
a. Stomach
b. Small intestine
c. Large intestine
d. Colon

36-2. A client who is immobile after surgery begins to continuously ooze liquid stool from the lower bowel. What is this condition?
a. Diarrhea
b. Incontinence
c. Valsalva maneuver
d. Impaction

36-3. A client has a colectomy and is going to undergo a bowel diversion. What will this client have?
a. No continency of the bowel
b. Permanent stoma
c. Possibly continent ostomy with an IAR procedure
d. Ostomy pouch, but no stoma if an IAR procedure is performed

36-4. A client is malnourished. Which lab test will be decreased?
a. Serum protein
b. Serum bilirubin
c. Serum amylase
d. Alkaline phosphatase

36-5. A client has a suspected chronic hemorrhage from a peptic ulcer. What test should the nurse perform?
a. Guaiac test
b. CEA test
c. Upper GI
d. Ultrasound

36-6. A client is given an opiate as an antidiarrheal. The opioids work by what process?
a. Decreasing segmental contractions that mix intestinal contents
b. Evacuating pathogens from the lower bowel
c. Inhibiting peristalsis
d. Softening the fecal mass in the GI system

36-7. A client is bloating from flatulence. What should the nurse administer?
a. Harris flush
b. Glycerin suppository
c. Oil retention enema
d. Cleansing enema

36-8. A client is concerned about her breastfed infant's stool, stating that it is yellow instead of brown. What should the nurse explain to her?
a. A change to formula might be necessary
b. Her infant is dehydrated, and she should increase the fluid intake
c. It will be necessary to send a stool specimen to the lab
d. The stool is normal for infants

36-9. The nurse instructs a client to take time to defecate 1 hour after meals. What is the rationale for this intervention?
a. A regular time develops a habitual pattern for the client
b. Neglecting the urge to defecate leads to diarrheal or constipation problems
c. The gastrocolic reflex normally occurs at this time
d. High fiber foods increase peristalsis

36-10. A client is over 50 years of age. What should be done to screen for colon cancer?
a. The stool should be guaiac tested each year
b. An endoscopy should be performed every 3 to 5 years
c. A digital rectal examination is required every other year
d. A radiographic study is necessary each year

36-11. A urinary catheter with a 30 ml balloon is inserted into the rectum as a test for what?
a. Dexterity
b. Anal sphincter function
c. Abdominal muscle contractility
d. Anorectal sensation

CHAPTER 37

47 **Immobility**

37-1. A client is immobile because of orthopedic injury. This causes pancreatic activity to do what?
a. Increase
b. Decrease
c. Lower blood glucose levels
d. Decrease nitrogen metabolism

37-2. A postsurgical client has cardiovascular changes because of immobility. What might one of these changes be?
a. Hypertension
b. Hypercoagulability of the blood
c. Orthostatic hypotension
d. Atelectasis

37-3. A client with rheumatoid arthritis develops skeletal changes related to the severely restricted physical movements. What is a likely skeletal alteration?
a. Pressure ulcerations
b. Muscle atrophy
c. Venous thrombi
d. Disuse osteoporosis

37-4. When assessing an immobilized client for edema, what is the most likely place for the edema to be found?
a. Face and neck
b. Sacrum
c. Arms and hands
d. Abdomen

37-5. A client is immobilized. What should the nurse do to maintain the respiratory system?
a. Turn the client every 4 hours
b. Maintain a maximum fluid intake of 1500 cc per day
c. Apply an abdominal binder continuously while in bed
d. Encourage the use of an incentive spirometer

37-6. A client experiences pain in the calf when the foot is dorsiflexed. This condition indicates what?
a. Positive Homan's sign
b. Deep tendon reflex
c. Developmental sign of neurological deterioration
d. Output of muscle skeletal impairment

37-7. A client is immobile after gallbladder surgery. To reduce orthostatic hypotension, what should the nurse encourage the client to do?
a. Perform isometric exercises
b. Participate in chest physiotherapy
c. Increase ankle pumps
d. Sit up in a chair

37-8. A client is recovering from pneumonia. To best prevent musculoskeletal system problems, the nurse should encourage what frequency of activity?
a. 2 hours every morning
b. 1 hour in the morning and 1 hour in the evening
c. Intermittently throughout the day
d. Passive range-of-motion exercises

37-9. A client experiencing DVT is wearing antiembolic stockings. How should the client wear them?
a. Remove them at night
b. Remove and reapply them every shift
c. Wear them no longer than 4 hours at a time
d. Roll them no lower than the upper thigh

37-10. A client is immobilized with a spinal cord injury. What is one effect on the renal system?
a. Thrombus formation
b. Decreased hemoglobin levels
c. Calculi formation
d. Decreased muscle mass

37-11. A client is asked to point the toes toward the floor. What is this movement?
a. Plantar flexion
b. Dorsiflexion
c. Abduction
d. Hyperextension

B C D B D A D C B C A
1 2 3 4 5 6 7 8 9 10 11

CHAPTER 38

Skin Integrity and Wound Care

38-1.   A client is experiencing ischemia to the lower sacral area. How is this condition described?
   a.   Increased tissue buildup during the healing process
   b.   Deficiency of blood supply to a part
   c.   Decreased fluid to the tissues
   d.   Increased irritability of the nerves

38-2.   To improve oxygen saturation, a client is placed in the reverse Trendelenburg position. The client frequently slides down in bed and must be repositioned once an hour. What is the cause of potential integument damage?
   a.   Friction
   b.   Shearing force
   c.   Maceration
   d.   Impaired peripheral circulation

38-3.   A client is recovering from a surgical incision, and collagen fibers have strengthened the wound area. This response is most likely what phase?
   a.   Inflammatory
   b.   Proliferative reconstruction
   c.   Maturation
   d.   Healing by secondary intention

38-4.   A client has a hyperemic area of skin from pressure to the area. How often should the nurse recheck that region?
   a.   15 minutes
   b.   30 minutes
   c.   45 minutes
   d.   60 minutes

38-5.   A client's draining wound is streaked with plasma and red blood cells. How is this drainage described?
   a.   Serous
   b.   Sanguinous
   c.   Serosanguinous
   d.   Purulent

38-6.   When cleansing a wound, the nurse cleans from the least contaminated to the most contaminated area. What is the rationale for this cleaning regimen?
   a.   Preventing contamination of previously cleaned areas
   b.   Promoting proper absorption of drainage
   c.   Reducing excess moisture that can harbor microorganisms
   d.   Preventing introduction of organisms into the wound

38-7.   A client has a clean wound that needs protection from secondary infection. What is the appropriate dressing material?
   a.   Occlusive hydrocolloid
   b.   Semiocclusive hydrogel
   c.   Transparent
   d.   Self-adhesive synthetic

38-8.   How does the nurse maintain client comfort during a wound irrigation?
   a.   Warming the irrigation solution
   b.   Wearing gloves when removing the dressing
   c.   Holding the irrigation syringe 1 inch above the wound
   d.   Drying the wound edges with sterile gauze when finished

38-9.   A client is asked to take a sitz bath twice daily. What is the rationale for this therapy?
   a.   Properly lower the pathogen buildup in the perineal area
   b.   Cause widespread vasodilation to the body
   c.   Reduce swelling of the perineum area
   d.   Increase circulation to the periphery

38-10.   A client has a moist dressing applied. What is the primary advantage of the moist application?
   a.   Less risk of burns to the skin
   b.   Avoidance of skin macerations
   c.   Longer retention of temperature
   d.   Deep penetration into tissue layers

38-11.   An older client has a wound in the healing process. What aspect of the aging process should the nurse keep in mind?
   a.   Thicker dermis layers and less subcutaneous fat
   b.   Faster epidermal cell renewal rates
   c.   Decreased elasticity of the integument
   d.   Increased number of sweat glands

CHAPTER 39

Sensory Alterations

39-1.   A client has lost the ability to sense the position of the extremities. This example is a loss of what sense?
   a.   Tactile
   b.   Gustatory
   c.   Kinesthetic
   d.   Visual

39-2. A client has been hospitalized for 6 days and has had no visitors. The nurse notices that the client appears bored, restless, and anxious. What type of alteration is occurring related to sensory deprivation?
a. Affective
b. Cognitive
c. Perceptual
d. Receptual

39-3. A 53-year-old client has experienced some ocular changes during the past 2 years. How often should this client have regular medical eye exams?
a. Every year
b. 1 to 2 years
c. 3 to 4 years
d. 5 to 6 years

39-4. What is an appropriate nursing intervention to assist a client who has a recent visual impairment?
a. Stand at the client's dominant side, approximately one step behind, to assist with walking
b. Keep bedside rails up at night
c. Provide a nightlight with a blue bulb
d. Keep necessary objects on the client's bedside table

39-5. A person has presbyopia. In whom does this condition typically occur?
a. Infants
b. Children
c. Adults
d. Older adults

39-6. A postsurgical client is receiving chloramphenicol to reduce the chances of infection. The client should be taught to possibly expect changes in which sense?
a. Hearing
b. Taste
c. Smell
d. Vision

39-7. A client with congestive heart failure requires furosemide to eliminate excess ECF fluid. Which sense might be affected?
a. Vision
b. Hearing
c. Touch
d. Taste

39-8. A client complains of distortion of vertical lines. This complaint is likely a symptom of what?
a. Senile macular degeneration
b. Diabetic retinopathy
c. Open-angle glaucoma
d. Cataract formation

39-9. For safety concerns, what is the maximum appropriate threshold level with the floor?
a. 1/2 inch in height
b. 3/4 inch in height
c. 1 inch in height
d. 2 to 3 inches in height

39-10. A client is told to avoid reading materials with shiny surfaces. What is the rationale for this intervention?
a. Too much illumination is damaging to the eyes
b. Glare will reduce visual acuity
c. Shiny surfaces reflect damaging ultraviolet rays
d. Glare causes headaches

39-11. In communicating with a client who has a hearing impairment, what should the nurse do?
a. Ensure that the client has glasses on if the client normally wears them
b. Repeat the conversation if it is not understood at first
c. Exaggerate lip movements to facilitate lip reading
d. Rely on the client's family to interpret for the client

CHAPTER 40

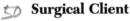

Surgical Client

40-1. A client with Crohn's disease is going to have palliative surgery. How is this type of surgery interpreted?
a. Surgical exploration that allows the surgeon to make a diagnosis
b. Relieving or reducing intensity of disease symptoms
c. Necessary or urgent to save the person's life
d. Necessary for the client's physical health

40-2.   A client has a history of cirrhosis of the liver related to alcoholism. Why is this information important preoperatively?
   a. Higher than normal amounts of anesthetic agents will be required
   b. Postoperative narcotic agonists should not be administered
   c. Surgery time will necessarily be prolonged
   d. The surgical procedure could require altering

40-3.   What might a preoperative CBC indicate?
   a. High potassium levels
   b. Low clotting times
   c. Increases in muscle damage
   d. Changes in blood urea nitrogen

40-4.   A client receives PCA after a resection of the bowel. What is the rationale for this form of analgesia?
   a. It is more long lasting
   b. It requires less health care provider input
   c. It keeps the pain levels in a narrower range
   d. It is more easily administered than IV bolus medications

40-5.   A client is awaiting surgery for a hernia repair, and the nurse takes vital signs. What is the rationale for this intervention?
   a. Identify the anxiety level of the client
   b. Determine the temperature level of the client
   c. Assess for any new conditions of the pulse and blood pressure
   d. Allow for a baseline of the vital signs that can be used in intraoperative comparisons

40-6.   A preoperative client receives an anticholinergic medication. What is the purpose of this medication?
   a. Decrease the amount of anesthesia that is required intraoperatively
   b. Partially sedate the client to decrease the stress level
   c. Decrease mucous secretions to prevent aspiration
   d. Relax skeletal muscles

40-7.   Intraoperatively, the first assistant contaminates a sterile field. Which professional is responsible for observing and rectifying this type of incident?
   a. Surgeon
   b. Scrub nurse
   c. Anesthesiologist
   d. Circulating nurse

40-8.   A surgical suite for a client undergoing a coronary bypass graft is kept at 69° F. What is the rationale for this temperature setting?
   a. Offset the potential malignant hyperthermia complication in the intraoperative setting
   b. Decrease the oxygenation demands of the client
   c. Reduce the chance of infection from prolific pathogen growth
   d. Increase the client's shiver response in order to facilitate normal blood pressure

40-9.   A PACU nurse is caring for a client who has had an appendectomy. The nurse is most concerned about what problem?
   a. Respiratory difficulties
   b. Potential for an evisceration or increased wound drainage
   c. Hypertensive crisis
   d. Electrophysiological changes resulting in cardiac arrhthymias

40-10.   A client is receiving phase II postanesthesia care. What should the client have?
   a. The same interventions as a phase I postanesthesia care client
   b. Encouragement to sit up and take sips of fluids early after the surgery
   c. No pain during this time of recovery
   d. No analgesics during this care period

40-11.   After having a partial gastrectomy, a client is performing leg exercises. What is the rationale for this movement?
   a. Promotion of venous return
   b. Maintenance of muscle tone
   c. Assessment of range of motion
   d. Exercise of fatigued muscles

40-12.   A client is at risk for developing an acute ileus related to decreased peristalsis. What should the nurse do?
   a. Notify the physician of this potential risk
   b. Encourage the client to ambulate early
   c. Auscultate the abdomen routinely
   d. Direct the client in the use of the bedpan or bedside commode

ANSWERS TO TEST BANK

CHAPTER 1
Health and Wellness

1-1. b

1-2. c

1-3. c

1-4. d

1-5. b

1-6. d

1-7. a

1-8. c

1-9. d

1-10. d

1-11. c

CHAPTER 2
The Health Care Delivery System

2-1. d

2-2. c

2-3. d

2-4. a

2-5. b

2-6. c

2-7. c

2-8. d

2-9. b

2-10. b

2-11. c

2-12. b

2-13. a

2-14. b

CHAPTER 3
Nursing Management of Client Care

3-1. b

3-2. c

3-3. d

3-4. b

3-5. b

3-6. c

3-7. d

3-8. c

3-9. d

3-10. c

3-11. a

3-12. b

CHAPTER 4
Critical Thinking and Nursing Judgment

4-1. c

4-2. b

4-3. c

4-4. b

4-5. b

4-6. d

4-7. d

4-8. b

4-9.   a

4-10.   c

CHAPTER 5
Nursing Assessment

5-1.   c

5-2.   d

5-3.   b

5-4.   a

5-5.   d

5-6.   c

5-7.   b

5-8.   a

5-9.   d

5-10.   b

5-11.   c

CHAPTER 6
Nursing Diagnosis

6-1.   a

6-2.   a

6-3.   d

6-4.   c

6-5.   d

6-6.   c

6-7.   d

6-8.   b

6-9.   d

6-10.   b

CHAPTER 7
Planning for Nursing Care

7-1.   d

7-2.   a

7-3.   d

7-4.   b

7-5.   b

7-6.   c

7-7.   b

7-8.   a

7-9.   c

7-10.   c

CHAPTER 8
Implementing Nursing Care

8-1.   d

8-2.   b

8-3.   d

8-4.   c

8-5.   b

8-6.   a

8-7.   a

8-8.   d

8-9.   d

8-10.   c

CHAPTER 9
Evaluation

9-1.   b

9-2.   d

9-3.   c

9-4.   d

9-5.   a

9-6.   b

9-7.   d

9-8.   c

9-9.   c

9-10. b

CHAPTER 10
Professional Nursing Roles

10-1.   c

10-2.   d

10-3.   b

10-4.   d

10-5.   d

10-6.   c

10-7.   c

10-8.   b

10-9.   a

10-10. d

CHAPTER 11
Ethics and Values

11-1.   c

11-2.   b

11-3.   c

11-4.   c

11-5.   b

11-6.   d

11-7.   b

11-8.   c

11-9.   b

11-10. d

CHAPTER 12
Legal Concepts in Nursing Practice

12-1.   b

12-2.   d

12-3.   b

12-4.   c

12-5.   b

12-6.   a

12-7.   c

12-8.   c

12-9.   d

12-10. a

12-11. c

12-12. d

CHAPTER 13
Communications

13-1.   c

13-2.   d

13-3.   b

13-4.   b

13-5.   a

13-6.   c

13-7.   a

13-8.   b

13-9.   a

13-10. d

13-11. c

CHAPTER 14
Documentation and Reporting

14-1.   c

14-2.   d

14-3.   a

14-4.   b

14-5.   b

14-6.   a

14-7.   c

14-8.   b

14-9.   c

14-10. c

14-11. d

14-12. b

CHAPTER 15
Client Education

15-1.   a

15-2.   c

15-3.   d

15-4.   b

15-5.   b

15-6.   d

15-7.   c

15-8.   c

15-9.   a

15-10. b

15-11. c

CHAPTER 16
Self-Concept and Sexuality

16-1.   b

16-2.   a

16-3.   b

16-4.   c

16-5.   d

16-6.   a

16-7.   c

16-8.   c

16-9.   b

16-10. d

16-11. c

CHAPTER 17
Spiritual Health

17-1.   d

17-2.   b

17-3.   a

17-4.   c

17-5.   b

17-6. b

17-7. c

17-8. b

17-9. c

17-10. a

17-11. d

CHAPTER 18
Cultural Care in Nursing

18-1. c

18-2. d

18-3. d

18-4. c

18-5. b

18-6. a

18-7. c

18-8. d

18-9. b

18-10. a

CHAPTER 19
Family Context in Nursing

19-1. c

19-2. a

19-3. c

19-4. d

19-5. c

19-6. a

19-7. c

19-8. b

19-9. c

19-10. d

CHAPTER 20
Growth and Development

20-1. a

20-2. a

20-3. b

20-4. b

20-5. c

20-6. a

20-7. d

20-8. b

20-9. a

20-10. b

20-11. c

20-12. b

CHAPTER 21
Loss and Grief

21-1. c

21-2. c

21-3. a

21-4. c

21-5. b

21-6. a

21-7. d

21-8. c

21-9. a

21-10. c

CHAPTER 22

Stress and Adaptation

22-1. a

22-2. d

22-3. c

22-4. b

22-5. b

22-6. c

22-7. d

22-8. b

22-9. d

22-10. c

22-11. b

CHAPTER 23

Vital Signs

23-1. d

23-2. a

23-3. d

23-4. c

23-5. b

23-6. d

23-7. c

23-8. a

23-9. d

23-10. b

23-11. c

CHAPTER 24

Health Assessment and Physical Examination

24-1. a

24-2. c

24-3. d

24-4. b

24-5. c

24-6. a

24-7. c

24-8. a

24-9. c

24-10. b

24-11. a

24-12. c

24-13. d

CHAPTER 25

Infection Control

25-1. a

25-2. d

25-3. c

25-4. a

25-5. b

25-6. d

25-7. b

25-8. b

25-9. b

25-10. c

25-11. b

CHAPTER 26

Administering Medications

26-1.   b

26-2.   c

26-3.   d

26-4.   b

26-5.   c

26-6.   b

26-7.   d

26-8.   c

26-9.   a

26-10. a

26-11. d

26-12. b

26-13. c

CHAPTER 27

Body Mechanics

27-1.   c

27-2.   a

27-3.   c

27-4.   b

27-5.   d

27-6.   d

27-7.   c

27-8.   d

27-9.   b

27-10. b

27-11. c

27-12. d

CHAPTER 28

Safety

28-1.   b

28-2.   d

28-3.   c

28-4.   a

28-5.   d

28-6.   c

28-7.   b

28-8.   c

28-9.   a

CHAPTER 29

Hygiene

29-1.   b

29-2.   a

29-3.   b

29-4.   c

29-5.   a

29-6.   d

29-7.   b

29-8.   d

29-9.   c

29-10. d

29-11. c

CHAPTER 30

Oxygenation

30-1.   b

30-2.   b

30-3.	a
30-4.	d
30-5.	c
30-6.	a
30-7.	b
30-8.	c
30-9.	b
30-10.	c
30-11.	d

CHAPTER 31
Fluid, Electrolyte, and Acid-Base Balances

31-1.	a
31-2.	c
31-3.	b
31-4.	d
31-5.	b
31-6.	a
31-7.	d
31-8.	b
31-9.	c
31-10.	b
31-11.	c

CHAPTER 32
Sleep

32-1.	d
32-2.	b
32-3.	c
32-4.	a

32-5.	b
32-6.	d
32-7.	c
32-8.	b
32-9.	c
32-10.	d
32-11.	a

CHAPTER 33
Comfort

33-1.	b
33-2.	c
33-3.	a
33-4.	d
33-5.	c
33-6.	c
33-7.	d
33-8.	d
33-9.	a
33-10.	c
33-11.	d

CHAPTER 34
Nutrition

34-1.	b
34-2.	c
34-3.	c
34-4.	d
34-5.	b

34-6. a

34-7. b

34-8. d

34-9. c

34-10. d

34-11. a

CHAPTER 35
Urinary Elimination

35-1. c

35-2. d

35-3. c

35-4. a

35-5. b

35-6. a

35-7. a

35-8. d

35-9. c

35-10. b

35-11. d

CHAPTER 36
Bowel Elimination

36-1. b

36-2. d

36-3. c

36-4. a

36-5. a

36-6. c

36-7. a

36-8. d

36-9. c

36-10. b

36-11. d

CHAPTER 37
Immobility

37-1. b

37-2. c

37-3. d

37-4. b

37-5. d

37-6. a

37-7. d

37-8. c

37-9. b

37-10. c

37-11. a

CHAPTER 38
Skin Integrity and Wound Care

38-1. b

38-2. b

38-3. b

38-4. d

38-5. c

38-6. d

38-7. a

38-8.   a

38-9.   a

38-10.   c

38-11.   c

CHAPTER 39
Sensory Alterations

39-1.   c

39-2.   a

39-3.   d

39-4.   b

39-5.   c

39-6.   d

39-7.   b

39-8.   a

39-9.   a

39-10.   b

39-11.   c

CHAPTER 40
Surgical Client

40-1.   b

40-2.   a

40-3.   b

40-4.   c

40-5.   d

40-6.   c

40-7.   d

40-8.   b

40-9.   a

40-10.   b

40-11.   a

40-12.   c